CAROTID ARTERY DISEASE - FROM BENCH TO BEDSIDE AND BEYOND

Edited by **Rita Rezzani**

Carotid Artery Disease - From Bench to Bedside and Beyond
http://dx.doi.org/10.5772/57002
Edited by Rita Rezzani

Contributors

Reza Mofidi, Foad Abdallah, Elias Skopelitis, Dimitrios Levisianou, Sofoklis Kougialis, Helen Lydataki, Antenor Tavares Junior, Masanori Kawasaki, Jose Milei, Andres Izaguirre, Ricardo Luis Beigelman, Eric Deshaies, David Padalino, Jeffrey Indes, Lindsay Gates

Published by InTech

Janeza Trdine 9, 51000 Rijeka, Croatia

Publishing Process Manager Iva Lipovic

Technical Editor InTech DTP team

Cover InTech Design team

First published January, 2014

Printed in Croatia

Additional hard copies can be obtained from orders@intechopen.com

Carotid Artery Disease - From Bench to Bedside and Beyond, Edited by Rita Rezzani

p. cm.

ISBN 978-953-51-1214-3

For EU product safety concerns:
IN TECH d.o.o., Prolaz Marije Krucifikse Kozulić 3, 51000 Rijeka, Croatia,
info@intechopen.com or visit our website at intechopen.com.

Meet the editor

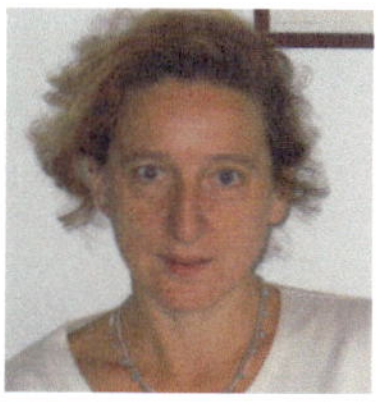

Dr. Rita Rezzani is Full Professor of Human Anatomy and Chair of Anatomy and Physiopathology Section at University of Brescia (Italy). Her scientific fields include the immunosuppressive effects of cyclosporine A, the oxidative stress and the morphological alterations induced by cardiovascular diseases. Recently her interest involves the beneficial effect of natural antioxidants, in particular of melatonin, in several diseases. She is interested in studying both the therapeutic and protective melatonin effects. For this purpose, she is working with important scientists around the world. She is an author of 165 full-length publications and she participated in writing of several books regarding cardiovascular diseases and atherogenesis.

Contents

Preface

Atherosclerosis is a multifactorial and dynamic disease which makes the process of prevention and management complex.

The clinical studies include the thickness of intima-media tunica, evaluation of the stenosis severity and plaque morphology. These points are important for monitoring plaque stabilization, and for development of therapeutic strategies.

The book consists of 8 chapters describing the cytoarchitecture of carotid plaques from morphological and physiopathological points of view. It includes clinical applications such as the effect of statin therapy and new updates for the benefit of the patients.

The book is written for all those working in the field of atherosclerosis, cardiovascular diseases and basic scientists. Moreover, it is important for linking basic scientists to clinicians.

This book will bring out the state of art of carotid stenosis in the basic and clinical approaches for better understanding of the mechanisms and useful therapies for these disease. We hope that would be a new "current trend" understanding new aspects regarding this scientific problematic involving not only anatomical, functional but also clinical questions.

Dr. Rita Rezzani
Full Professor of Human Anatomy
Chair of Anatomy and Physiopathology Section
University of Brescia
Italy

Chapter 1

Evaluation and Treatment of Carotid Artery Stenosis

Lindsay Gates and Jeffrey Indes

Additional information is available at the end of the chapter

http://dx.doi.org/10.5772/57258

1. Introduction

Stroke is the fourth leading causes of death in the United States. Annually, about 795,000 people suffer from a stroke with about 140,000 people, or 1 in 19, dying each year due to stroke related causes. [1] Between 1995-2005 overall stroke death rate fell 30%, even so, annual health care related costs for stroke patients in 2012 were up to 38.6 billion. [1] It is well recognized that cerebrovascular disease, specifically carotid atherosclerosis and subsequent stenosis, is a leading cause of ischemic stroke, which makes up 87% of all strokes. Due to the significant morbidity and mortality incurred by these patients the identification, management, and treatment of carotid disease is of paramount importance.

2. Epidemiology

Cerebrovascular disease does not appear to affect all races and genders equally. In addition to the usual cardiovascular risk factors of hypertension, diabetes, and smoking; age, gender and race have also been shown to have an additive effect on stroke risk. In a study by Rockman et al. they looked at a little over 3 million patients for evidence of carotid artery stenosis. After controlling for gender and age differences, they found that there was a marked variation in the prevalence of carotid artery stenosis with Native American subjects having the highest prevalence followed by Caucasians. [2] Yet, based on CDC data, African Americans' risk of having a first stroke is nearly twice that of Caucasians. Overall, as would be expected based on the prevalence of carotid disease, American Indians/Alaska Natives are more likely to have a stroke than other groups. [1] Gender differences have also been analyzed. In a large population based study carotid artery stenosis was detected in 3.8% of men and 2.7% of women. [3] The reasons for these differences are thought in part to be due to carotid plaque differences between men and women. Sangiorgi et al. evaluated plaque specimens from 457 patients and found that women, as compared to men of the same age, had a lower prevalence of thrombotic plaques and a smaller area of necrotic core and hemorrhage extension. Also, they found inflammatory features were less pronounced in women as compared to men. [4] These results correlate with similar studies done for evaluation of patients with coronary artery disease that showed that sex hormones seem to play a fundamental protective role in women. [5, 6] More studies still need to be conducted to determine the true role of gender in carotid artery disease. Age greater than 70 also appears to be a risk for stroke. In the Framingham study they found that seventy year olds with hypertension and the presence one additional risk factor, such as diabetes mellitus, cigarette smoking, cardiovascular disease, atrial fibrillation or electrocardiographic abnormalities had an increase in 10 year stroke risk from an average of less than 9% in women and 12.3% in men, to greater than 80%. [7].

3. Evaluation

Significant carotid artery atherosclerosis can put patients at a risk for stroke and/or transient ischemic attack (TIA) making it imperative that at risk populations be accurately evaluated and followed for disease progression. An ideal diagnostic imaging test could accurately and reproducibly determine the degree of luminal stenosis as well as plaque morphology in both a non-invasive and cost effective way. No one single imaging test encompasses all these traits however several have been shown to have benefit in the diagnosis and work up of carotid disease. At this time the most clinically effective first line imaging modality for identifying patients with carotid artery disease is duplex ultrasound (DUS). In 2006 Wardlaw et al published a meta-analysis looking at non-invasive imaging tests either alone or combined to determine if they could replace intra-arterial angiography for evaluation of carotid stenosis. They included 41 studies and found that contrast-enhanced magnetic resonance angiography (CEMRA) was the most accurate imaging modality for patients with 70-99% stenosis, however it was not cost-effective. Alternatively, DUS had a sensitivity of 0.89 and specificity of 0.84 for carotid stenosis between 70-90%, was cost effective and allowed for expedient diagnosis and treatment for patients recommending it as the diagnostic test of choice. In patients with lower degrees of stenosis around 50-69% the sensitivity of DUS dropped to 0.36. [8] Conversely, another meta-analysis performed by Jahromi et al found improved sensitivities and specificities of 0.98 and 0.88 for detecting greater than 50% ICA stenosis; and 0.94 and 0.90 respectively for detecting greater than 70% ICA stenosis. [9] Due to the potential risk of surgical intervention in patients with a questionable or 50-69% stenosis, a subsequent CEMRA or a multi detector computed tomographic angiogram (MDCTA), is highly recommended. [8] Principle limitations of ultrasound remain primarily operator experience. Occasionally, plaque calcification, shadowing and patient body habitus can also prevent accurate assessment of stenosis. Currently the indications for carotid duplex ultrasonography are cervical bruit, amaurosis fugax, focal or cerebral transient ischemic attacks, drop attacks, or syncope.

http://dx.doi.org/10.5772/57258

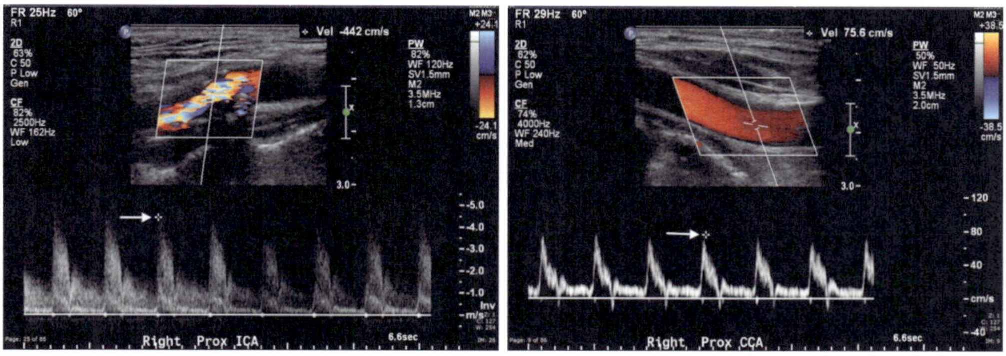

(a) (b)

Figure 1. 71 year old male presenting with history of transient ischemic attack presenting as left arm numbness and weakness. A. Ultrasound of the right internal carotid artery showing elevated velocities (arrow) up to 442 cm/s correlating with a greater than 70% stenosis by NASCET criteria. B. Same patient US of right proximal common carotid artery with baseline velocities (arrow) 75.6 cm/s.

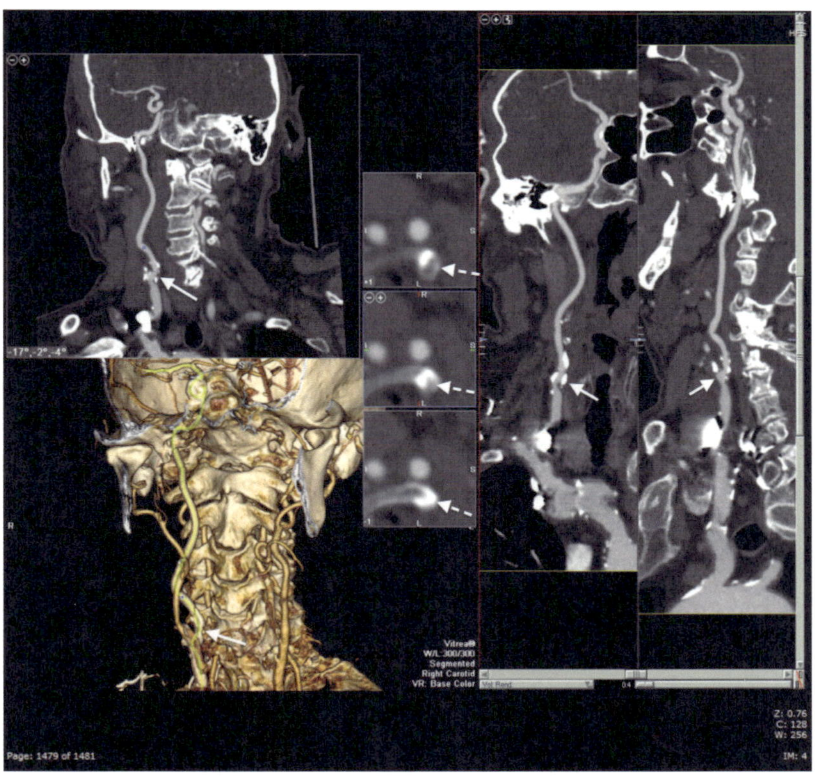

Figure 2. 79 year old male presented after transient ischemic attack. CTA obtained showing proximal right internal carotid artery stenosis (greater than 70%) with heavy calcification (arrow). Also shown cross-sectional view of area of greatest stenosis (dashed arrow).

The degree of luminal stenosis has traditionally been the most important element when considering the severity of carotid disease, however recently several studies have shown that plaque structure and composition may be an additional marker for future cerebrovascular events. [10, 11] DUS can provide only a basic view of plaque morphology, unable to consistently and accurately delineate characteristics of plaque vulnerability such as ulceration, a large lipid necrotic ore, and a thin fibrous cap. [12, 13]. Gray-Weale developed a scale, later modified by Geroulakos that identified 5 types of carotid artery plaques: type 1 (anechogenic with echogenic fibrous cap), type 2 (predominately anechogenic but with echogenic areas representing less than 25% of the plaque), type 3 (predominately hyperechogenic but with anechogenic areas representing less than 25% of the plaque), type 4 (echogenic and homogeneous plaque) and type 5 (unclassified plaques reflecting calcified plaques with areas of acoustic shadowing which hide the deeper part of the arterial layers). [14, 15]. Using this type of classification, a study by Polak et al. showed that asymptomatic elderly patients with a hypo-echoic plaque have relative risk of ipsilateral ischemic stroke of 2.78, this was independent from the degree of stenosis and other cardiovascular risk factors. [16]Another, similar investigation by Mathiesen et al. found comparable results with the relative risk of ipsilateral cerebrovascular events in patients with hypo-echoic plaques to be 3.52. [17] Nevertheless in the Asymptomatic Carotid Surgery Trial (ACST), there was no evidence that the Gray-Weale classification, or plaque echolucency, showed any influence on the risk of stroke over degree of stenosis. [18]. The emergence of multi-detector computed tomographic angiography (MDCTA) came with the increased advances of improved spatial and temporal resolution for evaluating different arterial regions but also the ability to further differentiate plaque morphology between smooth, irregular and ulcerated surfaces. [19] Density of a plaque can also be determined measured in Hounsfield units (HU). This can differentiate a "soft" plaque (<50 HU) which usually has a lipid-rich core and more likely to be associated with symptoms from a "calcified" plaque (>120 HU) which generally remains asymptomatic. [20]. Even so, it seems that MRA is probably the best modality for evaluating plaque morphology. Plaque components such as lipid cores, intraplaque hemorrhage, fibrotic tissue, fibrotic caps and calcifications can all be evaluated with MRA to distinguish unstable plaques from stable ones. [21-23] In a study by Sadat et al. MRA was used to evaluate plaque morphology in acute symptomatic, recently symptomatic and asymptomatic patients. Results showed that MRA was clearly able to identify plaque features including hemorrhage and thin fibrous caps in the acutely symptomatic group that varied from the recently symptomatic and asymptomatic groups. [23] The use of MRA for further risk stratifying symptomatic patients or predicting high-risk asymptomatic patients, however requires further evaluation to determine its role in the evaluation of carotid artery disease.

Even with all of the advances of DUS, MDCTA, and MDMRA, for many practitioners intra-arterial digital subtraction arteriography (IADSA) still remains the gold standard for imaging extra cranial and intracranial circulation. Although angiography allows for detailed evaluation of the aortic arch, origins of the great vessels and the distal ICA, it is still an invasive imaging modality potentially exposing patients to unnecessary complications and even possibly death. Complications rates do vary among studies from as low as 0.4% in the Veterans Affair Cooperative Study to 1.2% in the Asymptomatic Carotid Atherosclerosis Study and as high as

12.5% in patients with severe bilateral carotid obstructive disease. [24-26]. IADSA can be forgone in most situations where noninvasive diagnostic tests are available and now usually only utilized in conjunction with planned carotid artery stenting.

3. Asymptomatic carotid stenosis

Patients with cerebrovascular disease can be divided into asymptomatic and symptomatic disease. Patient's with asymptomatic carotid disease generally come to the attention of practitioners because they are found to have one or more risk factor for developing cerebrovascular disease (age, diabetes mellitus, coronary artery disease, peripheral vascular disease, hypertension, or hyperlipidemia) and/or signs on clinical exam, such as carotid bruit on auscultation, that warrant further diagnostic evaluation. About 5% of the general population over 65 years of age has an asymptomatic CAS of 50% or greater. [27-28]. This is increased in patients with peripheral arterial disease up to 15% and in patients with abdominal aortic aneurysms up to about 12%. [29] The overall annual risk of ipsilateral stroke for patients found to have asymptomatic carotid stenosis that are treated medically is about 2%. Asymptomatic carotid disease, in fact, seems to be a better indicator of generalized vascular disease than of stroke risks. In this population the average annual non-stroke death rates are generally higher than those of ipsilateral stroke with more than 50% of the non-stroke related deaths due to ischemic heart disease and its complications. [30] For patients who are found to have carotid disease, optimal medical management is the cornerstone to overall treatment. The goal of medical therapy is to reduce overall cardiovascular events as well as stroke by a five pronged attack including: treatment of hypertension, treatment of diabetes mellitus, treatment of lipid abnormalities, smoking cessation, and antithrombotic treatment. As mentioned previously, hypertension has been consistently found to be an independent risk factor for carotid artery atherosclerosis with each 10-mm Hg increase in blood pressure resulting in an increase in risk for stroke of 30-45%. Conversely each 10-mm Hg reduction in blood pressure in hypertensive patients decreases risk for stroke by 33%. [31] Currently recommendations are for blood pressures to be maintained less than 140 systolic and 90 diastolic. For patients with coronary artery disease the relationship between lipid abnormalities and ischemic heart events has also been clearly identified in the literature however at this time the relationship between elevated cholesterol and stroke risk remain unclear. [32,33] Nevertheless, studies have shown that patients with known atherosclerosis have demonstrated reduced stroke rates by 15-30% when treated with lipid lowering therapy. [34] Smoking cessation is important for all patients with vascular disease, and in carotid artery disease this is no different nearly doubling the overall risk for stroke. [35] Finally both antithrombotic and anticoagulant therapy can also be utilized for prevention in patients with carotid disease. There is more robust evidence for the use of antithrombotic treatment for secondary prevention of recurrent stroke in symptomatic patients than for prevention in asymptomatic patients, however it is still recommended that patients who are at risk, or have known vascular disease, take a daily aspirin for prophylaxis. [36] Anticoagulation with Coumadin is generally reserved for patients at risk for an embolic stroke from atrial fibrillation and is not used as prophylaxis for asymptomatic or symptomatic carotid disease. [37]

For asymptomatic patients who continue to have worsening carotid disease even with best medical management the next step in treatment is to consider operative intervention. The current recommendations from the Society for Vascular Surgery is for carotid endarterectomy in asymptomatic patients with carotid stenosis of greater than or equal to 60% as long as the expected combined stroke and mortality rate for the individual surgeon was not greater than 3%. [38] These recommendations are based on three major prospective, randomized trials the Veterans Administration Asymptomatic Carotid Stenosis Study (VA ACS), the Asymptomatic Carotid Atherosclerosis Study (ACAS), and the Asymptomatic Carotid Surgery Trial (ACST).

The VA ACS evaluated a total of 444 patients over an 8 year period randomizing them to a surgical group (211) or and a medical group (233). Both groups were treated with aspirin and best medical risk factor control. For the surgical arm, the 30-day mortality rate was 1.9% and the incidence of stroke was 2.4% with a combined stroke and mortality rate of 4.3%. In total, all neurologic events were 30 (14.2%). Conversely, the medical group had a total of 55 (23.6%) neurologic events recorded. These findings were found to be statistically significant with a P value of less than 0.006. [39] However, the study did not find any difference in overall survival rates between groups. This trial gave credence that best medical treatment plus carotid endarterectomy (CEA) would reduce stroke and TIAs versus medical treatment alone in asymptomatic patients.

The ACAS was a NIH-funded randomized trial which included 1662 patients between the ages of 40-79 years with greater than 60% asymptomatic stenosis. Patients were randomized to optimal medical management versus CEA and medical management. The 30-day combined mortality and stroke rate was 2.3%, which accounts for two preoperative deaths and seven preoperative strokes making the actual stroke rate 1.3% and mortality rate 0.1%. After a mean follow up of 2.7 years the overall 5-year risk for ipsilateral stroke, perioperative stroke and death was 5.1% for surgical patients and 11% for the medical group (P=0.004). [40] An absolute risk reduction for stroke and death in the surgical group was calculated to be 53%. [41] One drawback of the ACAS study is that all patients with 60%-99% carotid stenosis were analyzed together and there was no breakdown for event rates by deciles. Nevertheless, their results again favored CEA plus medical management over medical management alone.

Finally a group of European investigators embarked on an additional randomized trial, ACST, to try, in addition to validating CEA for asymptomatic patients with significant stenosis, to identify a higher-risk group of patients. They randomized 3129 patients, both men and women, with greater than 60% asymptomatic unilateral or bilateral carotid artery stenosis to CEA versus best medical therapy. The found a 5 year stroke or death rate to be 6.4% versus 11.8 % ($p<0.0001$) in the CEA versus medical group, respectively. Overall perioperative stroke or death rate was 3.1%. These results were found to be significant for bother males and females when analyzed separately [18].

4. Symptomatic carotid artery stenosis

When compared to asymptomatic patients the benefit of CEA with recent ipsilateral carotid territory symptoms and moderated to severe carotid stenosis is much greater. In patients who experience a TIA or minor stroke the risk of subsequent stroke or death is very high, especially during the first few days and weeks after an event. [42] Traditionally the mainstay of treatment for symptomatic disease in these patients is surgical intervention with CEA. Recently there has been literature advocating aggressive medical therapy alone may be adequate in certain patients, preventing early stroke after TIA and reducing the need for urgent CEA. The Stroke Prevention Aggressive Reduction of Cholesterol Levels (SPARCL) trail tested whether treatment with atorvastatin reduced strokes in subjects with recent minor stroke or TIA. The study included 4731 participants with a mean follow up of 4.9 years and found that high does Atorvastatin use after TIA or stroke was associated with a 16% relative reduction in risk of fatal or nonfatal stroke. Also patients treated were found to have a 56% reduction in later carotid revascularization compared with placebo. Researchers postulated that the use of statins might help stabilize the arterial wall decreasing events as well as reducing intraoperative complications as well for patients who did proceed with surgery. [43,44] Merwick et al. also evaluated early high dose statin use postulating that pretreatment at TIA onset would modify early stroke risk. They found that non-procedural 7-day stroke risk was 3.8% with statin treatment compared to 13.2% in those not pretreated. [45] Another study by Chimowitz et al. evaluated a different medical treatment looking at recently symptomatic patients with intracranial 79-99% stenosis who were treated with dual antiplatelet therapy versus percutaneous transluminal angioplasty and stenting (PTAS) (gold standard for intracranial lesions). This study found a 30-day rate of stroke or death was found to be 14.7% in the PTAS group and 5.8% in the medical-management group. At one year follow this study concluded that medical management with dual antiplatelet therapy was superior to PTAS and advocates belief this data can be extrapolated to severe, symptomatic extra cranial disease as well. [46,47]. Several other older studies have compared the use of platelet antiaggregants with placebo in treating patients with cerebral ischemia secondary to extra cranial atherosclerosis. [48-51] These results however proved inferior to surgery, which was highlighted in the landmark North American Symptomatic Carotid Endarterectomy Trial.

Two major randomized control trials have reported data to date advocating for CEA in symptomatic patients with 50%-99% stenosis: The North American Symptomatic Carotid Endarterectomy Trial (NASCET) and Medical Research Council European Carotid Surgery Trial (ECST). The NASCET trial was set up to evaluate two subsets of patients those with 70-99% stenosis and those with 30-69% stenosis. In the high-grade stenosis group the 30-day operative morbidity and stroke mortality rate for patients was 5%. In the surgical group at 2-year follow-up the incidence of ipsilateral stroke was 9% compared to 26% in the medical treatment group. This difference represented an absolute risk reduction of 17% in favor of surgical management and a relative risk reduction of 71% at the end of the 18-month follow up. Mortality rates were also measured at the end of 18 months yielding 12% mortality rate in the medical group compared to a significantly lower rate of 5% in the surgical group. [52,53]. The results for the moderate stenosis group were also reported. The 30-day combined mortality, disabling stroke rate, and non-disabling stroke rate was 6.7%. At 5 year follow up in this group the ipsilateral stroke rate was 22.2% in the medical patients and 16.7% in the surgical patients. [54]

The ECST trial was a European randomized control trial that enrolled patients over 10 years almost concurrently with the NASCET trial. There were 2518 patients with nondisabling ischemic stroke, TIA or retinal infarct due to a stenotic lesion in the ipsilateral carotid artery randomized to either medical management with aspirin or surgery. At 3 years, the risk of stroke was found to be 26.5% in the medical group compared to 7% in the surgery group with an absolute reduction of 14.9%. The actual incidence of ipsilateral stroke was 2.8% in the surgery group versus 16.8% in the medical group. [55] ECST trial also evaluated gender, age, severity of stenosis, plaque morphology, and time since last event. They found that risk of events increased with age and with male gender. They did not find any benefit for surgery over medical treatment in the mild stenosis group (10%-29%) unlike the severe stenosis group, which showed a 6-fold reduction in subsequent strokes over 3 years. [56]

Based on these randomized studies there seems to be a consensus on which patients would benefit from operative intervention after an ischemic event, however the timing of intervention has been much debated. The risk of recurrent stroke after TIA or minor stroke is the highest within the first 7-10 days. According to a meta-analysis by Giles et al the risk of stroke after TIA is 6.7% at 48 hours and 10% at 7 days with more than half of the strokes occurring within the first 7 days doing so within the first 24 hours after the inciting event. [57,58] In another study by Ois et al. the rate of recurrent stroke in symptomatic patients with greater then 50% stenosis was determined to be 20.9% in the first 72 hours, 6.7% between 72 hours and 7 days and 3.7% between 7 and 14 days. [59] These results support early intervention in the first 48 hours because the risk of recurrent stroke appears to outweigh the operative risk in patients who are medically stable and have relatively small or no infarcts on imaging studies. Alternatively, for a completed stroke researchers advocate delayed surgical intervention for at least 4-6 weeks due to the risk of converting an ischemic cerebral infarction into a hemorrhagic one. Giordano et al reported on 49 CEAs done after a completed acute stroke. 27 of these were performed within 5 weeks of the event and 22 were done between 5 and 20 weeks. The early intervention group had a morbidity and mortality of 18.5% compared to nothing for the later group. [60] These results seem to corroborate with observations in both the NASCET and ECST trials.

5. Carotid artery stenting

Along with CEA, carotid artery stenting (CAS) has emerged as an alternative treatment strategy for patients with carotid artery disease. Initially proponents of angioplasty and stenting projected that this procedure could overcome the risks associated with CEA and provide a minimally invasive alternative for patients. However at this time the utility of CAS is highly debated with CEA remaining the standard of care in most asymptomatic and symptomatic patients.

There have been very few studies that have specifically addressed CAS in asymptomatic patients and most of the data available comes from high-risk registries which include patients with lesions located at or above the level of C2, contralateral carotid occlusion, severe ulceration and tandem intracranial stenosis, age over 80, active coronary artery disease or congestive heart failure, and patient's with "hostile necks" (immobile neck, previous irradiation, previous surgery on the ipsilateral side or previous surgery on the contralateral side with vocal cord paralysis). In the SAPPHIRE trial, which population included 70% asymptomatic high-risk patients, their results found cumulative perioperative incidence of death, stroke, and MI of

5.4% for CAS and 10.2% for CEA. [61] Their results found that CAS with cerebral protection was not inferior to CEA. This study, however had several limitations including failure to randomize >50% of patients, unaccounted for elevated incidence of perioperative stroke, and possible reporting bias. The Carotid Revascularization Endarterectomy versus Stent Trial (CREST) enrolled more than 1000 asymptomatic patients. Stroke and death rates after CAS were 2.6% and 1.1% respectively with a difference between CAS and CEA in asymptomatic patients for any periprocedural stroke being 2.5% versus 1.4%. [62-64] These results did not show significant difference between CAS and CEA. The results from this study, however, were based on procedures performed by highly experienced operators and have not been replicated by other trials. [65]

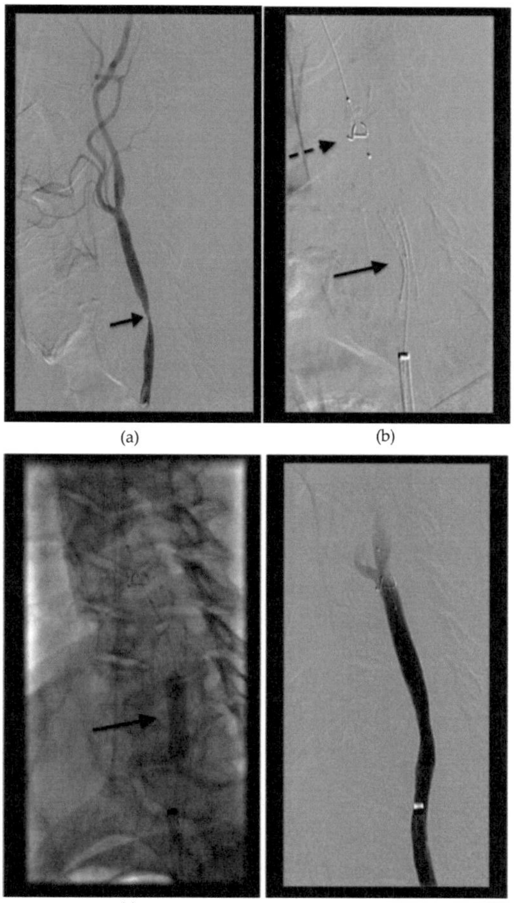

(a) (b) (c) (d)

Figure 3. 70 year old Male with a history of squamous cell carcinoma status post neck radiation and hemiglossectomy found to have a 90% asymptomatic left common carotid artery stenosis. A: Angiogram of left common carotid artery stenosis (arrow) B. Angiogrom showing cerebral protection device located in the left internal carotid artery (dashed arrow) and stent placed in common carotid artery stenosis (black arrow). C. Post stent placement angioplasty balloon inflated (arrow) D. Completion angiogram showing minimal residual stenosis after stent placed.

For symptomatic patients several major randomized trials comparing CEA versus CAS have been completed. These include the International Carotid stenting Study (ICSS), the Stent-Supported Percutaneous Angioplasty of the Carotid Artery Versus Endarterectomy (SPACE) trial, the Endarterectomy versus Angioplasty in Patients with Symptomatic Severe Carotid Stenosis (EVA-3s) trial, the Stenting and Angioplasty with Protection in Patients at high risk for Endarterectomy (SAPPHIRE) trial and the Carotid Revascularization Endarterectomy Versus Stenting Trial (CREAST).

Trial	Methods	Results	Conclusions
ICSS	1713 patient with symptomatic stenosis >50% CEA vs CEA -Primary endpoint at 120 days was stroke, death or MI	-Primary endpoints: Stroke: 7.7% CAS vs 4.1% CEA Death: 2.3% CAS vs. 0.8% CEA MI: 8.5% CAS vs. 5.2% CEA	-CAS higher rates of any stroke and all cause death -No significant difference between groups in disabling stroke
SPACE	European study 1196 patients with symptomatic stenosis randomly assigned 180 days after TIA or stroke to CAS vs. CEA -Primary endpoint: ipsilateral stroke or death at 30 days	-Stroke or Death: -6.9% CAS vs. 6.5% CEA -2 year follow up showed no significant difference btw CAS and CEA - 9.5% CAS vs. 8.8% CEA	-failed to prove noninferiority of CAS vs. CEA -2 year restenosis more frequent in CAS group -10.7% vs 4.6%
EVA-3S	French multicenter study 259 patients with severe symptomatic stenosis >60% CAS vs. CEA -Evaluate hypothesis that CAS in not inferior to CEA (similar to SPACE) -Primary endpoint: stroke or death at 30 days	- Stroke and/or Death: -9.6% CAS vs. 3.9% CEA -RR 2.5 -4 year follow up Stroke and/or Death - 11.1% CEA vs. 6.2% CAS	-Stopped premature 2/2 deaths in CAS group -CEA needs to be safer before it can be alternative to CEA *CPD were optional
CREST	RCT largest comparing CAS vs. CEA in both symptomatic and asymptomatic patients -2502 enrolled; 47% asymptomatic	- Death: 0.7% CAS vs. 0.3% CE - Stroke: 4.1% CAS vs. 2.3% CEA - MI: 1.1% CAS vs. 2.3% CEA - Combined endpoints: 7.2% CAS vs. 6.8% CEA -4 year follow up combined endpoints:	-overall effectiveness and safety were similar -similar results male vs. female and symptomatic vs. asymptomatic -Periprocedural higher risk of stroke with CAS and higher risk MI with CEA -Subanalysis: - No difference in primary endpoint based

Trial	Methods	Results	Conclusions
		6.4% CAS vs. 4.7% CEA	on symptomatic status - Periprocedure stroke and death lower in CEA in symptomatic
SAPPHIRE	Multicenter RCT comparing CAS vs. CEA in both symptomatic and asymptomatic patients -334 patients randomized ->70% of patients asymptomatic -CPD used in about 95%	-30 day Death stroke and MI: 5.4% CAS and 8.4% CEA -1 year follow up death, stroke and /or MI -12.2% CAS vs. 20.1% CEA	- CAS with use of CPDs is not inferior to CEA Limitations: -Mostly high risk patients enrolled -747 patients enrolled only less then ½ randomized -High periprocedural death rate compared to other trials

The ICSS was a randomized prospective, multicenter trial in 2010 composed of 1713 subjects with recently symptomatic carotid artery stenosis greater than 50% who were randomized to either CEA or CAS. At this time the 120-day reported results show that the CAS group had a stroke, death, and MI rates of 7.7%, 2.3% and 8.5%, respectively. These were significantly higher than rates in the CEA group, which were 4.1%, 0.8%, and 5.2% respectively. Also there was an additional group that was analyzed by MRI. This analysis showed a greater number of patients in the CAS group that had a new ischemic brain lesion compared to the surgery counterpart. [66] The EVA-3S and SPACE trial had similar protocols as the ICSS trial. EVA-3S study divided 259 patients to CAS with cerebral protection devices (CPD) and CEA. This study found a significant, 2.5, higher risk for 30-day stroke and death in the CAS group than in the CEA group (9.6% versus 3.9%). At 4 year follow-up the risk of periprocedural stroke or death, and nonperiprocedural ipsilateral stroke was also higher in the CAS group (11.1% versus 6.2%). [67] This trial however was limited by operator experience were physicians were only required to perform a minimum of two procedures with any device to qualify for enrollment. In the SPACE trial, which was larger with 1196 patients, the rate of death or ipsilateral ischemic stroke was 6.9% in the CAS group and 6.5% in the CEA group. At the end of two years results showed a greater probability of recurrent carotid stenosis of more than 70% in the CAS group Similar concerns were raised against the SPACE trial concerning the inexperience of the operators. The inconsistent use of CPDs was another concern raised by opponents of this trial. [68,69] Nevertheless, all three of these trials strongly favor CEA over CAS.

The SAPPHIRE trial previously mentioned was another one of the initial trials comparing CAS versus CEA. This corporate sponsored study had a high proportion of patients who were asymptomatic and at high risk for CEA. Results at one year found primary end-points of ipsilateral stroke or death to be lower in the stenting group than in the CEA group (12.2% versus 20.1%; P=0.5) supporting the superiority of CAS over CEA. The clinical correlation to symptomatic patients however is unclear. The CREST trial, alternatively, was a randomized, prospective, multicenter trial, which included 2502 patients. This trial had about an equal inclusion of symptomatic and asymptomatic patients. The primary endpoint of any stroke, MI or death at 30-days were similar between CAS and CEA (6.8% versus 7.2%). Upon further examination, patients in the CAS group had a lower rate of MI within 30 days (1.1% versus 2.3%) and patients in the CEA group had a lower 30-day rate of stroke (2.3% versus 4.1%). At one-year follow up quality of life measurements were examined. Investigators found that patients who had strokes reported significantly lower quality of life scores than those who had MI or cranial nerve palsy. After one year, however, these measurements did not show any significant difference. [62,64]The improved outcomes found in the CREST trial may reflect the increased experience of vascular surgeons with endovascular procedures and stent placement as well as the improvement in stents and device designs. This data supports that CAS is not inferior to CEA and both procedures can be safely offered to patients for the treatment of carotid artery disease.

Current overall recommendations by the Society of Vascular Surgery for intervention in patients with carotid artery disease are:

1. For symptomatic patients with stenosis <50% or asymptomatic patients with stenosis <60% optimal medical therapy is indicated
2. In patients who have >50% symptomatic lesions or >60% asymptomatic lesions CEA is preferred to CAS
   a. Asymptomatic patients >60% stenosis should be considered for CEA if that have a 3-5 year life expectancy and perioperative stroke/death rates are <3%
   b. In patients with symptomatic stenosis >50% CEA is preferred, especially if patient is >70, has a long lesion (>15mm), preocclusive stenosis, lipid-rich plaque that can be completely removed, and have not had previous neck operations or radiation
3. CAS is preferred over CEA in symptomatic patients with >50% stenosis when
   a. Patient has a tracheal stoma, scarred and fibrotic tissue from previous ipsilateral surgery or radiation, prior cranial nerve injury, and lesions that extend proximal to the clavicle or distal to the C2 vertebral body
   b. Patient has severe uncorrectable CAD, CHF or COPD
4. Asymptomatic patients with >60% stenosis deemed "high risk" for CEA should be managed with optimal medical therapy
   a. Insufficient data to recommend CAS for asymptomatic patients that are normal or high risk for CEA. [38]

Author details

Lindsay Gates and Jeffrey Indes

Yale University School of Medicine, New Haven CT, USA

References

[1] Roger, VL, Go AS, Lloyd-Jones DM et al. "Heart disease and stroke statistics-2012 update: a report from the American Heart Association." Circulation 125.1 (2012): E2-220.

[2] Rockman C, Hoang H, Guo Y, et al. "The prevalence of carotid artery stenosis varies significantly by race." J Vasc Surg 57 (2013): 327-337.

[3] Mathieson E, Joakkimsen O, Bonaa K, et al. "Prevalence of and risk factors associated with carotid artery stenosis: the Troms Study." Cerebrovasc Dis 12 (2001): 44-51.

[4] Sangiorgi G, Roversi S, Zoccai G, et al. "Sex-related differences in carotid plaque featuresand inlammation." J Vasc Surg 2013 57 (2013): 338-344.

[5] Kardys I, Vliegenthart R, Oudkerk M, et al. "The female advantage in cardiovascular diseae: do vascular beds contribute equally?" Am J Epidemiol 166 (2007): 403-412.

[6] Agrinier N, Cournot M, Dallongeville J, et al. "Menopause and modifiable coronary heart disease risk factors: a population based study.." Maturitas 65 (2010): 237-243.

[7] Wolf P, D'Agostino R, Belanger A, et al. "Probability of Stroke: A risk profile from the Framinham Study." Stroke 22 (1991): 312-318.

[8] Wardlaw J, Chappell F, Best J, et al. "Non-invasive imaging compared with intra-arterial angiography in the diagnosis of symptomatic carotid stenosis: a meta-analysis." Lancet 367 (2006): 1503-1512.

[9] Jahromi A, Cina C, Liu Y, et al. "Sensitivity and specificity of color duplex ultrasound measurements in the estimation of the interval carotid artery stenosis: a systemic review and meta-analysis." J Vasc Surg 41 (2005): 962-972.

[10] Saba L, Sanfilippo R, Sannia S et al. "Association between carotid artery plaque volume, composition, and ulceration: a retrospective assessment with MDCT.." AJR Am J Roentgenol 199.1 (2012): 151-156.

[11] Saba L, Sanfilippo R, Sannia S, et al. "Imaging of the carotid artery." Atherosclerosis 220.2 (2012): 294-309.

[12] Hermus L, Van Dam G, Zeebregts C, et al. "Advanced carotid plaque imaging." Eur J Vasc Endovasc Surg 39 (2010): 125-133.

[13] Tahara N, Imaizumi T, Virmani R, et al. "Clinical feasibility of molecular imaing of plaque inflammation in atherosclerosis." J Nucl Med 50 (2009): 331-334.

[14] Gray-Weale A, Graham J, Burnett J, et al. "Carotid artery atheroma: comparison of pre-operative B-mode ultrasound appearance with carotid endarterectomy specimen pathology." J Cardiovasc Surg 29 (1988): 676.

[15] Geroulakos G, Ramaswani G, Nicolaides A, et al. "Characterization of symptomatic and asymptomatic carotid plaques using high resolution real time ultrasound.." Br J Surg 80 (1993): 2171-2177.

[16] Polak J, Shemanski L, O'Leary D, et al. "Hypoechoic plaque at US of the carotid artery: an independent risk factor for incient stroke in adults aged 65 years or older.." Radiology 208 (1998): 649-654.

[17] Mathiesen E, Bonaa K, Joakimsen O et al. "Echolucent plaques are associated with high risk of ischemic cerebrovascular events in carotid stenosis: The Tromso Study." Circulation 103 (2001): 2171-2175.

[18] Halliday A, Mansfield A, Marro J et al. "Prevention of disabling and fatal stroked by successful carotid endarterectomy in patients without recent neurological symptoms: a randomised controlled trial." Lancet 363 (2004): 1491-1502.

[19] DeWeert T, Cretier S, Groen H, et al. "Atherosclerotic carotid plaque surface morphology in the carotid bifurcation assessed with multi-detector computed tomography." Stroke 40 (2009): 1334-1340.

[20] De Weert T, Ouhlous M, Meijerling E, et al. "Characterisation and quantification of atherosclerotic plaque components with multidetector computed tomography and histopathological correlation." Arterioscler Thromb Vasc Biol 26 (2006): 2366.

[21] Yuan C, Mitsumori L, Beach K, et al. "Carotid atherosclerotic plaque: noninvasive MR characterization and identification of vulnerable lesions.." Radiology 221.2 (2001): 285-299.

[22] Chu B, Kampschulte A, Ferguson M, et al. "Hemorrhage in teh atherosclerotic carotid plaque: a high-resolution MRI study." Stroke 35.5 (2004): 1079-1084.

[23] Sadat U, Weerakkody R, Bowden D, et al. "Utility of high resolution MR imaging to assess carotid plaque morphology: a comparisnon of acute symptomatic, recently symptomatic and asymptomatic patients with carotid artery disease." Atherosclerosis 207 (2009): 434-439.

[24] Hobson R, Weiss D, Fields W et al. "Efficacy of carotid endarterectomy for asymptomatic carotid stenosis: the Veterans Affairs Cooperative Study Group.." N Engl J Med 328 (1993): 221-227.

[25] Executive Committee for the Asymptomatic Carotid Atherosclerosis Study. "Endarterectomy for asymptomatic carotid artery stenosis." JAMA 273 (1995): 1421-1428.

[26] Theodotou B, Whaley R, Mahaley et al. "Complication following transfemoral cerebral l angiography for cerebral ischemia: report of 159 angiograms and correlation with surgical risk.." Surg Neurol 28 (1987): 90-92.

[27] The European Carotid Surgery Trialists Collaborative Group. "Risk of stroke in the distribution of an asymptomatic carotid artery." Lancet 345 (1995): 209-212.

[28] Mineva P, Manchev I, Hadijiev D et al. "Prevalence and outcome of asymptomatic carotid stenosis: a population-based ultrasonographic study." Eur J Neurol 9 (2002): 383-388.

[29] Goessens B, Visseren F, Algra A, et al. "Screening for asymptomatic cardiovascular disease with noninvasive imaging in patients at high-risk and low-risk according to the European Guidelines on Cardiovascular Disease Prevention: the SMART study." J Vasc Surg 43 (2006): 525-532.

[30] Pickett C, Jackson J, Hemann B, et al. "Carotid bruits as a prognostic indicator of cardiovascular death and myocardial infarction: a meta-analysis." Lancet 371 (2008): 1587-94.

[31] Lawes C, Bennett D, Feigin V, Rodgers A. "Blood Pressure and stroke: an overview of published reviews." Stroke 35 (2004): 1024.

[32] Iso H, Jacobs D, Wentworth D, et al. "Serum cholesterol levels and six-year mortality from stroke in 350,977 men screened for the multiple risk factor intervention trial." N Engl J Med 320 (1989): 904-910.

[33] Bots M, Elwood P, Nikitin Y, et al. "Total HDL cholesterol and risk of stroke. EUROSTROKE: a collaborative study among research centres in Europe." J Epidemiol Comm Health 55 (2002): i19-24.

[34] Bucher H, Griffith L, Guyatt G. "Effect of HMGCoA Reductase Inhibitors on stroke. A meta-analysis of randomized, controlled trials." Ann Intern Med 128 (1998): 89-95.

[35] Shinton R, Beevers G. "Meta-analysis of relation between cigarette smoking and stroke." BMJ 298 (1989): 789-794.

[36] Wolff T, Miller T, KoS. "Aspirin for the primary prevention of cardiovascular events: an update of the evidence for the U.S. Preventive services Task Force." Ann Intern Med 150 (2009): 405-410.

[37] Mohr J, Thompson J, Lazar R, et al. "A comparision of warfarin and aspirin for the prevention of recurrent ischemic stroke." N Engl J Med 345 (2001): 1444-1451.

[38] Ricotta J, AbuRahma A, Ascher E, et al. "Updated Society for Vascular Surgery guideline for management of extracranial carotid disease." J Vasc Surg 54 (2011): e1-e31.

[39] Veterans Administration: A Veterans Administration Cooperative Study. "Role of carotid endarterectomy in asymptomatic carotid stenosis." Stroke 17 (1986): 535-539.

[40] Moore W, Young B, Baker W. "Surgical results: A justification of the surgeon selection process for the ACAS Trial." J Vasc Surg 23 (1996): 323-328.

[41] Asymptomatic Carotid Artery Stenosis Group. "Study design for randomized prospective trial of carotid endarterectomy for asymptomatic atherosclerosis." Stroke 20 (1989): 844-849.

[42] P, Rothwell. "Medical and surgical management of symptomatic carotid stenosis." Int J Stroke 1 (2006): 140-149.

[43] McFarlane, Sammy. "High-Dose Atorvastatin AFter Stroke or Transient Ischemic Attack: The Stroke Prevention by Aggressive Reduction in Cholesterol Levels (SPARCL) investigators." J Cardiometab Syndr 3.1 (2008): 68-69.

[44] Goldstein L, Amarenco P, Zivin J, et al. "Statin treatment and stroke outcome in the Stroke Prevention by Aggressvie Reduction in cholesterol Levels (SPARCL) trial." Stroke 40.11 (2009): 3526-3531.

[45] Merwick A, Albers G, Arsava M, et al. "Reduction in early stroke risk in carotid stenosis with transient ischemic attack associated with statin treatment." Stroke 44 (2013): Epud August 1 2013.

[46] Chimowitz M, Lynn M, Derdeyn C, et al. "Stenting versus aggressive medical therapy for intracranial arterial stenosis." N Engl J Med 367.1 (2012): 93.

[47] Chaturvedi, S. "Aggressive Medical Therapy Alone is Adequate in Certain Patients with Severe Symptomatic Carotid Stenosis." Stroke 44 (2013).

[48] S, Jonas. "Anticoagulant therapy in cerebrovascular disease: Review and meta-analysis." Stroke 19 (1988): 1043-1048.

[49] Canadian Cooperative Study Group. "A randomized trial of aspirin and sulfinpyrazone in threatened strokes." N Engl J Med 299 (1978): 53.

[50] Bousser, et al. "AICLA controlled trial of aspirin and dipyridamole in the secondary prevention of arteriothrombotic cerebral ischemia." Stroke 14 (1983): 5-14.

[51] Sorenson P, Pedersen H, Marquardsen J et al. "Acetylsalicylic Acid in the prevention of stroke in patients with reversible cerebral ischemic attacks: A Danish cooperative study." Stroke 14 (1983): 15-22.

[52] North American Symptomatic Carotid Endarterectomy Trial (NASCET) Steering Committee. "North American Symptomatic Carotid Endarterectomy Trial: Methods, patient characteristics, and progress." Stroke 22 (1991): 711-720.

[53] North American Symptomatic Carotid Endarterectomy Trial Collaborators. "Beneficial effect of carotid endarterectomy in symptomatic patients with high-grade carotid stenosis." N Engl J Med 325 (1991): 445-453.

[54] Barnett M, Taylor D, Eliasziw M, et al. "Benefit of carotid endarterectomy in patients with symptomatic moderate or severe stenosis." N Engl J Med 339 (1998): 1415-1425.

[55] European Carotid Surgery Trialists'Collaborative Group. "MRC European Carotid Surgery Trial: Interim results for patients with severe (70-99%) or with mild (0-29%) carotid stenosis." Lancet 337 (1991): 1235-1243.

http://dx.doi.org/10.5772/57258

[56] Alqadri S, Qureshi A. "Treatment of Symptomatic Carotid Stenosis: Carotid Stent Placement Versus Endarterectomy." Curr Atheroscler Rep 15 (2013): 345-350.

[57] Giles M, Rothwell P. "Risk of stroke early after transient ischemic attack: a systematic review and meta-analysis." Lancet Neurol 6 (2007): 1063-1072.

[58] Chandratheva A, Mehta Z, Geraghty O, et al. "Population-based study of risk and predictors of stroke in the first few hours after a TIA." Neurology 72 (2009): 1941-1947.

[59] Ois A, Cuadrado-Godia E, Rodriguez-Campello A, et al. "High risk of early neurological recurrence in symptomatic carotid stenosis." Stroke 40 (2009): 2727-2731.

[60] Giordano J, et al. "Timing of carotid arterial endarterectomy after stroke." J Vasc Surg 2 (1985): 250.

[61] Yadav J, Wholey M, Kuntz R, et al. "Protected carotid-artery stenting versus endarterectom in high risk patients." N Engl J Med 351 (2004): 1493-1501.

[62] Brott T, Hobson R, Howard G, et al. "Stenting verss endarterectomy for the treatment of carotid-artery stenosis." N Engl J Med 363 (2010): 11-23.

[63] Bonati L, Dobson J, Algra A, et al. "Short-term outcome after stenting versus endarterectomy for symptomatic carotid stenosis: a preplanned meta-analysis of individual patient data." Lancet 376 (2010): 1062-1073.

[64] Silver F, Mackey A, Clark W, et al. "Safety of stenting and endarterectomy by symptomatic status in the Carotid Revascularization Endarterectomy Versus Stenting Trial (CREST)." Stroke 42 (2011): 675-680.

[65] Hobson R, Howard V, Roubin G, et al. "Credentialing of surgeions as interventionalist for carotid artery stenting: experience from the lead-in phase of CREST." J Vasc Surg 40 (2004): 952-957.

[66] Ederle J, Dobson J, Featherstone R, et al. "Carotid artery stenting compared with endarterectomy in patients with symptomatic carotid stenosis (International Carotid Stenting Study): an interim analysis of randomised controlled trial." Lancet 375 (2010): 985-997.

[67] Mas J, Chatellier G Beyssen B, et al. "Endarterectomy versus stenting in patents with symptomatic severe carotid stenosis." N Engl J Med 19.2 (2007): 201-203.

[68] Ringleb P, Allenberg J, Bruckmann H, et al. "30-day result from the SPACE trial of stent-protected angioplasty versus carotid endarterectomy in symptomatic patients: a randomised non-inferiority trial." Lancet 368 (2006): 1239-1247.

[69] Stingele R, Berger J, Alfke K et al. "Clinical and angiographic risk factors for stroke and death within 30 days after carotid endarterectomy and stent-protected angioplasty: a subanalysis of the SPACE study." Lancet Neurol 7 (2008): 216-222

Chapter 2

Tissue Characterization of Carotid Plaques

Masanori Kawasaki, Shinichi Yoshimura and Kiyofumi Yamada

Additional information is available at the end of the chapter

http://dx.doi.org/10.5772/57155

1. Introduction

Carotid plaque vulnerability has been reported to be associated with stroke and other cerebrovascular events [1, 2]. Therefore, tissue characterization of carotid plaques is important to evaluate the risk of cerebrovascular disease and outcome of treatment for carotid arterial stenosis. Stabilization of vulnerable plaques rather than regression of plaque volume is considered the major contributor to beneficial effects on cerebrovascular events [3].

With respect to the ultrasound technique, ultrasonic tissue characterization of the myocardium with an integrated backscatter (IBS) analysis was developed, which is capable of providing both conventional two-dimensional echographic (2DE) images and IBS images. In studies of the myocardium, calibrated myocardial IBS was significantly correlated with the volume fraction of interstitial fibrosis [4, 5]. In preliminary *in vitro* studies, IBS values reflected the structural and biochemical composition of atherosclerotic lesion and could differentiate fibrofatty, fatty and calcification of arterial walls [6-8]. However, it is not precise, because IBS values of lipid pool and intimal hyperplasia were similar. Discrimination of intimal hyperplasia, fibrous cap and thrombus, and sensitivity and specificity of these measurements were not studied in these papers. Furthermore, extent evaluation of each composition, that is, two-dimensional (2D) tissue structure, in entire plaque has not been examined. Therefore, we measured IBS values in carotid arteries in patients compared before and immediately after death, and compared these IBS values with their histopathological features. Subsequently, we constructed 2D color-coded maps of arteries with plaque to assess visually the arterial tissue characteristics.

2. Comparison between IB values and histological images in carotid arteries

Conventional echo images and IBS images were acquired using an ultrasonic imaging system (Sonos 5500, Philips Medical Systems) to characterize the carotid arterial tissue at the bedside conveniently using a 5-12 MHz multifrequency transducer for all studies. This software enabled the acquisition, storing and retrieving of a sequence of continuous 2D conventional and IB images, forming a continuous loop digital recording of two seconds (60 frames in two seconds). Off-line analysis of the 2D IBS images was performed by retrieving the previously stored data from the built-in optical disc drive in the system. IBS value was calculated as the average power of the ultrasound backscattered signal from a small volume of tissue measured in decibels (dB). We used an 11 x 11 pixels (0.6 mm x 0.6 mm) rectangle shaped ROI and set the time gain compensation at 0 dB and the lateral gain compensation at 50 dB at every measurement in both *ex vivo* and *in vivo* study. At this setting, IBS values of stainless steel at a distance of one to two centimeters from the transducer were 50 dB, which was within the dynamic range of the system. IBS values of the posterior arterial wall were corrected (corrected IBS) by subtracting the IBS values of the vessel lumen.

Carotid arteries were excised at autopsy and were fixed with 10% neutral buffered formalin. Ring-like arterial specimens obtained at a similar level to the ultrasound study were decalcified in a standard K-CX solution for five hours, and were embedded with paraffin and cut into 4 μm thick transverse sections perpendicular to the longitudinal axis of the artery. They were stained with hematoxylin-eosin, elastic van Gieson and Masson's trichrome. In addition, immunohistochemical analysis using anti-actin antibody was performed for detection of smooth muscle cells.

Histology of these sampling sites was divided into thrombus (n=5), lipid pool (n=31), intimal hyperplasia (n=7), fibrosis (n=25), mixed lesion (n=12) and calcification (n=17) in the intima, and the media (n=24). Each corrected IBS value of these tissues after fixation at autopsy was 7.3 ± 1.5, 13.0 ± 3.2, 10.9±1.0, 19.3 ± 2.4, 28.2 ± 3.3 and 39.3 ± 3.6 in the intima, respectively, and 11.3 ± 1.9 dB in the media. Also each corrected IBS value during lifetime was 4.9 ± 1.0, 10.0 ± 2.4, 8.0±0.8, 16.0 ± 2.0, 23.5 ± 3.4 and 30.5 ± 2.5 in the intima, respectively, and 8.4 ± 1.8 dB in the media. The difference among thrombus, fibrosis (category-3), mixed lesion, calcification and lipid pool, intimal hyperplasia or media were statistically significant. However, lipid pool, intimal hyperplasia and media had similar IBS values (category-2) [9]. In category-2, the media and intima were differentiated using conventional 2DE. Generally, the lipid pool (category-2) is anatomically located under a fibrous cap consisting of fibrosis (category-3). Therefore, the presence of ROIs with category-2 under a layer of ROIs with category-3 was defined as the lipid pool, but not as intimal hyperplasia.

Based on the above definitions using *in vivo* 2DE and IBS color-coded maps of tissue characterizations were constructed in *in vivo* images. These also reflected the pathology well (Figure 1).

http://dx.doi.org/10.5772/57155

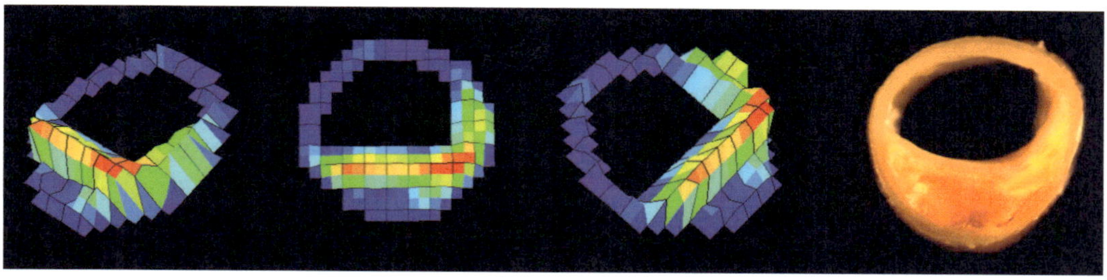

Figure 1. Integrated backscatter ultrasound color-coded maps of the carotid plaque. Left: color-coded maps (red: calcification, orange: mixed lesion, green: fibrosis, blue: lipid pool). Right: pathological specimen.

3. Effects of statin on carotid atherosclerotic plaques

Several large clinical trials have demonstrated that lipid-lowering therapy with HMG-Co-A reductase inhibitors, (statins), reduces cerebrovascular events [10, 11]. Stabilization of vulnerable plaques rather than regression of plaque volume is considered the major contributor to this beneficial effect (5). Stabilization of vulnerable plaques rather than regression of plaque volume is considered the major contributor to this beneficial effect [3].

We assessed the effect of a strong lipophilic statin (atorvastatin) on the stabilization of carotid plaques with ultrasound IBS color imaging by calculating the relative lipid volume. We enrolled patients who were diagnosed with asymptomatic carotid artery stenosis (30-60%) based on carotid ultrasonography and MR angiography. The patients were randomized to a statin (atorvastatin 20mg/day) treatment group (n = 20) or a diet group (n = 20). Transverse and longitudinal scans of carotid plaques were performed using an ultrasound imaging system (SONOS 7500, Philips Medical Systems). The plaques which have unstable component such as lipid core or necrotic core were also imaged with a 1.5-T magnetic resonance imaging (MRI) system (Intera Achieva Nova Dual, Philips Medical Systems) equipped with standard neck array coils. T1-weighted (T1W), proton density-weighted (PDW), and T2-weighted (T2W) images as well as time-of-flight (TOF) images of the plaques were obtained by standardized protocol. The components of plaque were assessed using previous established criteria [12]. We calculated the ratio of the signal intensity of carotid plaques to that of sternocleidomastoid muscle and defined this as the signal intensity ratio (SIR).

At baseline, clinical parameters did not differ between groups. After initiating statin therapy, the lipid profile significantly improved in the statin group, but remained unchanged in the diet group. Baseline IBS values and other characteristics and parameters were similar between the study groups. At baseline, no significant differences were found in these parameters between the statin and diet groups. The relative lipid volume significantly increased in the statin group after 6 months (Figure 2). However, IBS values did not change significantly in the diet group.

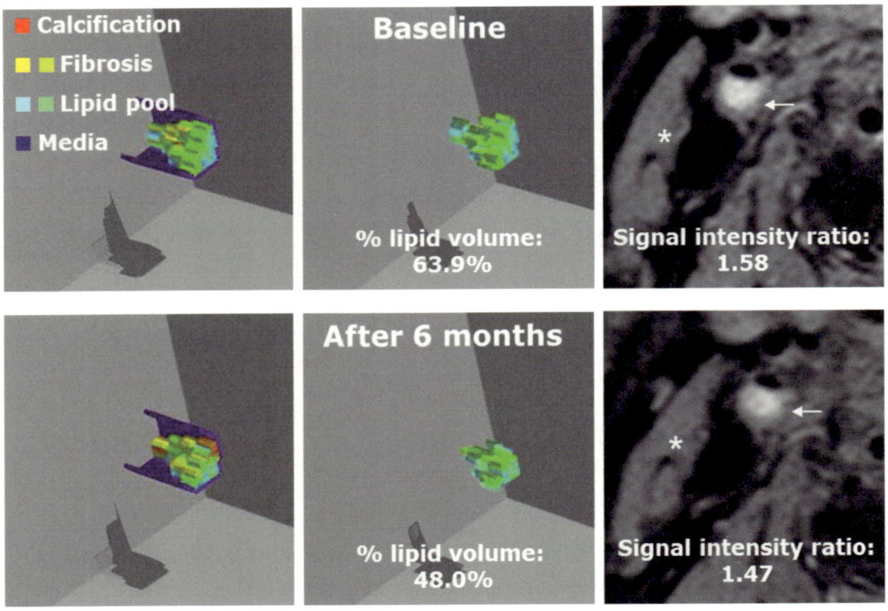

Figure 2. Representative images of three dimensional IBS color-coded maps. Left: Three-dimensional cut out images of color-coded maps of carotid arteries. Middle: Three-dimensional images of lipid pool. Right: High resolutional magnetic resonance images of carotid plaques.

4. Prediction of silent ischemic lesions after carotid artery stenting using IBS and MRI

Carotid artery stenting (CAS) has recently emerged as a potential alternative to carotid endarterectomy (CEA) [13] because it is a less invasive procedure and results in a shorter duration of hospitalization. Although many advantages of CAS have been reported, one of its disadvantages is the considerably high incidence of distal emboli during CAS, even though they are subclinical. Asymptomatic or silent ischemic lesions were detected by diffusion-weighted magnetic resonance imaging (DWI) more often in CAS than in CEA patients [14]. We and other investigators reported that analysis of carotid plaques using IBS ultrasound or black-blood magnetic resonance imaging (BB-MRI) can identify the histological components of carotid plaques [9, 12, 15].

We evaluated carotid lesion with stenosis with a symptomatic carotid stenosis of > 70% or an asymptomatic carotid stenosis of > 60% assessed with angiography, as recommended by the North American Symptomatic Carotid Endarterectomy Trial collaborators [16]. In IBS analysis, relative unstable component area (%UCA: area of intra-plaque hemorrhage and lipid pool / area of plaque) were automatically measured in each plaque by computer software (T3D, Fortner Research LLC, Sterling, Virginia). IN MRI analysis, we calculated the ratio of the signal intensity of carotid plaques to that of sternocleidomastoid muscle and defined this as the signal

http://dx.doi.org/10.5772/57155

intensity ratio (SIR). We assessed newly appearing ipsilateral silent ischemic lesions (NISIL) detected by diffusion-weighted magnetic resonance imaging (DWI) before and after CAS. At the same time, we performed quantitative analysis of plaque characteristics using IBS ultrasound and BB-MRI before CAS in all patients.

After CAS, DWI showed 94 silent ischemic lesions in 19 patients (38%) (diffusion positive group; P group). There were no differences in baseline patient characteristics between the P group and diffusion negative group (N group). In the P group, %UCA analyzed by IBS was significantly higher than in the N group (60.2 ± 23.4% and 35.3 ± 19.2%, respectively, $p<0.001$). Also, the SIR of most stenotic lesions of carotid plaques analyzed by T1WI of BB-MRI was significantly higher in the P group than in the N group (1.40 ± 0.19 and 1.18 ± 0.25, respectively, $p<0.01$) (Figure 3). In multivariate logistic regression analysis, the independent predictors of NISIL were SIR ($p = 0.030$), the CRP level ($p = 0.041$) and the %UCA measured by IBS ($p = 0.049$). In the analysis of receiver operating characteristic curves, 50% of the %UCA measured by IBS analysis and an SIR of 1.25 measured by BB-MRI analysis were determined as the most reliable cutoff values for predicting NISIL. Using these cutoff values, the respective positive and negative predictive values were 76% and 82% in the IBS analysis and 62% and 88% in the BB-MRI analysis.

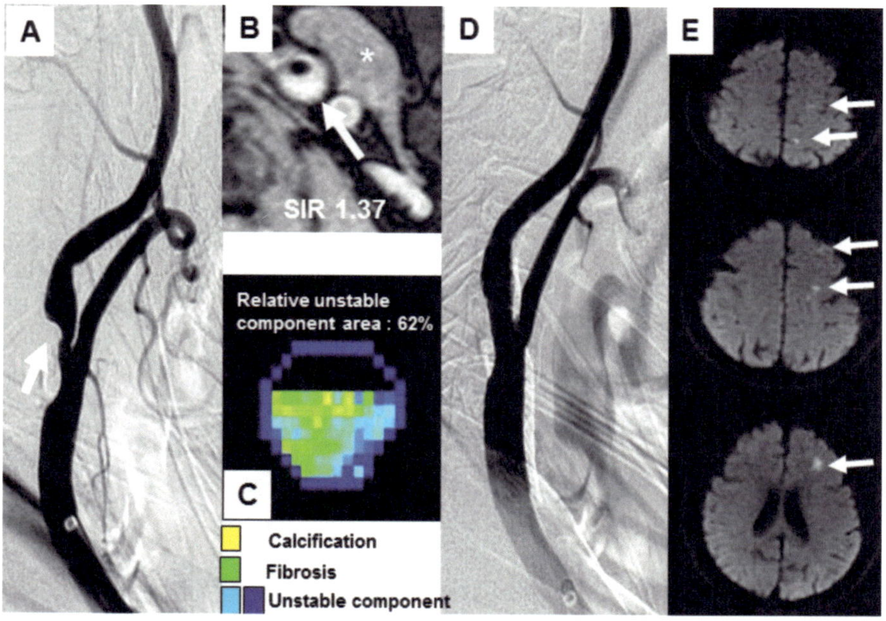

Figure 3. Representative images of CAS for an internal carotid plaque that consisted of less unstable component. (A) Pre-steting angiogram of the left internal carotid artery stenosis. (B) White arrow: Axial image of the most stenotic lesion of the plaque on T1WI of BB-MRI. *: sternocleidomastoid muscle. The SIR was 1.37 (C) Cross-sectional color-coded map of the most stenotic lesion of the plaque on IBS. Relative unstable component area was 62%. (D) Post-stenting angiogram of the left internal carotid artery stenosis. After carotid artery stenting, the lumen of the right internal carotid artery was successfully dilated. (E) Diffusion-weighted magnetic resonance imaging. White arrows: multiple silent ischemic lesions are detected in the left cerebral hemisphere after the post-stenting procedure.

5. Plaque feature of the internal carotid plaques evaluated by optical coherence tomography

Recently, intravascular optical coherence tomography (OCT) provides high-resolution, cross-sectional images of tissue in situ and has an axial resolution of 10 μm and a lateral resolution of 20 μm [17, 18]. The OCT images of human coronary atherosclerotic plaques obtained in vivo provide additional, more detailed structural information than intravascular ultrasound [19].

By applying this technique to carotid plaques, we previously reported the first case of cerebral infarction due to plaque rupture that could be visualized by OCT in the internal carotid artery [20]. An 83-year old male was admitted to our hospital due to newly developed motor weakness of the left hand. MRI-DWI showed multiple high intensity spots in the territory of the middle cerebral artery, and an initial MRA revealed significant stenosis at the origin of the right internal carotid artery. After angiography, a 9-F guiding catheter with an occlusion balloon was navigated to the right common carotid artery and a guidewire with an occlusion balloon (Guardwire, Medtronic Japan Co., Ltd., Tokyo, Japan) was introduced into the external carotid artery. Carotid angiography revealed apparent changes of the wall morphology of the stenotic site, suggesting an enlargement of intraluminal thrombus (Figure 4), which is considered a risk

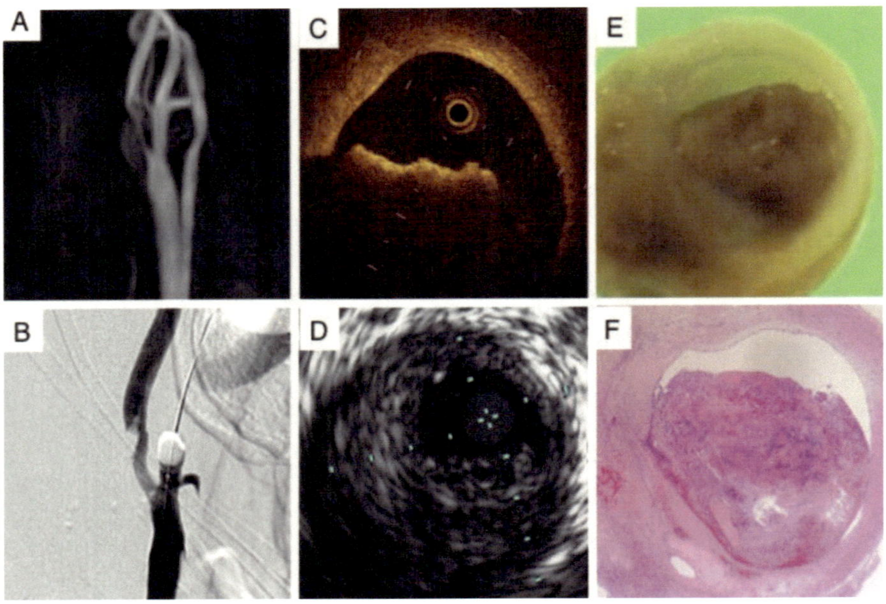

Figure 4. Optical coherence tomography of the internal carotid artery and pathological findings. A: An initial magnetic resonance angiography revealed severe stenosis of the internal carotid artery and high intensity plaque. B: The carotid angiogram showed internal carotid artery stenosis and enlargement of an intraluminal protrusion in the internal carotid artery. C: Cross-sections by the optical coherence tomography (OCT) demonstrated intraluminal thrombus with shadowing in the internal carotid artery. D: Cross-sections by intravascular ultrasound showed only eccentric and low-echoic plaque in the internal carotid artery. E: Macroscopic view of surgical specimen revealed intraluminal thrombus formed at the ruptured site of the soft plaque. F: Pathological analysis with Hematoxylin-Eosin staining confirmed soft plaque and intraluminal red thrombus which coincided with OCT findings.

factor for stenting. To confirm the presence of intraluminal thrombus, the stenotic site was imaged with OCT (Image Wire, Light-lab imaging, Goodman, Co, Ltd, Nagoya, Japan) using an automatic pull-back device from the distal portion at 1 mm/s. OCT clearly revealed an intraluminal thrombus (Figure 4-C), and a tear of a fibrous cap with ulceration at the more proximal internal carotid artery. Carotid artery stenting was cancelled due to enlarged thrombus being considered a high risk factor, and carotid endarterectomy was performed the next day. The specimen obtained during endarterectomy showed soft plaque and intraluminal thrombus which coincided with OCT findings performed preoperatively (Figure 4-E, F).

6. Assessment of arterial medial characteristics in carotid arteries using integrated backscatter ultrasound

In general, atherosclerotic changes consist of two components: atherosis and sclerosis. According to a pathological study, these changes are recognized as thickening of intima-media thickness (IMT) which is associated with structural atheromatous changes and decreased

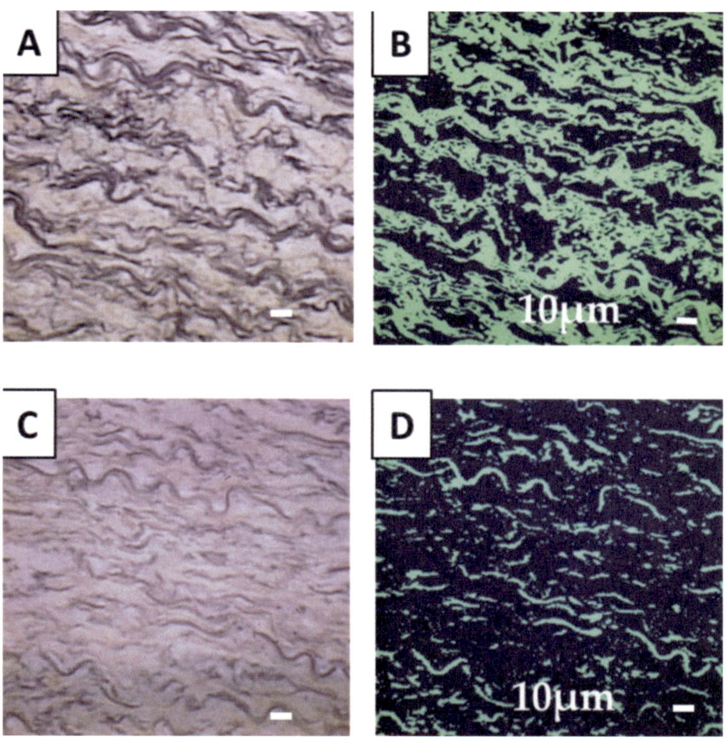

Figure 5. Representative histological images of carotid media. (A) (C) Histological images stained by elastic van Gieson staining. (B) (D) Digitized images, in which elastic fibers were selected by the following thresholding of the digital image LUZEX F (Nireco, Kyoto, Japan). (B) Elastic fiber index: 59.3 %, Elastic fragmentation index: 57.7 % and IBS value: 9.1 dB. (D) Elastic fiber index: 18.9 %, Elastic fragmentation index: 79.3 % and IBS value: 14.4 dB.

extensibility which is associated with functional sclerotic changes in elastic and collagen fibers. There are several ultrasound parameters to evaluate atherosclerosis, such as IMT, which is associated with atheromatous plaque formations and stiffness ß, which are associated with decreased extensibility of the arterial wall. IMT measurement is widely performed for the detection of atheromatous lesions and associated with age and coronary risk factors [21, 22]. However, IMT is not always associated with the severity of arterial sclerosis in patients with hypertension [23]. This may be due to the degenerative changes in the medial smooth muscle cells and variably increased amount of elastin and collagen in hypertensive vessels [24].

The elasticity of major arteries is also affected by cardiovascular risk factors such as hypertension, hyperlipidemia, diabetes and aging. Stiffness ß, which was defined by Hayashi et al was found to be independent of blood pressure in the physiological range and associated with the severity of coronary atherosclerosis [25-27]. An increase in arterial stiffness has been reported as an early sign of atherosclerosis [28]. Therefore, it is very important to evaluate arterial sclerosis non-invasively. We showed that IBS values of carotid media were correlated with the stiffness of carotid arteries, and those were also correlated with elastic fiber fragmentation index (Figure 5) [29].

7. Conclusion

Recently, many techniques for the tissue characterization of human carotid arteries have been established. IBS, MRI and OCT are promising techniques to assess the degree of atherosclerotic lesions in carotid artery and predict cerebrovascular disease.

Author details

Masanori Kawasaki[1*], Shinichi Yoshimura[2] and Kiyofumi Yamada[2]

*Address all correspondence to: masanori@ya2.so-net.ne.jp

1 Department of Cardiology, Gifu University Graduate School of Medicine, Gifu, Japan

2 Department of Neurosurgery, Gifu University Graduate School of Medicine, Gifu, Japan

References

[1] Polak JF, Shemanski L, O'Leary DH, Lefkowitz D, Price TR, Savage PJ, Brant WE, Reid C. Hypoechoic plaque at US of the carotid artery: An independent risk factor for incident stroke in adults aged 65 years or older. The Cardiovascular Health Study. Radiology 1998;208:649–654.

[2] Gronholdt ML, Nordestgaard BG, Schroeder TV, Vorstrup S, Sillesen H. Ultrasonic echolucent carotid plaques predict future strokes. Circulation 2001;104:68-73.

[3] Libby P, Aikawa M. Stabilization of atherosclerotic plaques new mechanisms and clinical targets. Nat Med 2002;8:1257-1262.

[4] Picano E, Pelosi G, Marzilli M, Lattanzi F, Benassi A, Landini L, L'Abbate A. In vivo quantitative ultrasonic evaluation of myocardial fibrosis in humans. Circulation. 1990; 81:58-64.

[5] Naito J, Masuyama T, Mano T, Kondo H, Yamamoto K, Nagano R, Doi Y, Hori M. Ultrasound myocardial tissue characterization in the patients with dilated cardiomyopathy: Value in noninvasive assessment of myocardial fibrosis. Am Heart J. 1996;131:115-121.

[6] Barziliai B, Shffitz JE, Miller JG, Sobel BE. Quantitative ultrasonic characterization of the nature of atherosclerotic plaques in human aorta. Circ Res.1987; 60: 459-463.

[7] Urbani MP, Picano E, Parenti G, Mazzarisi A, Fiori L, Paterni M, Pelosi G, Landini L. In vivo radiofrequency-based ultrasonic tissue characterization of the atherosclerotic plaque. Stroke. 1993;24:1507-1512.

[8] Picano E, Landini L, Lattanzi F, Salvadori M, Benassi A, L'Abbate A. Time domain echo pattern evaluation from normal and atherosclerotic arterial walls: a study in vitro. Circulation. 1988;77:654-659.

[9] Kawasaki M, Takatsu H, Noda T, Ito Y, Kunishima A, Arai M, Nishigaki K, Takemura G, Morita N, Minatoguchi S, Fujiwara H. Non-invasive tissue characterization of human atherosclerotic lesions in carotid and femoral arteries by ultrasound integrated backscatter. -Comparison between histology and integrated backscatter images before and after death- J Am Coll Cardiol. 2001;38:486-492

[10] Amarenco P, Bogousslavsky J, Callahan A 3rd, Goldstein LB, Hennerici M, Rudolph AE, Sillesen H, Simunovic L, Szarek M, Welch KM, Zivin JA; Stroke Prevention by Aggressive Reduction in Cholesterol Levels (SPARCL) Investigators. High-dose atorvastatin after stroke or transient ischemic attack. N Engl J Med 2006;355:549-559.

[11] Waters DD, Schwartz GG, Olsson AG, Zeiher A, Oliver MF, Ganz P, Ezekowitz M. For the MIRACLE study investigator. Effects of atorvastatin on stroke in patients with unstable angina or non-Q-wave myocardial infarction. A Myocardial ischemia reduction with aggressive cholesterol lowing (MIRACLE) substudy. Circulation 2002;196:1690-1695.

[12] Yuan C, Mitsumori LM, Ferguson MS, Polissar NL, Echelard D, Ortiz G, Small R, Davis JW, Kerwin WS, Hatsukami In vivo accuracy of multispectral magnetic resonance imaging for identifying lipid-rich necrotic cores and intraplaque hemorrhage in advanced human carotid plaques. Circulation 2001;104:2051-2056.

[13] Diethrich EB, Ndiaye M, Reid DB. Stenting in the carotid artery: initial experience in 110 patients. J Endovasc Surg. 1996;3:42-62.

[14] Schnaudigel S, Gröschel K, Pilgram SM, Kastrup A. New brain lesions after carotid stenting versus carotid endarterectomy: A systematic review of the literature. Stroke 2008;39:1911-1919.

[15] Kawasaki M, Ito Y, Yokoyama H, Arai M, Takemura G, Hara A, Ichiki Y, Takatsu H, Minatoguchi S, Fujiwara H. Assessment of arterial medial characteristics in human carotid arteries using integrated backscatter ultrasound and its histological implications. Atherosclerosis 2005;180:145-54.

[16] North American Symptomatic Carotid Endarterectomy Trial Collaborators: Beneficial effect of carotid endarterectomy in symptomatic patients with high-grade carotid stenosis. N Engl J Med 1991;325:445-453.

[17] Tearney GJ, Brezinski ME, Bouma BE, Boppart SA, Pitris C, Southern JF, Fujimoto JG. In vivo endoscopic optical biopsy with optical coherence tomography. Science. 1997; 276:2037–2039.

[18] Brezinski ME, Tearney GJ, Bouma BE, Izatt JA, Hee MR, Swanson EA, Southern JF, Fujimoto JG. Optical coherence tomography for optical biopsy: properties and demonstration of vascular pathology. Circulation. 1996; 93:1206–1213.

[19] Jang IK, Tearney GJ, MacNeill B, Takano M, Moselewski F, Iftima N, Shishkov M, Houser S, Aretz HT, Halpern EF, Bouma BE. In vivo characterization of coronary atherosclerotic plaque by use of optical coherence tomography. Circulation. 2005;111:1551-1555.

[20] Yoshimura S, Kawasaki M, Yamada K, Enomoto Y, Hattori A, Nishigaki K, Minatoguchi S, Iwama T. Determination of intraluminal thrombus in the carotid artery by optical coherence tomography: a case report. Neurosurgery 2010;67:onsE305.

[21] Hadjiisky P, Peyri N, Grosgogeat Y et al. Tunica media changes in the spontaneously hypertensive rat (SHR). Atherosclerosis. 1987;65:125-137.

[22] Mannami T, konishi M, baba S et al. Prevalence of asymptomatic carotid atherosclerotic lesions detected by high-resolution ultrasonography and its relation to cerdiovascular risk factors in the general population of a Japanese city. Stroke. 1997;28:518-525.

[23] Rossi M, Cupisti A, Perrone L et al. Carotid ultrasound backscatter analysis in hypertensive and in healthy subjects. Ultrasound Med Biol. 2002;28(9):1123-1128.

[24] Wolinsky H. Response of the rat aortic media to hypertension. Circ Res. 1970;26:507-522.

[25] Ebrahim S, Papacosta O, Whincup P et al. Carotid plaque, intima media thickness, cardiovascular risk factors, and prevalent cardiovascular disease in men and women. The British regional heart study. Stroke. 1999;30:841-850.

[26] Hirai T, Sasayama S, Kawasaki T et al. Stiffness of systemic arteries in patients with myocadial infarction. A noninvasive method to predict severity of coronary atherosclerosis. Circulation. 1989;80:78-86.

[27] Hayashi K, Handa H, Nagasaka S et al. Stiffness and elastic behavior of human intracranial and exracranial arteries. J Biomech. 1980; 13: 175-184

[28] Ferrier KE, Muhlmann MH, Baguet JP et al. Intensive cholesterol reduction lowers blood pressure and large artery stiffness in isolated systolic hypertension. J Am Coll Cardiol. 2002; 39: 1020-1025.

[29] Kawasaki M, Ito Y, Yokoyama H, Arai M, Takemura G, Hara A, Ichiki Y, Takatsu H, Minatoguchi S, Fujiwara H. Assessment of arterial medial characteristics in human carotid arteries using integrated backscatter ultrasound and its histological implications. Atherosclerosis. 2005;180:145-54.

Chapter 3

Carotid Artery – Pathology, Plaque Structure – Relationship between Histological Assessment, Color Doppler Ultrasonography and Magnetic Resonance Imaging – Dolichoarteriopathies – Barorreceptors

Ricardo Luis Beigelman, Andrés María Izaguirre,
Francisco Azzato and José Milei

Additional information is available at the end of the chapter

http://dx.doi.org/10.5772/57157

1. Introduction

Carotid artery atherosclerosis is a major cause of disabling stroke and death [1] and it is thought to be the predominant etiology of stroke in Western society [2]. Moreover, stroke is the third leading cause of death and the primary cause of disability in the world [2].

Compared with medical therapy, surgical endarterectomy or carotid stenting have been proven to decrease stroke in symptomatic patients with severe stenosis[3-7] and in a very selective group of asymptomatic patients suffering of this pathology[8-9]

Nevertheless, clinical assessment of stroke risk had not progressed beyond the use of luminal stenosis in spite of evidence to suggest that this is an inadequate predictor of stroke. [10]

More recently, imaging studies have suggested plaque composition as an independent risk factor for ischemic stroke. [11]

Because of this, many efforts have been made to correlate symptoms and cerebral events with histological studies, color doppler ultrasonography (CDU) and magnetic resonance imaging (MRI).

Carotid dolichoarteriopathies were have also been proposed as a source of cerebral vascular insufficiency but this issue remains very controversial in the literature.[12-14]. In this chapter, our experience on CDU of neck vessels in 885 individuals with carotid dolichoarteriopathies (age 1-day-old infants to 90-year-old adults),[15-16], the correlation of plaque appearance between B ultrasonography and pathology, [17] and the histological assessment in 281 carotid endarterectomy specimens [18] will be widely described and discussed.

In this connection, in a pioneer study we made a complete immunohistochemical characterization in complicated carotid plaques. [18] The cellular components of carotid endarterectomy specimens were analyzed to assess their role in the pathogenesis of plaque rupture and intraplaque hemorrhage without rupture. The site of plaque rupture is associated with the presence of an extensive infiltrate of macrophages, T-lymphocytes, scarce B-lymphocytes, mast cells, and smooth muscle cells. Both the plaques showing these features and those with large amounts of lipid and thin fibrous caps, should be considered as "plaques at risk". Intraplaque hemorrhages without plaque rupture may be caused by the breakdown of neoformed vessels in the core, base, and periphery of the plaques. [18]

This paper emphasized the importance of the detection of vulnerable plaque for preventing future cerebral events. The main factors in advanced plaque that are most likely to lead to complications are the thickness of the fibrous cap, the size of the necrotic core and intraplaque hemorrhage, and the extent of inflammatory activity within the plaque.

Later on, we analyzed the relation between the anatomy of the carotid plaques and the presence of symptoms in 281 carotid endarterectomy specimens. [19] Almost 70% of plaque specimens demonstrated thrombus, intraplaque hemorrhage, or both. Thrombosis was observed in one fourth of specimens, and intraplaque hemorrhage in almost two thirds of specimens. Sixty four percent of plaques demonstrated neovascularization. In spite of findings in some published articles, [20] it was not possible to demonstrate that complicated plaques (plaque rupture, thrombosis, intraplaque hemorrhage) are associated with symptoms, and it appears that complicated plaques may occur at any time, irrespective of symptoms. [19]

Regarding the biology of the unstable atherosclerotic carotid plaque, an expression of c-fos, p53 and PCNA was demonstrated by us. [21]

On the other hand, MRI has excellent soft tissue contrast and is able to quantify carotid plaque size and composition with good accuracy and reproducibility and provides an opportunity to prospectively examine the relationship between plaque features and subsequent cerebrovascular events. [22] In a paper by Takaya et al [23] 154 patients with an asymptomatic 50% to 79% carotid stenosis by ultrasound with > or =12 months of follow-up were included for multicontrast-weighted carotid MRIs were included. Over a mean follow-up period of 38.2 months, arteries with thinned or ruptured fibrous caps, intraplaque hemorrhage, larger maximum %lipid-rich/necrotic cores, and larger maximum wall thickness were associated with the occurrence of subsequent cerebrovascular events. [23]

MRI imaging techniques have permitted serial monitoring of atherosclerotic disease evolution and the identification of intraplaque risk factors for accelerated progresión. [22]

At last, based upon our research, carotid barochemoreceptor involvement in old patients who died from stroke and suffering obstructive carotid atheromatosis will be discussed. [24]

2. Pathology

Carotid atherosclerosis is commonly associated with symptoms of cerebral ischemia. However little attention has been directed to intraplaque factors that precipitate the onset of symptoms. [25] On the other hand, the treatment of coronary and carotid atherosclerosis, requires an understanding of the pathogenesis of plaque fissure. [26] Advances in molecular biology, coronary diagnostic techniques and cardiac treatments have suggested new factors leading to plaque fissure. [26-28] It was suggested that the risk of plaque fissure depends on plaque composition rather than plaque size, because only plaques rich in soft extracellular lipids are prone to rupture. [27] Also, it was demonstrated that ruptured plaque caps have much larger transverse gradients of connective tissue constituents than non-ruptured plaque caps, and that the development of these transverse gradients may be critical in determining the propensity of a plaque to rupture. [28] It was also shown that the site of rupture of thrombosed coronary atherosclerotic plaques is marked by an inflammatory infiltration where the macrophages are the dominant cells. [29]

However, the exact mechanisms causing plaque rupture are yet not complete known. [29] In this connection, papers dealing with rupture of carotid plaque surface are few in spite of the growing importance of the subject. [18,19,30] We analyzed in pioneer papers[18,19,30] the cellular and vascular components of surgically excised carotid endarterectomies. Thus, the cell populations involved in the inflammatory activity in atherosclerotic lesions were further characterized with cell specific monoclonal antibodies in order to obtain information about their role in the pathogenesis of plaque rupture and intraplaque hemorrhage.[30] In brief, 76 surgical specimens of 74 patients who were submitted to carotid endarterectomy were used for these studies. There were 55 males and 19 females. Age ranged from 40 to 83 years (mean 69.4 years).Patients were divided into three clinical subgroups: asymptomatic (carotid lumen obstruction > 70%), symptomatic (stable) and symptomatic (unstable). The usual unifying pathologic feature in the plaques was the presence of large lipid cores with a fibrous cap overlying the lipid core and a band of fibrous tissue of varying thickness separating the plaque from the atrophic media (Figure 1). This collagen rim was in general extensively vascularized. Exceptionally the plaque was composed of fibrocellular tissue without a clear lipid core. In most cases, widespread chronic inflammatory infiltrates were observed either in the cap or in the lipid core (Figure 2). In all cases the carotid bifurcation and the first 1.5 cm of the internal carotid were involved.

The result of immunophenotyping of the cellular constituents of the plaques were described in relation to the different layers (from the lumen to the media), namely: Endothelial lining (Anti-CD31 and anti-CD34). The fibrous cap at the site of the rupture/erosion had an eroded surface characterized by loss of the endothelial lining (Figure 3). On the other hand in the remaining surface a continuous, not damaged row of endothelial cells stained with anti-CD31 and anti-CD34 was observed in all cases

Fibrous cap: the collagenous fibrous cap at the site of erosion was attenuated and the phenotypic characterization of the cells showed inflammatory components consisting mainly of macrophages (CD68 positive), approximately 2/3 of the total infiltration (Figure 4). The remaining 1/3 was composed of T-lymphocytes and rare B-lymphocytes. This pattern was observed in 34/ 41 (83%) of ruptured plaques. A close interaction between macrophages and the abundant capillaries of the lipid cores (Figure 4) and macrophages and T-lymphocytes was commonly observed. Some foamy macrophages showed not only brown staining corresponding to the expression of CD68 but also weak red staining for CD31, thus suggesting that these cells also contain this adhesion molecule. Plaques "at risk" (attenuated fibrous cap, large lipid core and extensive macrophage infiltration) are represented in Figure 1.

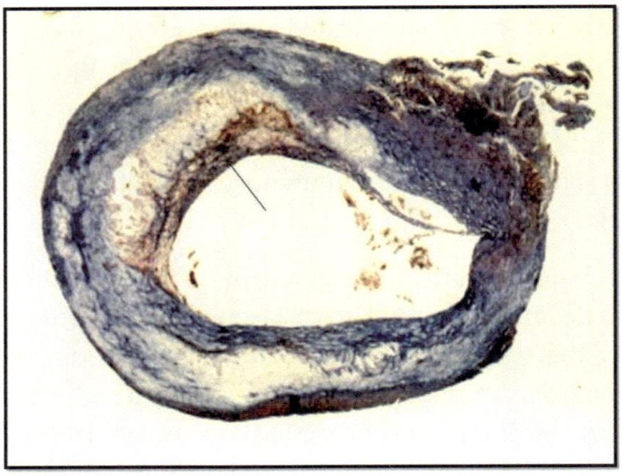

Figure 1. A large lipid core with a thin fibrous cap (arrow) overlying the lipid core is observed.

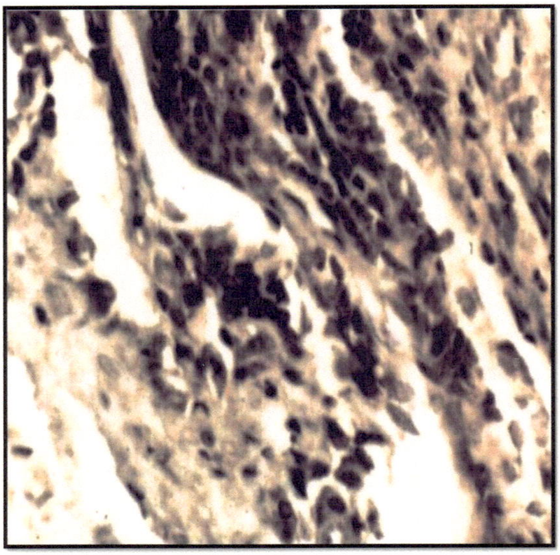

Figure 2. A neoformed thin-walled vessel is shown with lymphocytes migrating to the highly vascularized lipid. Magnification ´250

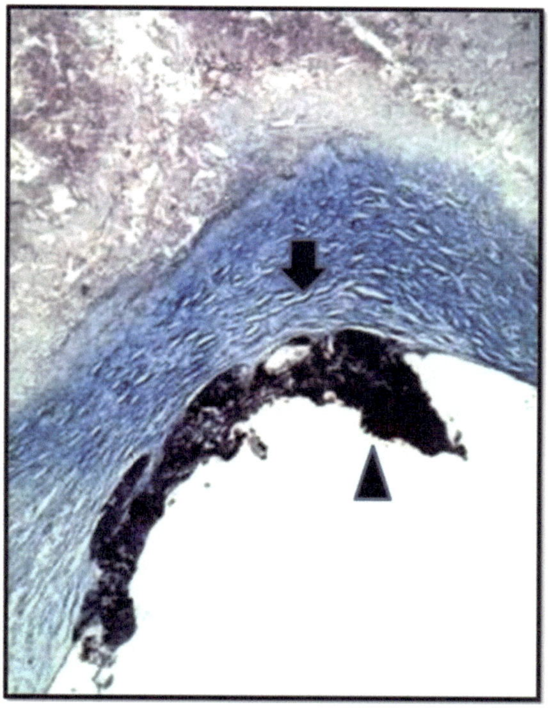

Figure 3. Intraplaque hemorrhage without plaque rupture. Superimposed parietal thrombus. A continuous non ruptured thick cap is shown (arrow). A parietal thrombus is implanted in an eroded surface (arrowhead), and a rich lipid core is heavily embedded by intraplaque hemorrhage(LC).Trichrome-stained collagen, *blue*; hemorrhage, *light red*; thrombus *blue-red* (original magnification _200).

Lipid cores: two different types of lipid cores could be depicted, avascular or mildly vascularized lipid cores and highly vascularized, with neoformed vessels stained with CD34 and CD31(Figure 5 and 6). These vessels varied from proliferated small, thin walled blood vessels to bigger ones, in some cases presenting a hemangioma-like aspect. CD34 stained endothelia of all kind of vessels; conversely, neoformed vessels showed a weak stain with CD31.T-lymphocytes were found to be in contact with neoformed vessels, and in some cases, migrating through the endothelial cells

Media: this tunic was composed of 5 to 12 rows of smooth muscle cells, with their long axes oriented circumferentially, as the edge of the endarterectomy passed through that level. Some thin walled normal capillaries oriented longitudinally to the long axis of the smooth muscle cells were fairly showed by the CD34 and CD31 (Figure 8). Although this tunic did not belong to the plaque itself, it is herein described because of its peculiar vascularization. It is therefore necessary to make a clear distinction regarding the neoformed vessels of the base and periphery of the plaque, and the adjacent capillaries of the media originating from the vasavasorum.

Deeper layers of the plaque: the base and the shoulder of the plaques showed in 28/76 cases neoformed vessels, thin or thick walled, CD34 positive (Figure 7), generally surrounded by mild to extensive mononuclear infiltrates.

Basically atherosclerotic plaques were found to be-long to six different lesions, namely: plaque rupture plus thrombosis (18/76, 23.6%), plaque rupture plus intraplaque hemorrhage plus thrombosis (18/76, 23.6%), intraplaque hemorrhage without plaque rupture (16/76, 21.0%), plaque rupture plus intraplaque hemorrhage (5/76, 6.5%), stable calcified non complicated plaque (14/76, 18.4%) and unstable, soft, non complicated plaque (5/76, 6.5%). The first four lesions were considered as "complicated lesions".

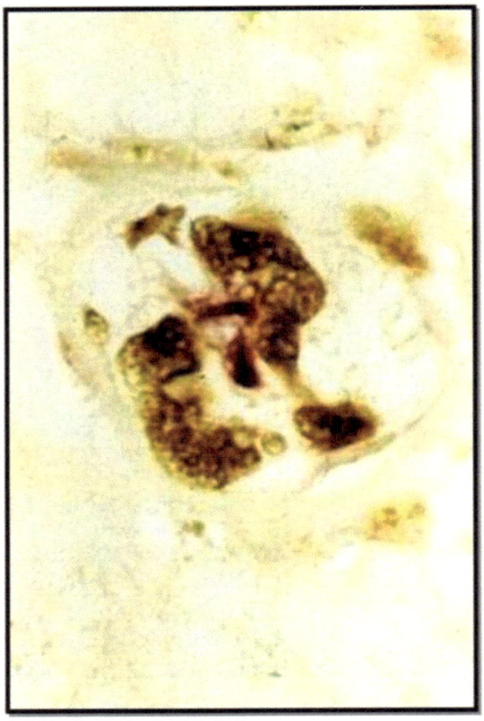

Figure 4. Foamy macrophages show brown staining corresponding to the expression of CD68 and weak red staining for CD31.

- **Plaque rupture plus thrombosis (PR+T).** The fibrous cap overlying the lipid core was highly variable in thickness and cellular constituents. Plaques presented ulcerations with break-down of the surface of the cap. Their-regularity had a punched-out characteristic or was simply a tear with borders; in rare cases plaques contained virtually no fibrous cap. The rupture was covered by a thrombus, and in many cases the thrombus was found directly overlying the lipid core of the lesion, entering a large pool of extracellular lipids. As said the borders of the rupture presented a mononuclear infiltration with a high density of macrophages.

- **Plaque rupture plus intraplaque hemorrhage plus thrombosis (PR+IPH+T).** (Figure 9)The histological findings were similar to the ruptured-thrombosed plaques, but there was also extensive disruption of the plaque by an intraplaque hemorrhage.

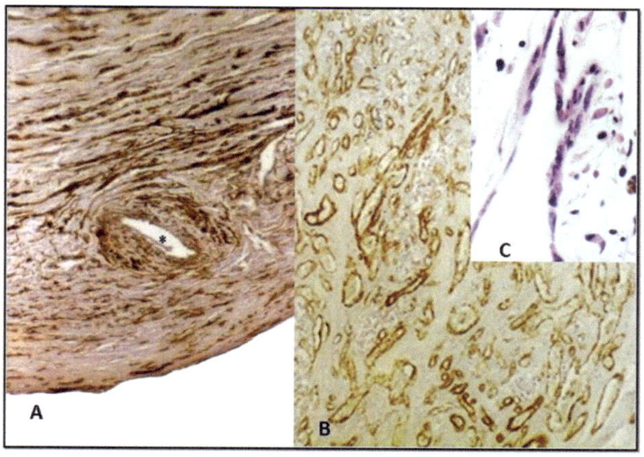

Figure 5. Intense neovascularization of the lipid core. Immunoperoxidase technique for smooth muscle cells (α-actin). In panel A, the asterisk indicates a thick neovascularization vessel. Panel B shows the middle arterial layer. In panel C:,a central neoformed vessel outgrowth in "glove finger" is seen into the lipid core. Endothelial pyknotic cells surrounded by scarse pericytes, macrophages, and lymphocytes in the periphery are shown.

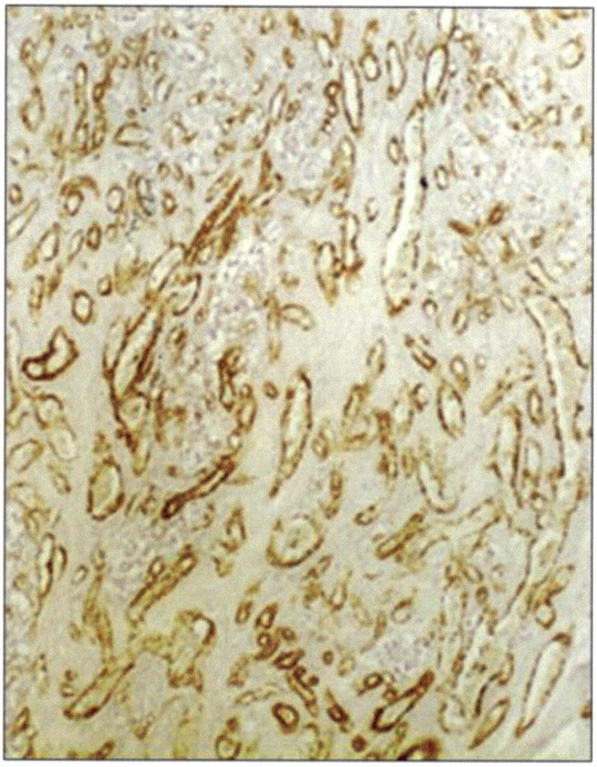

Figure 6. Lipid-rich core is heavily vascularized by great number of thin-walled, neoformed,CD34-positive vessels. Magnification ´250.

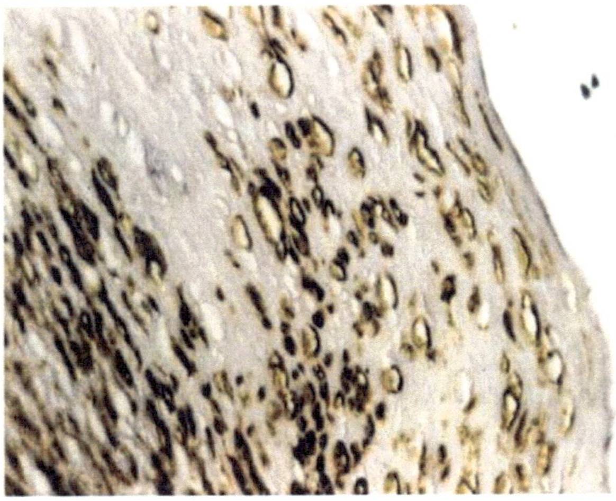

Figure 7. Vascularization of the shoulder of the plaque. Note thin-walled neoformed vessels of different shapes and sizes. Outer zone shows media and an extensive quantity of thin-walled normal capillaries,longitudinally oriented *(brown).* Antiactin monoclonal antibody(HHF35) was used to demonstrate vascular structures (original magnification _250).

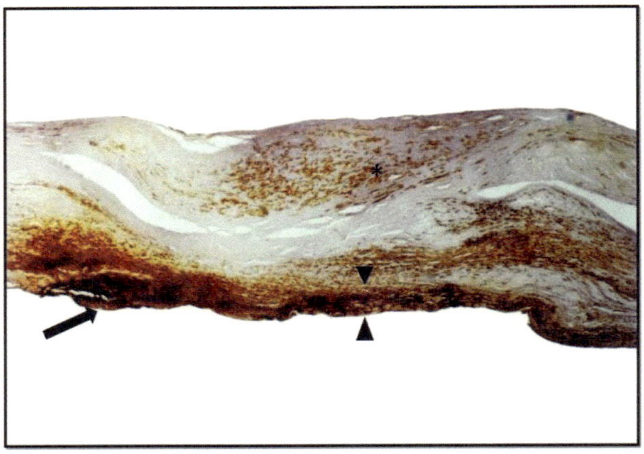

Figure 8. Low magnification view of an entire endarterectomy specimen shows actin-positive vessel walls (HHF35) and hyperplastic smooth muscle cells (asterisc). Media (arrowheads) shows normal arrangement and at this level is composed of only 5 to 10 layers of smooth muscle cells (arrow). Magnification x25.

Intraplaque hemorrhage without plaque rupture (IPH) (Figure 10). None of them had a connection between the hemorrhage and the arterial lumen, in spite of a careful search in serial sections. Conversely the intimal surfaces were clean and none showed evidence or platelet or fibrin deposition. Hemorrhages varied from microscopic, microfocal or slitlike foci of recent hemorrhage, with no evident changes in the overall makeup of the plaque to massive hemorrhage, elevation and disruption of the intima to massive hemorrhage,elevation and disruption of the intima and occlusive stenosis. Only these massive lesions were considered. Of note, slitlike hemorrhages distant to the main lesion were found in 12 cases, in 5 of them without the presence of a massive intraplaque hemorrhage.

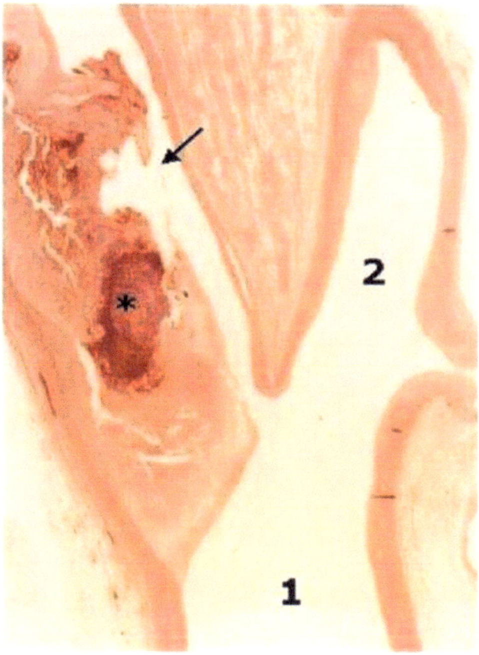

Figure 9. Plaque rupture (arrow) plus intraplaque hemorrhage and parietal thrombosis. An entire specimen from a carotid endarterectomy frontally cut is shown. 1, Common carotid artery; 2,external carotid artery. *Large lipid core with huge intraplaque hemorrhage with thrombotic components, and small parietal thrombus are observed. Fibrous cap is extremely thin (hematoxylin-eosin; original magnification 3).

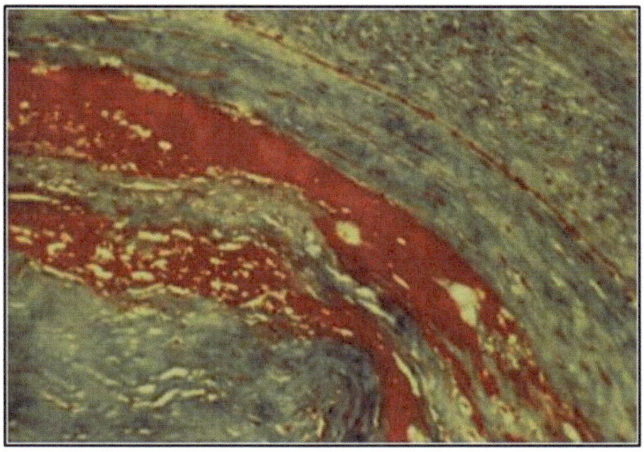

Figure 10. Sample of carotid endarterectomy. Laminar hemorrhage, distal to the main lesion Trichrome-stained collagen, *blue*; hemorrhage, *light red*; Magnification ´250.

Plaque rupture plus intraplaque hemorrhage (PR+IPH) (Figure 11). It was characterized by an extensive hemorrhage within the plaque with separation of its varying components and disruption of the intima.

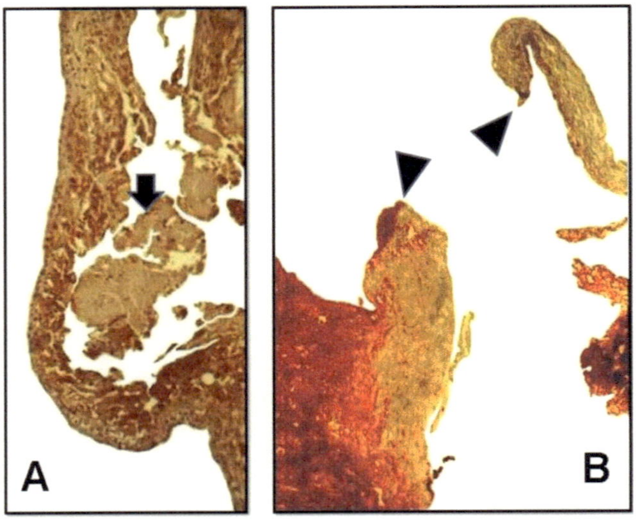

Figure 11. Plaque rupture. A intraplaque hemorrhage (arrow) B-. Breakdown of cap is clearly shown (between arrow-heads)

- **Stable, calcified, non complicated plaque (S+C)** (Figure 12).These plaques contained neither thrombosis nor hemorrhages and consisted of laminated fibrous connective tissue and irregular masses of calcified material. These areas appeared as acellular, roughly circular masses of pale-staining debris.

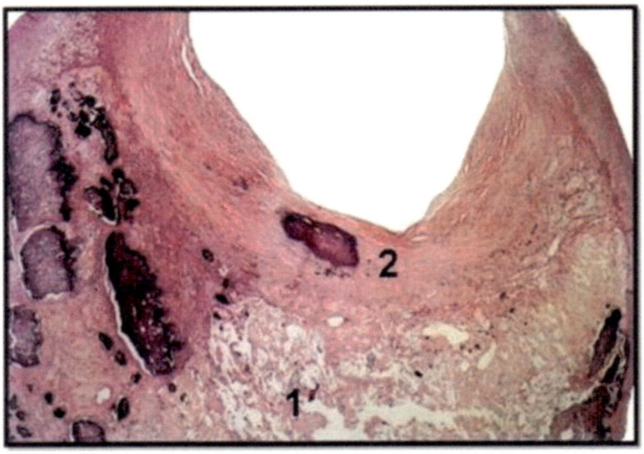

Figure 12. Stable calcified plate. Lipid core (1), thick cover (2), and abundant calcified areas in black

Unstable, soft, non complicated plaque (U+NC). These plaques consisted of thin fibrous caps covering a lipid-rich core with extensive vascularization. As these are the ingredients of a plaque "at risk", those may be plaques in which rupture hemorrhage and/or thrombosis might have occurred in the future.

Complicated vs stable calcified, non complicated plaques. Complicated plaques presented neoformed vessels in the periphery, shoulder and base of the plaque in 22/57 (38.5%) cases. Conversely only 1/14 (7.1%) of non complicated, stable calcified plaques presented this type of vessels ($p < 0.05$). Of note, the 5 cases of unstable, soft non complicated plaque presented neoformed vessels surrounding the plaque. In 10/57 (17.5%) complicated plaques unequivocal histological signs of old hemorrhages were found surrounding those vessels. Irrespective of presenting no rupture, 11/35 plaques showed a mononuclear in-filtrate in the fibrous cap.

Clinical-pathological correlation. The risk factor variables (age, gender, hypertension, left ventricular hypertrophy, diabetes, weight, smoking and uric acid) could not be correlated with any of the pathological and immunohistochemical findings. Hypertension (70%) and smoking (59%) were the risk factors more frequently found irrespective of the morphological findings.Therefore, carotid endarterectomies provided the material for phenotypic characterization of vascular and cellular components of the plaque. This permitted to known the topography and the distribution of mononuclear infiltrates as well as endothelial cells. Although the cellular composition of advanced atherosclerotic plaques is known to be heterogeneous, [31] it can be summarized as:

Intimal plaque rupture-inflammatory process. We demonstrated for the first time[30] that rupture of carotid plaques is characterized by the presence of a macrophagic infiltration of the caps. The presence of a large number of foamy macrophages in plaque fissuring in human coronary thrombosis had been reported previously [29,32-34] and it was suggested that inflammation through enzymatic degradation of the fibrous cap by macrophages might destabilize the plaque, causing weakening at the immediate site of rupture. In carotid endarterectomies although the fibrous cap overlying the plaque was variable in thickness, the area of rupture was dominated by macrophages as the main cellular component, T-lymphocytes and scarce B-lymphocytes and granulated and/or degranulated mast cells. Complete rupture of the fibrous cap was found to be the cause of thrombosis in 18 cases, intraplaque hemorrhage plus thrombosis in 18 and intraplaque hemorrhage in 5 cases. It means that approximately 50% of carotid endarterectomies have the plaque fissure as the anatomic substratum. Of note, only 23/41 (56%) of these cases have been symptomatic. Our studies in carotid plaques showed direct apposition of T-lymphocytes to macrophages and a close relation of these cells to endothelial cells. This highly suggests a cell-to-cell interaction, which results in an inflammatory process mediated by cellular adhesion molecules (such as CD31), cytokines, growth factors and other substances as described in coronary arteries[29] and aorta. [35] Therefore, the possibility of autocrine, juxtacrine or paracrine secretion was evident. [36]

Intraplaque hemorrhage without plaque rupture-plaque vascularization. Intraplaque hemorrhage without rupture was present in 21% of the endarterectomies. This subset of carotid lesions was not related to cap erosion, but to plaque vascularization. Most lipid cores were highly vascularized with neoformed vessels with macrophages and T-cells in close contact and some cases disrupting the endothelium The abrupt growing of the lipid cores and/or an overproduction of oxygen free radicals could lead to the breakdown of core vessels and intraplaque hemorrhage. This seems to be the most plausible mechanism. The periphery and shoulder of the plaques had in 30% of the cases neoformed vessels surrounded by extensive mononuclear infiltrates. Theseneoformed vessels showed a weak stain with CD31. Considering that CD31 (PECAM-1) is a molecular adhesion molecule, the lack of expression could be pointing out a functional difference between normal and neoformed vessels. PECAM- 1 is required for transendothelial migration of leucocytes.

The same mechanism postulated for the vessels of the core may operate in neoformed vessels. The presence of histological signs of old hemorrhages and the existence of slitlike hemorrhages at that level strongly suggest that a local origin of bleeding may operate. Lusby et al[25] demonstrated that the resultant angiogenesis associated with hemorrhages might make those lesions prone to mechanical stress and subsequent hemorrhages. Accordingly, our observations and those by other authors suggest that intraplaque hemorrhages may occur at any time in the history of carotid plaque. [37] Hypertension may be a predisposing factor in the rupture of neoformed vessels and the development of the hemorrhage within the plaque.

Our results in 76 endarterectomies suggest that the site of plaque rupture is associated with the presence of a large macrophagic infiltration, [38] as well as T-lymphocytes rare B-lymphocytes and mast cells and lack of smooth muscle cells. These peculiar type of plaque should be considered as a "plaque at risk"[29] in addition to plaques containing large amounts of lipid pools and a thin fibrous cap. [34] Conversely, intraplaque hemorrhages without plaque rupture might be due to the breakdown of neo-formed core vessels and/or neoformed vessels of the base and shoulder of the plaque.

The decision of whether to perform endarterectomy in patients with asymptomatic disease should be made on the basis of data including degree of stenosis and activity of the carotid lesion, as well as issues of medical and surgical morbidity. [39]

The relationship between anatomy of carotid plaques and the presence or not of symptoms. For this purpose we carried out an investigation[19] in order to analyze in a large sample the relation between the anatomy of carotid plaques and the presence of symptoms in 281 endarterectomy specimens. To avoid an excessive number of plaque subtypes that might blur the relationship with symptoms, [31] only complicated and non-complicated plaques and ruptured and nonruptured plaques were used for statistical analysis. Patients (mean age, 68 +/-8 y.o.,range,40-84 y.o.) were 213 men (mean age, 68 y.o.s; range, 45-83 y.o.) and 68 women (mean age,68.7 y.o.; range, 40-84 y.o.).[19] In all cases the bifurcation and the first 10 to 15 mm of the internal carotid artery were involved. In 196 plaques, large lipid cores with a fibrous cap and a band of fibrous tissue separating the plaque from the remainder of the media were observed. The cap was frequently vascularized. In most cases, extensive inflammatory infiltrates consisting of macrophages, smaller numbers of T lymphocytes, a few B lymphocytes, and mast cells were observed. In the remaining cases, the plaque was composed of fibrocellular tissue only.[19]

For statistical purposes, plaques were divided into two subsets: **complicated** (types PR+T, PR +IPH+T, PR+IPH, ulcerated calcified plaques and IPH) vs. **non-complicated**, and **ruptured** (types 1 through 4) vs **non-ruptured** (types IPH,S+C and U+NC).

Complicated plaques (205 of 281) exhibited mononuclear infiltrates in the periphery, shoulders,and bases in 137 of 205 (67%) plaques, compared with only 22 of 76 (29%) noncomplicated plaques (p< 0.001). Complicated plaques demonstrated neoformed vessels in the periphery, shoulders, and bases in 146 of 205 (71%) plaques, compared with only 38 of 76 (50%) noncomplicated plaques (p<0.001). Twelve of 18 unstable, soft, non complicated plaques exhibited neoformed vessels surrounding the plaques. The remaining 6 plaques had huge lipid cores without evident neoformed vessels, suggesting very recent development. In 34 of 205(17%) complicated plaques, old hemorrhages were found surrounding neoformedvessels. Ruptured versus non-ruptured plaques. Infiltrates were noted in the caps and shoulders in 108 of 130 (83%) ruptured plaques and 22 of 151 (15%) unruptured plaques (p< 0.0001).External carotid arteries arteries exhibited typical histopathologic findings of advanced atheromatosis in 51 of 281 cases(18%).Only 2 of 51 affected cases demonstrated complicated plaques.This resulted in a significant difference when compared with the internal carotid artery ruptures (1of40 vs 85 of 165 p< 0.001).Risk factors could not be associated with any pathologic findings. Hypertension (74%), smoking (61%), hyperlipidemia (61%), and diabetes mellitus (24%) were the risk factors most frequently noted. No correlation could be established between plaque type and symptoms (Table I). Of note, although 99 of 205 (48%) complicated plaques were found in patients with symptomatic disease, a high percentage (106 of 205, 52%) were also found in patients with asymptomatic disease. The same was observed for ruptured plaques; 67 of 130 (52%) were found in patients with symptomatic disease, compared with 63 of 130 (48%) in patients with asymptomatic disease. No relation could be found between symptomatic versus asymptomatic disease with regard to old hemorrhage (18 [12%] vs 26 [19%]), distal IPH(19 [13%] vs 13 [10%]), laminar hemorrhage (14 [9%] vs 22 [16%]), and parietal thrombosis (14 [9%] vs18 [13%]).

Differences in flow velocity profiles and wall shear stress might explain the lower atherosclerotic involvement and rare complications of the external carotid artery as compared with the internal carotid artery (205 of 281 vs 2 of 281; P<0.0001). Areas of carotid plaque rupture were characterized by macrophagic infiltration at the rupture. This finding suggests that inflammation, through enzymatic degradation of the fibrous cap by macrophages, might destabilize the plaque, causing weakening at the site of rupture.[25,30,40] Complete rupture of the cap (46% of cases) was the cause of thrombosis in 7%, IPH plus thrombosis in 18%, and IPH in 19%. Therefore plaque rupture was the cause of thrombosis in only 25% of cases. Many factors can modulate the development of thrombus. Long-term preoperative administration of aspirin and use of heparin during surgery may explain the relatively low frequency of thrombosis observed in ruptured plaques. Other possibilities are that fibrin or platelet deposition was missed at previous embolization orduring microscopic examination because of sampling. However, inasmuch as excisionwas *in bloc*, without "touching" the lesion, thrombus displacement seems unlikely. IPH without rupture represented 27% of endarterectomy specimens in the present study. This subset of lesions was not related to rupture of the cap, but to plaque neovascularization. Lipid cores were highly vascularized with heterogeneous neoformed vessels and with macrophages and T cells in close contact with the endothelial wall. An increase in the amount of lipid in the core, mechanicalstresses,[25] and overproduction of oxygen free radicals by macrophages could lead to breakdown of core neoform vessels and IPH production.[27] The same mechanisms might also act in neoform vessels in the periphery of the plaques. Old hemorrhages in 17% of complicated plaques and presence of distant slitlike hemorrhages strongly suggest that the bleeding may be of local origin.[30,41] Hemorrhages were attributed to mechanical stress of turbulent flow and to wall vibration secondary to stiffness of the carotid wall,[30] and have also been associated with an increase in matrix metalloproteinase 1 expression in the macrophages of the fibrous cap, suggesting a role for inflammatory mediators in vessel disruption.[31] Therefore, IPH may occur at any time in the course of a carotid plaque.[18,30,37,38]

Complicated and noncomplicated plaques versus symptomatic and asymptomatic disease. Plaque rupture was present in 46% of endarterectomy specimens. However, only 67 of 130 (52%) of these were found in patients with symptomatic disease. On the other hand, a high proportion of patients with asymptomatic disease (48%) demonstrated complicated plaques.Coronary plaque ruptures have been identified in patients who died of noncardiac causes.[18] Accordingly, occurrence of carotid plaque rupture or hemorrhage without symptomatic manifestation seems likely.The frequency of plaque hemorrhage and plaque disruption varied greatly among the various series from both symptomatic and asymptomatic specimens In a review of several studies,[25,37,42-46] Fisher et al observed that the pooled frequency of plaque hemorrhage and rupture demonstrated a significantly increased frequency in the symptomatic group. However,pooling data from multiple sources when methods of analysis are different (histologicvs macroscopic) is hazardous.[47] Therefore studies in which only macroscopic assessment was performed[25,37,48-53] must be discarded. Some authors stress that IPH indicates only the severity of atherosclerosis;[50,51,54-57] others suggest IPH has a direct role in pathogenesis of transient ischemic attack or stroke. [25,35,44,46,57] When most studies are considered, the incidence of IPH in symptomatic and asymptomatic disease spreads considerably In the symptomatic group, incidence varied from 17% to 97%, compared with 2% to 91% in the asymptomatic group. In the European Carotid Plaque Study, [58] a high incidence of IPH was observed in symptomatic (94%) and asymptomatic (71%) groups A higher incidence of IPH was reported in patients without symptoms.[55,59,60] Lennihan et al[54] scored the occurrence of IPH only in patients with symptoms, and found ipsilateral symptoms in 57% of patients with IPH and 65% of patients without IPH, indicating little difference between the two groups. IPH seems to be more common in plaques causing high-grade stenosis.[47,54,55] Carr et al[52] found patients with symptomatic plaques to have more frequent plaque rupture, fibrous cap thinning, and cap foam cell infiltration, compared with patients with asymptomatic plaques. IPH was also seen in all specimens from symptomatic specimens and in 68% of asymptomatic specimens. However, this study included too few patients to be significant. Despite a close relationship between IPH and symptoms,[37,61-63] and carotid plaque rupture, thrombosis, and symptoms, [25,60,61] it has also been claimed that patients with symptomatic plaques typically have large necrotic cores within the carotid arteries.[31] Some studies indicate that the association of complicated plaque and symptomatic disease does not exist.[55,62-64] It is conceivable that patients presumed to have no symptoms might have had embolic episodes and that emboli became impacted in silent cerebral areas or occurred during sleep.[25,37,44,57] Also, symptoms may not be recalled by patients, who are often elderly or frail. Of note, in a high-risk subgroup of patients with asymptomatic carotid stenosis the annual stroke rate was more than 4%.[33] Inzitari et al[10] confirmed that cardioembolic and small vessel stroke can occur, in addition to large vessel atherothrombotic stroke, in patients with asymptomatic carotid stenosis. Finally, NASCET[3] demonstrated that most carotid strokes occur without warning symptoms, and only 5% to 15% of patients have a transient ischemic attack as an impending symptom of stroke. Nevertheless nowadays carotid endarterectomy or stenting should not be performed in asymptomatic patients except those in which some clinical conditions are present, as recommended by the American Heart Association/American Stroke Association. [65]

Patients with asymptomatic carotid artery stenosis should be screened for other treatable risk factors for stroke with institution of appropriate lifestyle changes and medical therapy (Class I; Level of Evidence C).

1. Selection of asymptomatic patients for carotid revascularization should be guided by an assessment of comorbid conditions and life expectancy, as well as other individual factors, and should include a thorough discussion of the risks and benefits of the procedure with an understanding of patient preferences (Class I; Level of Evidence C).

2. The use of aspirin in conjunction with carotid endarterectomy (CEA) is recommended unless contraindicated because aspirin was used in all of the cited trials of CEA as an antiplatelet drug (Class I; Level of Evidence C).

3. Prophylactic CEA performed with <3% morbidity and mortality can be useful in highly selected patients with an asymptomatic carotid stenosis (minimum 60% by angiography, 70% by validated Doppler ultrasound) (Class IIa; Level of Evidence A). It should be noted that the benefit of surgery may now be lower than anticipated based on randomized trial results, and the cited 3% threshold for complication rates may be high because of interim advances in medical therapy.

4. Prophylactic carotid artery stenting (CAS) might be considered in highly selected patients with an asymptomatic carotid stenosis (≥60% on angiography, ≥70% on validated Doppler ultrasonography, or ≥80% on computed tomographic angiography or MRA if the stenosis on ultrasonography was 50% to 69%). The advantage of revascularization over current medical therapy alone is not well established (Class IIb; Level of Evidence B).

5. The usefulness of CAS as an alternative to CEA in asymptomatic patients at high risk for the surgical procedure is uncertain (Class IIb; Level of Evidence C).

6. Population screening for asymptomatic carotid artery stenosis is not recommended (Class III; Level of Evidence B).

Other points to consider is the necessity of interventionally treating an asymptomatic carotid artery disease are: age 80 years or less, life expectancy higher tan 5 years, hemispheric hypoperfusion, significant intracerebral vascular disease,unstable carotid plaque, rapid progression of the stenoses, presence of silent cerebral infarcts, neck radiotherapy and the necessity of a coronary by pass surgery. [66-74]

As it can be seen, up to date criterium for percentage stenoses in this group of patients are higher than in the ACAS study (60%). [75]

Finally and taking into consideration the mechanisms of atherosclerosis: cells component behavior, IPH, biology and gene expression, it can be seen in the literature a new tendency of treatment in animal models. However, attention should therefore focus on the processes of plaque breakdown andt hrombus formation in humans, whereas the use of animal models should probably be reserved for studying the function of particular genes and for investigating isolated features of plaques,such as the relationshipbetween cap thickness and plaque stability. [76] In this connection, Peter et al [77] described a ApoE(-/-) mice mouse model reflecting human atherosclerotic plaque instability in which atorvastatinwas used aimed at preventing plaque rupture. They concluded that distinctly expressed genes andmicroRNAscan be linked to plaque instability.On the other hand, Forte et al described the role of polyamines in reducing carotid arteriotomy-induced (re)stenosis s in vitro and in a rat model suggesting a novel therapeutic approach for this pathophysiological process. [78]

3. Plaque morphology

The atherosclerotic process in the carotid arteries begins with a thickening of the intima-media complex and, according to factors of disease progression can reach arterial occlusion, through-out intermediate stages of mild, moderate and severe stenosis. Moreover, depending on several factors, the structure of the plaque can show different evolutionary behaviors, from simple stable plaque, fibrotic, and non stenotic, to that hemorrhagic, ulcerated, with rupture that produces severe stenosis and strokes. Carotid risk factors are identical to those mentioned for coronary disease.[79,80]

3.1. Correlation between plaque morphology and cerebral symptoms

The incidence of cerebrovascular events depends primarily on the degree of carotid stenosis but plaque structure is also relevant, as well as the speed of progression of plaque, and consequent carotid disease stenosis and also the presence of systemic thrombogenic factors. [81-83]

Several studies have described a good correlation between intraplaque hemorrhage (IPH) with ulceration and cerebrovascular symptoms.[25,53] According to Bluth the plaque structure is even more important than the degree of stenosis, in predicting neurologic events. [84]

Bearing in mind than more than 40 % of the patients with transient ischemic attacks later may suffer a stroke some authors believe that these stroke occur because plaques with IPH are unstable.[25,28,53] Embolization of fibrin and platelets and/or atherosclerotic material from the plaque itself will continue.

As was mentioned, Geroulakos et al[81] classified ultrasonographic carotid plaques in 5 different types of stenosis, and correlated plaque type with symptomatology (not with pathology), showing the predominance of echolucent plaques in symptomatic patients with stenosis > 70 percent (see below) From the histologic point of view it was found that 50 % of the IPH had connections with the lumen while 20 % had not.[30] Lusby et al[25] showed that "haemorrhage in carotid atheromatous plaques plays a unique and major role in the development of cerebrovascular disease". IPH was not only identified in most symptomatic patients but also a close relationship was established between the onset of symptoms and the presence of plaque haemorrhage. Seeger et al[81-85] reported that the composition of plaques from symptomatic patients is significantly different from those asymptomatic. The former contains more total lipid and cholesterol, and less collagen and calcium.

Johnson et al [86] classified asymptomatic plaques according to ultrasonographic characteristics into calcified, dense and soft. At the end of a 3 year follow-up a large proportion of asymptomatic patients with soft plaques had become symptomatic, while a small proportion of those with calcified plaques have developed symptoms. Hennerici et al [87] reported that patients with fibrous carotid plaques had a tendency to remain stable while plaque progression was common in those with soft and complex calcified plaques. Spontaneous regression of minor carotid atheroma occurred in soft plaques corresponding to a reduction in plaque volume while fibrous and calcified plaques did not regress. [87]

Despite that currently the presence of symptoms and percentage of luminal narrowing remain the most useful predictors of transitory ischemic cerebral attacks or stroke risk, [3,75,88,89] there is a body of evidence that plaque morphology is crucial in the development of its natural history.

Regarding the relationship of IPH with a higher prevalence of symptoms or hemorrhagic stroke, the results are contradictory. [23-64] However, current guidelines recommend reporting the plaque structure in question and that in occasions define therapeutic behaviors. [82-83]

There are several reasons that make knowledge of plaques structure very important. It is well known that fibrous plaques, are predominantly collagen in content, showing a highly echogenic quality and being generally homogeneous in texture. When lipid content of the plaque increased, the plaque turns more echolucent. [84] Complex plaques protrude more frequently into the lumen presenting high incidence of surface irregularities and ulcers. [60] Several authors found that the incidence of IPH, histologically assessed, in symptomatic carotid stenosis is higher than 90 %. [25,44,53,99] Imparato et al, prospectively studied 376 carotid artery plaques concluding that IPH was strongly associated with the presence of cerebrovascular symptoms and it was the main characteristic of the carotid plaque that correlated statistically with the presence of symptoms. [44] O'Donnel theorized that IPH is the most common morphologic characteristic in symptomatic patients. [60]

3.2. B-mode ultrasound and pathology correlation

In the 80′s, several authors attempted to describe plaque morphology and the presence of ulceration by ultrasonographic imaging. However, results were not convincing [90,91]. Other authors mentioned only relevant the percentage of carotid stenosis [92,93].

The accuracy of the carotid ultrasonography procedure in assessing the percentage of luminal diameter narrowing is well established [94,95].Percentage of stenosis has been the main point of interest for noninvasive carotid testing due to its correlation with stroke risk.[96,97]

Developed technics in ultrasound (US) permit a more detailed analysis and accurate information about the plaque morphology. This technique is useful to evaluate the natural history and the stroke risk associated to the lesions.

High-resolution B-mode ultrasonography (B-mode) seems advantageous over arteriography for characterizing atherosclerotic plaque. [53] The method can identify those lesions that place the patient at risk for transient ischemic attacks.

It was suggested that echolucent plaques have increased lipid and cholesterol levels, making them unstable and prone to rupture and hemorrhage. On the other hand, the echogenic plaques which contain significantly more fibrin and collagen are more stable and therefore less likely to cause complications. [81,85] There is a paper correlating these two ultrasonic types of plaques with whole frontal and/or transverse histological sections, correlating the B mode ultrasonographic diagnosis of at carotid arteries with their respective pathological examinations assessing US accuracy. [98]

According to Lehay, [99] Bluth, [84] Goes [100] and the recommendations from the Committee on Standards in Non - invasive Vascular Testing, [101] carotid plaques were classified as homogeneous or heterogeneous. But these two groups arose from categorizing the plaques into 4 types according to the scale of l to 4 based on the Geroulakos' classification [81]. In this classification, Type 1 corresponded to uniformly sonolucent; type 2, predominantly sonolucent; type 3 predominantly echogenic and type 4 uniformly echogenic. In this way types l and 2 corresponded to heterogeneous plaques and types 3 and 4 to homogeneous plaques. (Figures 13 and 14)

The analysis of the complex plaque structure regards defining histological types [98]:

- Thrombus, described “a brightly eosinophilic mass of compacted fibrin and degenerating erythrocytes sometimes accompanied by evidence of organization".
- Ruptured plaque was defined as "disruption of the fibrous cap of a lesion that provoked exposure of the thrombogenic lipid core region to the flowing blood and was classified histologically as an irregular plaque surface with breaks in of loss of the fibrous cap often associated with surface thrombus directly overlying the lipid~rich necrotic core of the lesion"[26]
- Inflammation was described as chronic inflammatory infiltrates (lymphocytes, histiocytes, macrophages and mast cells) within the plaque itself. Hemorrhage was identified by a

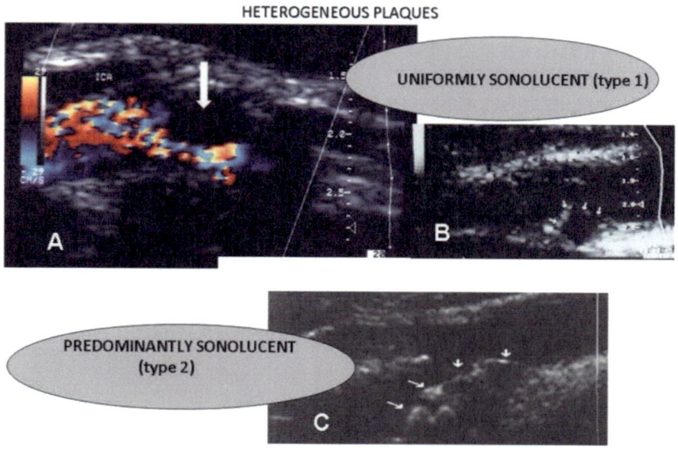

Figure 13. Panels A and B correspond to type 1 plaques-. The arrows indicate fully anechoic stenotic plaques which may correspond to fatty tissue and / or blood which indicate the instability of the same. Panel C Carotid plaque type 2 showing dense echoes (white color) alternating with most hypoechoic or anechoic areas(in black) which indicate plaque instability

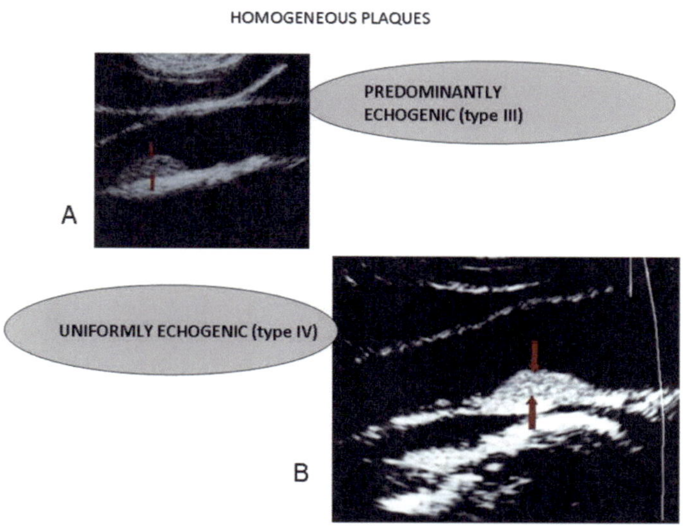

Figure 14. Panel A: it can be seen between arrows a carotid plaque containing predominantly echogenic areas (type 3)that generally correspond to fibrous tissue which gives it stability Panel B.This carotid plaque (type 4) is practically composed by echogenic areas (between arrows).

macroscopic hematoma within the arterial wall with or without extension through the luminal surface.

- Hemorrhage is identified by disruption of red blood cells and macrophage engulfment of hemosiderin, to distinguish it from surgical related hemorrhage consisting in preserved erythrocytes.

Plaque morphology analyzed by US, identifying those unstable or complicated plaques found a very good correlation unless calcium deposits exist. [98]

Ultrasonographically, calcium deposits are characterized by a highly echoreflective area with acoustical shadowing masking the real plaque structure below, resulting in a worse correlation between US and pathology.

Carotid plaques having calcium deposits correspond to a third classification (stable, unstable and calcium), as their evolution can be unpredictable. The presence of "acoustic shadows" that mask the true tissue structure is characteristic of this type of plaque on ultrasonography, making morphological interpretation difficult. [81] (Figure 15)

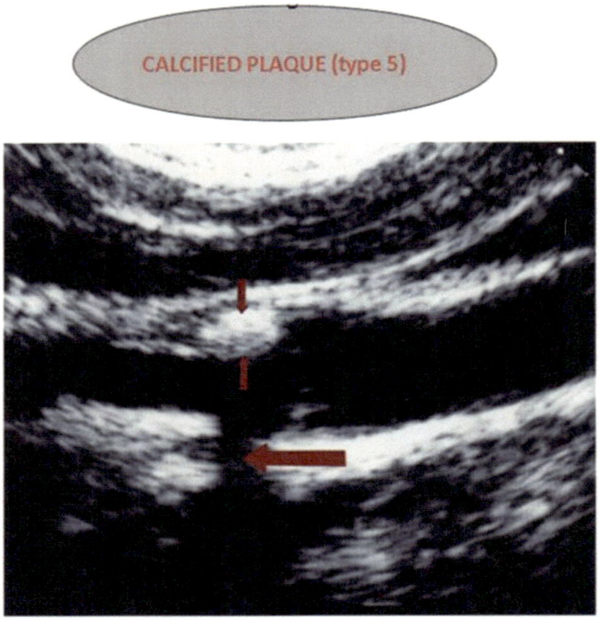

Figure 15. A type 5 calcified carotid plaque significantly reduces the lumen in the carotid bulb (between small arrows) The typically acoustic shadowing is clearly seen (big arrow)

In this sense, we published the results of an investigation showing ultrasonic vs pathologic correlation of carotid atheromatous plaques. This manuscript involved two ultrasonographers and one pathologist. [98] This work implied seventy-four carotid ultrasonographic studies randomly selected from a registry of 250 carotid endarterectomy specimens. (Thirteen of them had poor quality images and were excluded). The remaining 61 studies, belonging to 59 patients (2 bilateral endarterectomies) had been sent from five different laboratories and were analyzed blindly and independently by two different observers. There were 17 females and 42 males. Age ranged from 52 to 83 years (mean 68 years). A very good interobserver correlation was observed and, in turn, with histopathological findings. However, calcium plaques produced less agreement.

In our research regarding interobserver agreement, there were 2 non-coincidences vs. 59 coincidences (efficacy 98%), K = 0.956, demonstrating very good agreement.

Regarding the strictly classification in heterogeneous, homogeneous and calcified plaques, there were 59 coincidences, (96.7%) and 2 non-coincidences (3.3%), accuracy 98 %, K = 0.95 (very good agreement).

Coincidences not always were total. If we consider the fourth group in which operators agreed in plaques being heterogeneous but with difficulties in distinguishing IPH, calcium and lipids as non-coincidences, then the accuracy falls to 88.5 %.

When we considered agreement between observers and pathologist and taking into consideration the overall results from both observers, there was an agreement of 84% with the pathologist. When calcified plaques were not considered it is expected with 95% of confidence that US will agree with pathology in 70-93% of the cases (CI0,95).

When calcified plaques were considered, the percentage of coincidence fell to 67% (CI 0,95 54-79%). In others words calcified plaques clearly blurred the diagnosis of plaque structure. Operator 1 had an agreement of 67% with 18% of calcified plaques. Operator 2 had an agreement of 79% with 8% of calcified plaques.

Regarding the coincidence of IPH between B - mode and pathology, operator 1 had an agreement of 50% (11/22) while operator 2 agreed in 65 % of the cases (11 / 17). The pathologist diagnosed IPH in 33 cases, therefore both observers, together were able to detect IPH in only 1 / 3 of the cases.

This investigation has correlated the ultrasound aspect of carotid atheromatous plaques with pathology demonstrating the highest incidence of intraplaque hemorrhage (IPH) in those complex, irregular and heterogeneous producing stenosis 98. (Figure 16)

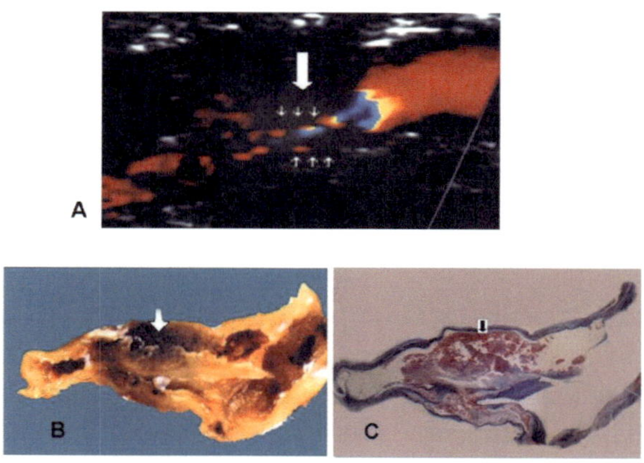

Figure 16. A.Two dimensional and color ultrasound image displays a very tight stenosis (between arrows) caused by an anechoic plaque (large arrow) B. The corresponding gross morphology shows an irregular stenotic plaque composed by a brownish tissue (arrow). C. Microscopically this plaque belongs to an intraplaque hemorrhage (arrow). Mallory Trichrome

Correlation with histology shows that lipid rich regions are the least echogenic on US and calcified areas are the most. [81,98] Dense collagen is also very echogenic not associated with acoustic shadowing. For example O´Donnel [60] emphasized that plaque haemorrhage could be differentiated from lipid-laden plaque because the former was more irregular, echolucent, frequently associated with irregular borders, and randomly distributed through the plaque producing a non-homogeneous texture. The surface of the plaque with hemorrhage is usually irregular and ulcerated. Surface ulceration is unusual in lipid plaques. By contrast, plaque hemorrhage produces an echolucent area within the plaque, in which its degree may be correlated with the age of hemorrhage. [60]

The anechoic or highly echolucent qualities of fresh hemorrhage are comparable with those of the lumen, being irregular and randomly distributed through the plaque (heterogeneous shape).

On the other hand, Bluth et al [84] found that the incidence of IPH in theheterogeneous type was 81 % vs. 3 % in the homogeneous plaques. Thus, the sensitivity and specificity of US to detect this lesion was 94 % and 88 % respectively.

Ultrasonography fails in detecting plaque ulceration even using color-flow Doppler assisted duplex, as was recently demonstrated by Sitzer et al. [102]

Hartmann et al [103] reported poor results between US and pathology concluding that visual assessment of B-mode images is not reliable. Lehay et al [99] found that plaques that caused a narrowing greater than 50% in the carotid lumen were more likely to be heterogeneous, suggesting that plaque appearance is a more relevant finding on preoperative duplex scanning than the percentage of carotid narrowing.

Taking all these concepts into consideration, decreased echogenicity would correspond either to lipid deposits or to hemorrhage within a plaque being both of them characteristic of instability. Lipid deposits appear more uniform and are less randomly distributed throughout the plaque.

Julian et al [104] divided plaques into two categories: "simple" composed of fibrous material and that do not generally cause stenosis greater than 50 %, and "complex" consisting of an atherosclerotic material, calcified deposits, surface fibrin, platelet material and hemorrhagic areas.

The European Carotid Plaque Study Group [105] correlated B-mode imaging studies with histology in 270 patients undergoing carotid endarterectomy. They concluded that US appearance of carotid plaque is related to histological composition being the echogenicity inversely related to the relative amount of soft tissue.

Backscattered radiofrequency derived signals devices have been applied for better characterization of the different components of plaque structure[106-108].But this technique is more expensive and not always available in most laboratories so we consider that conventional good quality B-mode images allow a reliable differentiation between the three types of plaques.

3.3. Magnetic resonance imaging – Patholgy correlation

Although carotid ulltrasound is the method of choice to study the structure of carotid plaques MRI also plays a significant role. Singh et at, [109] in an interesting paper describing structural MRI findings in 98 asymptomatic carotid arteries with moderate stenosis (50-70%) and subsequent one year evolution to symptomatic status: 36 (36.7%) had IPH on NMR, with 6 cerebrovascular events, ie 16%, (2 stroke and 4 AIT) related to carotid IPH showed, compared to the absence of events in the carotid without IPH. Their statistical analyzes confirmed that the detection of IPH on NMR was associated with an increased risk of cerebrovascular events. In another relevant work involving MRI, Cheung et al [110] investigated the presence of IPH in the carotid arteries of 217 patients who had symptomatic stenosis less than 50%. IPH was detected in 13% related to the hemisphere ipsilateral symptoms and 7% contralateral.

In summary, we believe necessary to describe and report the B-mode characteristic of carotid plaques together with the percentage of luminal stenosis. Ultrasonic plaque description correlates with histogy. The adoption of plaque characterization despite of the degree of carotid stenosis would allow recognition of a high-risk subset of patients that may benefit from carotid intervention.

4. Carotid artery dolichoarteriopathies

Atherosclerosis is the most frequent cause of extracranial carotidartery disease. [111] However, although atheromatous pathology of the carotid bulb and bifurcation is a major causes of stroke, other causes of carotid disease may also cause vessel occlusion, such as fibrodysplasia, trauma (with subsequent dissection of carotid arteries), aortic arch pathology as in Takayasu disease, and aortic dissection. [112]

Among nonatheromatous alterations of the carotid arteries, interest has long been placed on specific anatomical abnormalities called dolichoarteriopathies.

Carotid dolichoarteriopathies can be classified into three different types [113](Figure 17).Type 1: tortuosity – a nonrectilinear stretch of an artery with an angulation >90; type 2: loop – a 360 angulation of an artery on its transverse axis (''coil'' configuration) (Figure 18); type 3: kinking – the inflection of 2 or more segments of an artery with an internal angle of 90° or less. (Figures 19 and 20).

Dolichoarteriopathies of carotid arteries are frequent, ranging between 10% and 45%. [114] For type 3, a prevalence of 5% to 25% has been described.[115,116]

Published studies have reached disparate conclusions with regard to the origin or cause of carotid dolichoarteriopathies, as well as their hemodynamic and prognostic significance. [114-119] Mukherjee and Inahara [119] proposed that carotid kinking would induce turbulent flow, thus favoring intimal ulceration, platelet deposition, and distal thrombus embolism. Other investigators similarly believe that a causal connection exists between cerebral flow alteration and severe carotid dolichoarteriopathies, to the point of proposing surgical correction of kinking and coiling to prevent stroke. [14,120,121]

Conversely,other authors consider carotid dolichoarteriopathies as a mere anatomical variety, devoid of clinical consequences. [122]

Establishing the clinical impact of dolichoarteriopathies is further complicated by the fact that the mechanisms responsible for their formation are still debated.

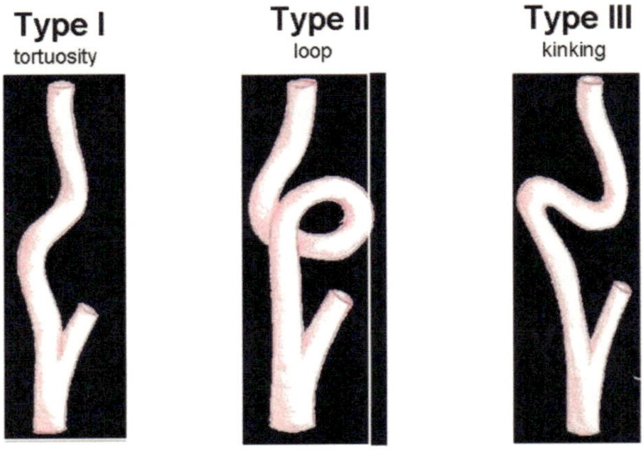

Figure 17. The different types of dolichoarteriopathies, according to the definition of Weibel and Fields.

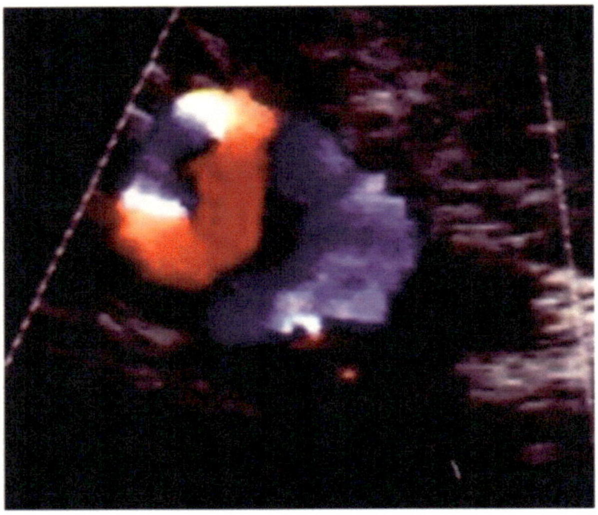

Figure 18. Color flow Doppler imaging shows circular-shaped internal carotid artery

http://dx.doi.org/10.5772/57157

A

B

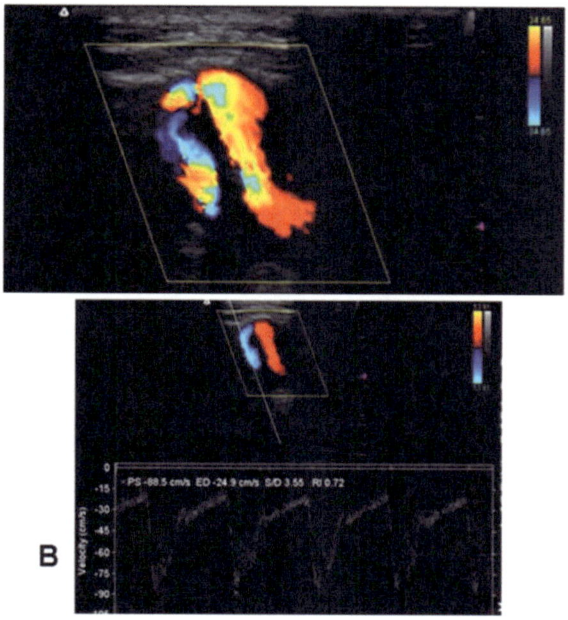

Figure 19. A: Color flow Doppler imaging discloses an internal carotid artery kinking.B: Color and pulsed-wave Doppler showed turbulences at the site of the kinking. However, both maximum systolic velocity and end-diastolic velocity of internal carotid arteries were substantially unaffected by kinking

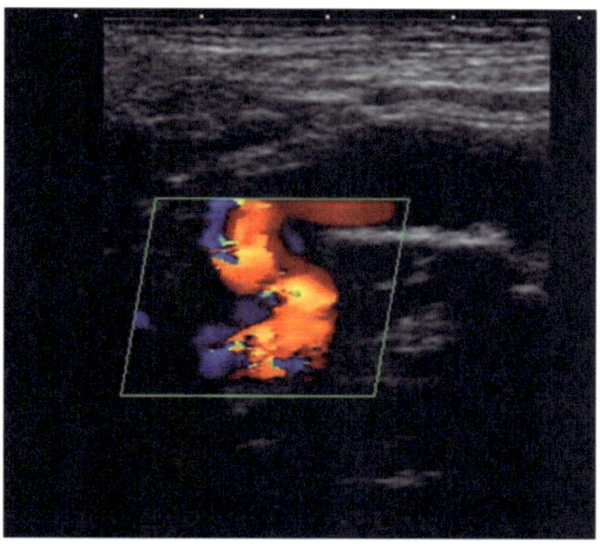

Figure 20. A double angled internal carotid artery showing a S shaped configuration (image corresponding to color Doppler ultrasound)

4.1. Origin of carotid dolichoarteriopathies — Congenital or acquired?

One theory maintains that they are pathological alterations caused by arterial aging and/or changes induced by atherosclerotic remodeling, which would cause the vessel to bend, [114,123-126] while other reports do not support an association between dolichoarteriopathies and cardiovascular risk status. [122,127,128] Alternatively, it has therefore been postulated that they have an embryological origin. Indeed, Kelly [129] observed that carotid arteries may be kinked or show loops at some point during intrauterine development, when the descent toward the mediastinum occurs enabling the union of the third aortic arch with the dorsal aorta.

Obviously, as these 2 etiological theories are so different from each other, they may also entail different implications both clinically and prognostically. Part of the uncertainty derives from the fact that previous observations had been made in small studies or in selected populations. [122-128] Therefore, it would be important to establish which theory has more solid basis.

Prevalence varies according to different diagnostic methodology and patients' inclusion criteria, but in aggregate they concur to indicate that this is a rather frequent finding. In contrast, lack of consensus exists over the clinical and prognostic significance of these alterations or even about their etiology. Much of the controversy revolves around a "nature- or-nurture" type of issue, that is, whether carotid dolichoarteriopathies develop late in life as a manifestation of vessel remodeling, particularly in individuals at risk of atherosclerosis, or rather they originate from alterations of embryological development.

With regard to the possibility that dolichoarteriopathies may be the result of a degenerative process, over the years several hypotheses have been put forward trying to explain how they may develop. Some of these seem quite unlikely, such as the possibility that carotid kinking could be due to kyphosis or lordosis of the spine, which might deviate the carotid axis, [130] or that inflammation of the tissues around the carotid arteries would cause them to retract. [131] Other investigators have proposed that arterial hypertension would produce alterations in the wall over time, which would favor its weakening withsubsequent kinking of the artery, [121-123] while other authors hypothesized a relationship between aging and arterial anatomical abnormalities. [114,126]

Data gathered in modern times also do not help in establishing firm conclusions. Two rather large reports by Ghilardi et al [125] and Del Corso et al [132] described a great prevalence of hypertension and atherosclerosis in patients with carotid dolichoarteriopathies; however, both studies lack a group of normal participants, and deal with a population of patients selected for vascular pathology, and in whom predominance of such cardiovascular risk factors is expected. Pancera et al [127] have reported an association between carotid artery kinking and age and with hypertension as well. However, in that study, prevalence of carotid abnormalities was actually identical across the age groups from 60 to>80 years, which represented 87% of their cohort: younger patients, in whom prevalence was apparently lower, were instead too few to make a solid comparison. This same reasoning applies to the effect of hypertension reported in that study, which was actually based on about a dozen patients. [127]

The possibility that carotid dolichoarteriopathies may have an embryological origin had also been suggested in the past. Again, however, those reports were not conclusive. Sometimes, this was because of the small numbers of cases studied. In this respect, Weibel and Fields [113] described at angiography 14 cases of anatomical abnormalities in patients aged between1 and 20 years, while Sarkari et al [133] reported 8 children (aged 9 months to 16 years) with symptomatic carotid kinkings and coilings. In a substantially largerstudy, there may have been a selection bias [134] in that case, 282 angiographies of neck vessels were obtainedin patients aged between 6 months and 82 years. The authors found that prevalence ofcarotid abnormalities in adults was 24% and even greater (43%) in children. Although that finding may seemingly support the view that in fact there is no association with aging and that dolichoarteriopathies have an embryological origin, the significance of such a high frequence in children might have been restricted to the peculiar population studied, as it is quite conceivable that children who were subjected to an invasive procedure such as angiography underwent it because of a high clinical suspicion of carotid abnormalities.

Togay-Isikay et al,through noninvasive Doppler ultrasonography assessment, observed carotid dolichoarteriopathies in 24.6% of a consecutive patient series, with no apparent relation between carotid alterations and cardiovascular risk factors. [122] In 1924,Cairney [135] had already reported autoptic findings in fetuses from the fifth month in whom morphological carotid arteries abnormalitieswere observed. In this respect, it is important to notice that the vascular wall in fetus develops from mesenchymal cells islets; in any artery, the tunica muscularis develops first in the main trunk and later in its branches. The proximal portion of the internal carotid artery originates from the third aortic arch while the more distal parts originate from the left dorsal aorta. [130] Harrison and Dávalos [130] suggested that development of carotid arteries and of skeletal system might be asynchronous, the different velocity explaining the tortuous path.Ochsner et al [136] proposed that fibromuscular dysplasia occurring during fetal life, located in a sector of the carotid artery, would be responsible for subsequent weakening and kinking of the wall at that level. Contrary to this specific hypothesis, however, is the fact that presence of fibromuscular dysplasia in areas with dolichoarteriopathies is very rare.[137-139]

Regarding the issue of congenital or adquired condition of dolichoarteriopathies, our group conducted an observational study involving 885 participants of either sex, aged between newborn(4 hour 30 minutes) to 90 years old. [16]

Patients were divided into 2 groups (G): G1 (control, healthy participants) n = 245. It consisted of infants, children, and adolescents up to 15 years of age (mean 6 + 3 years) from a town of 43 000 inhabitants just outside of Buenos Aires; these children participated in a voluntary screening health program, approved by their parents, under the patronage of the local municipality that was performed in the hospital and different schools. Group 2 (G2; n = 640) consisted of patients from 16 to 90 years of age (mean 57+8 years) in whom diagnostic color Doppler ultrasonography investigation of neck vessels had been requested for clinical suspicion of atherosclerotic disease. Patients were assessed with regard to presence of cardiovascular risk factors (hypertension, dyslipidemia, smoking). Presence of atheromatous plaques in the regions affected by dolichoarteriopathies was also evaluated.

Coiling prevalence was similar in healthy participants (G1 4%; n ¼ 10) and in patients (G2 3%; n = 19; NS;). At the same time, kinking prevalence in G1 was 27% (n = 67), and it was 22% (n = 143) in G2, which did not show any statistically significant association either Atheromatous plaques intrakinking were only observed in 3 G2 patients (0.47%). In this group, 56.2% of patients presented carotid atherosclerotic disease. Within G2 patients, prevalence of cardio-vascular risk factors evaluated individually was similar when patients were divided according to presence or absence of kinking and/or coiling.

We observed that the dolichoarteriopathies, namely, kinking and coiling of carotid arteries, had similar frequency across all ages, from newborn infants to elderly individuals. Furthermore, their prevalence was unrelated to the presence of cardiovascular risk factors or of frank atherosclerotic pathology of carotid artery. Collectively, these findings suggest that carotid dolichoarteriopathies are a result of alterations in embryological development rather than of vascular remodeling secondary to aging and/or atherosclerosis. [16]

5. Hemodinamical behavior of dolichoarteriopathies: Ischemic or not?

As was previously mentioned, there a wide span of clinical consequences have been atributed to the presence of carotid dolichoarteriopathies, ranging from asymptomatic carotid anatomical variety to carotid induced cerebral ischemia. [122] As referred, Mukherjee et al [119] proposed that carotid kinking would generate distal thrombus embolism, by means of the turbulent flow, intimal ulceration and platelet deposition. Surgical correction of kinking and coiling carotid arteries has been proposed to prevent stroke. [14,121]

The prevalence of cerebrovascular symptoms in patients with carotid dolichoarteriopathies varies between 15 and 23%. [140-141] But, there is not uniform criterion about the role of carotid dolichoarteriopathies in the development of neurological symptoms. If dolichoarteriopathies were certainly responsible for these events, cerebral ischemia could be demonstrated by functional hemodynamic tests.

In 1997, Oliviero et al. [128] demonstrated, in 36 patients suffering from hypertension and with kinks, that the percentage of neurological events was similar to the other 36 patients with hypertension but without kinks. The same author published new results of the follow-up of these patients, confirming the former conclusions as in the group of hypertensive patients with kinkings there were 10 neurological events registered, whereas 14 occurred in the control group (hypertensive patients without kinkings). [142]

Several previous papers [62,120,121,143-157] considered that carotid dolichoarteriopathies can produce neurological symptoms and proposed surgery and furthermore, they describe different surgical techniques.

A recent report of 7 kinkings of internal carotid arteries, defined five asymptomatic, one syptomatic for odynophagia and another symptomatic for pharyngeal bulge considering that no typical clinical symptoms were shown in the malformation of cervical segment of internal carotid artery. Pharyngeal bulge with pulsation could be encountered.

Grego et al. [156] assured that natural history of carotid dolichoarteriopathies is practically unknown but in some cases surgery would be justified, such as: a) transient ischemic attack (hemispheric symptoms); b) asymptomatic patients with a kinking angle less than 30° together with contralateral carotid occlusion; c) patients with non-hemispheric symptoms after evaluating that there were no other possible neurological or non-neurological causes through positive results of the following studies: 1) Doppler ultrasonography of neck vessels with increase in circulatory velocity; 2) computerized cerebral tomography and MRI angiography of ischemic lesions in the ipsilateral hemisphere and 3) Inversion of the circulatory flow in the anterior cerebral artery and its reduction in the middle cerebral artery, in both cases in relation to the rotation and flexo-extension maneuvers of the head.

Recent papers regarding surgical intervention on carotid arteries kinking, totalizing roughly 150 patients, flaw to show convincing evidence on the benefits of intervention.[158-160]

Up to now, there are no guidelines nor is there consensus (with a level of recommendation) for surgical treatment of dolichoarteriopathies.

Taking into account the pitfalls in measuring stenotic percentage in bended arteries, it is our point of view that manuscripts reporting big number of operated patients with carotid dolichoareriopathies failed in the diagnostic ultrasonographic criterions of stenotic kinkings and coils, furthermore, there is no mention about which method for angiographic measures were used. Also, most of their patients had cardiovascular risk factor which could have been the responsible of the neurological symptoms remaining doubts about their true relation with carotid abnormalities. [157,161]

Our group conducted an investigation study regarding the clinical implications in the genesis of neurological complications related to kinking and looping (coiling) of the carotid arteries. [162] Sixty patients with non-atheromatous carotid kinkings were subjected to head rotation tests, and were studied by carotid artery B-mode, color Doppler ultrasonography, and scanning the ophthalmic artery in order to assess the hemodynamic behavior of carotid dolichoarteriopathies. Results suggested that carotid dolichoarteriopathies are not the cause of neurological events or symptoms taking into account that no events were recorded during the study, and registering significant reduction in the velocities in the ophthalmic artery in only 3 of the 60 cases studied, in performing the head rotation tests.in the patient cohort. 23 % (n=14) were asymptomatic as only 6 patients were referred for stroke or transient ischemic attack. Consecuently we concluded that carotid dysembryoplasias, would not cause neurological events nor symptoms.

Computerized tomography angiography (CTA) and magnetic resonance angiography (MRA) showed excellent ability to depict the malformation of cervical segment of internal carotid artery and its relationship with surrounding structures, which could protect carotid artery from unintended damage. [163]

It may be concluded that dolichoartheriopathies recognize a congenital origin other than an acquired condition, based on controlled studies regarding juvenile control cases. Additionally, in the current state of knowledge, it unlikely appears that these dolichoartheriorpathies induce relevant symptomatic cerebral ischemia

6. Carotid sinus baroreceptor

The significance of the ability of the carotid sinus baroreceptor to sense and regulate blood pressure has been known since Hering's publications in 1927. [164]. Later, in1930, Heymans unequivocally demonstrated the chemoreceptor activity of the carotid (or glomus) bodies. [165] However, there have been few human necropsies and therefore, evidence relies on case patients with damage to the carotid sinus and glomus following surgery, radiotherapy and carotid endarterectomy. [166,167] Therefore, little information is available on the morphology of barochemoreceptor structures in disease. [168]

The baroreflex is very important for the maintenance of arterial pressure, particularly during orthostatic stress. Chemoreflexes play an important role in maintaining blood gas homeostasis. [169] Thus, barochemoreflex failure is a disabling and potentially life-threatening condition. Data on the long-term effect of human bilateral carotid sinus denervation on arterial blood pressure are limited and controversial. [166,170-173]

In patients submitted to bilateral tumoral carotid glomus resection it was found a long-term effect on the level, variability and rapid reflex control of arterial pressure included increased daytime and nighttime blood pressure variability, unopposed sympathetic activation in response to physical and mental stress, and the elimination of orthostatic hypotension and normocapnic hypoxic drive as a result of peripheral chemoreflex failure. [174] Barochemoreceptors are compromised in diseases such as diabetic autonomic neuropathy, Guillain-Barré syndrome, arterial hypertension and heart failure. [175] Fatal complications in most stroke patients likely result from baroreceptor malfunction. [175]

The available experimental and clinical evidence suggests that a pattern of chronic intermittent hypoxia, with short episodes of hypoxia followed by normoxia, selectively enhances the chemosensory and ventilatory responses of the carotid body to hypoxia, suggesting this sensor has an essential role in the enhanced ventilatory and cardiovascular responses observed in animals and obstructive sleep apnea patients. [176]

In a previous study we found a strong involvement of the chemoreceptor structures and corresponding supplying arterioles in a selected group of elderly patients who had died from cerebral vascular disorders with critical carotid artery lesions. [177] Despite the accepted dogma that the amount of connective tissue separating the glomic lobules increases with age, [166] the significant fibrotic involvement and the unquestionable reduction in the vascularity, could not merely be explained by the aging process. However, a possible limitation to the interpretation of those results was the superposition of arterial hypertension, atherosclerosis and aging in the patients.

Due to these facts, and to characterize the potential damage of the carotid glomus related to hemodynamic stress alone, we performed experiments using spontaneously hypertensive rats (SHRs), an animal model with arterial hypertension, in which other factors such as dyslipidemia, high blood sugar or aging were absent. In SHRs, we found a significant increase in extracellular matrix expansion in the carotid glomus and autonomic nerves, along with a decreased number of neurons in autonomic ganglia compared with normotensive controls.

All these findings were highly correlated with high blood pressure and an increase in plasminogen activator inhibitor 1 (PAI-1) and transforming growth factor beta-1 (TGF-β-1) deposits in the carotid glomus and autonomic ganglia. Additionally, SHRs presented a higher wall to lumen arteriole ratio in small periglomic vessels, a higher number of S100 protein-positive cells (sustentacular or type 2 cells) and a decreased number of type 1 cells in the carotid glomus. Interestingly, extracellular matrix expansion was highly correlated with the blood pressure level. Because of this, these structures must be considered as target organs in the model of systemic hypertension. [178]

Our group carried out an investigation in which the objective was to morphometrically characterize the alterations of the carotid barochemoreceptor structures and their supplying arteries in patients who died from stroke with complicated versus noncomplicated internal carotid atheromatosis. [179] For this purpose, samples consisting of bilateral or unilateral carotid segments were obtained at autopsy from 23 elderly patients who died from ischemic neurological disorders. Transient ischemic attacks preceding their strokes, with extensive cerebral damage precipitated their deaths.

Plaques were pathologically characterized) into seven categories (see page 3). [18]

Patients were also divided arbitrarily by age. Group 1 was older than 80 years, Group 2 was 65 to 80 years and Group 3 was younger than 65 years of age. The carotid bifurcation and the first 10 mm to 15 mm of the internal carotid artery were involved in all cases by atherosclerotic lesions. Large lipid cores with a fibrous cap and a band of fibrous tissue of variable thickness separating the plaque from the extensively damaged media were observed in all plaques. In one-third of cases, extensive calcified deposits were also found. The collagen border was frequently vascularized. In most cases, extensive chronic inflammatory infiltrates were observed, consisting of macrophages and minor numbers of lymphocytes as well as extensive neoangiogenesis and calcified deposits. Complicated plaques presented with mononuclear infiltrates in the periphery, shoulders and bases in two-thirds of the cases. In contrast, only one-third of noncomplicated plaques had inflammatory infiltrates ($P<0.0001$).

The carotid glomus was located in the carotid fork, measuring approximately 3 mm X 1.5 mm, and formed by lobules compactly arranged, separated by connective tissue [177,180-182] (Figure 21). The functional units consisted of numerous small groups of cells arranged in clusters. They were grouped to form lobules organized as compact nests that were embedded in a fibrous stroma through which numerous nerve fibrils and small blood vessels were observed (Figure 22). Parenchymal cells consisted of two types: the 'chief cells' (epithelioid or type 1 cells), which were large cells with a round nucleus and a large amount of cytoplasm containing vesicles and granules stained by the Grimelius silver reaction; and elongated cells, known as 'sustentacular cells' or type 2 cells. Chief cells were arranged in the centre and sustentacular cells at the periphery. [177] Complex arrangements of afferent nerves and postganglionic sympathetic nerves, as well as autonomic ganglion cells, were found surrounding the lobules. [181] The carotid glomus showed moderate atrophy and fibrosis to severe atrophy with extensive fibrosis (cirrhotic appearance) (Figure 23).

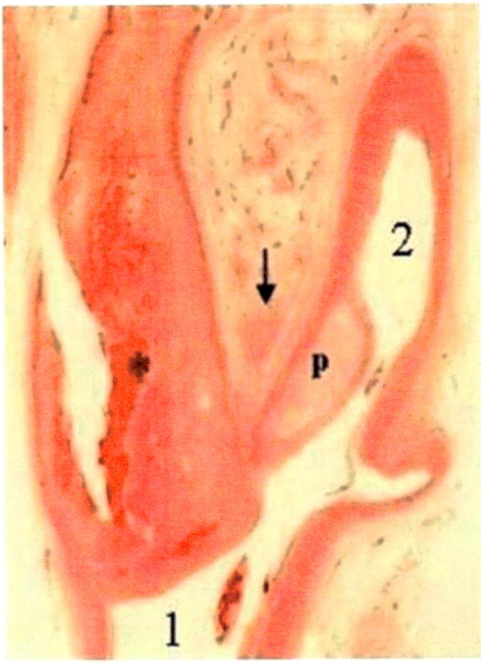

Figure 21. Whole specimen of a frontally cut carotid segment. The arrow points to the glomus located in the interstitial tissue between the internal and external carotid arteries and its corresponding nerves. Multiple nonstenotic fibrolipidic and fibrotic plaques are observed along the carotid axis.Also an intraplaque hemorrhage is shown (asterisk)Hematoxylin and eosin stain; ×20 objective lens. 1 Common carotid artery;2 External carotid artery showing an atheroma inside (P)

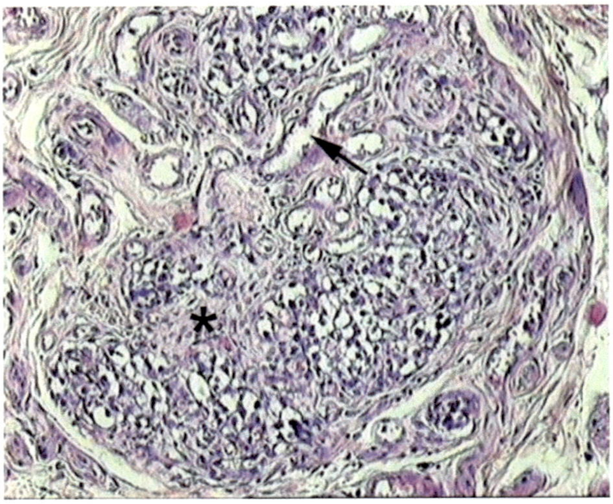

Figure 22. Carotid glomus showing almost normal structure and vascularization.Veins are dilated (arrow) and there is a mild increase in interstitial fibrosis (asterisk). Hematoxylin and eosin stain; ×100 objective lens

http://dx.doi.org/10.5772/57157

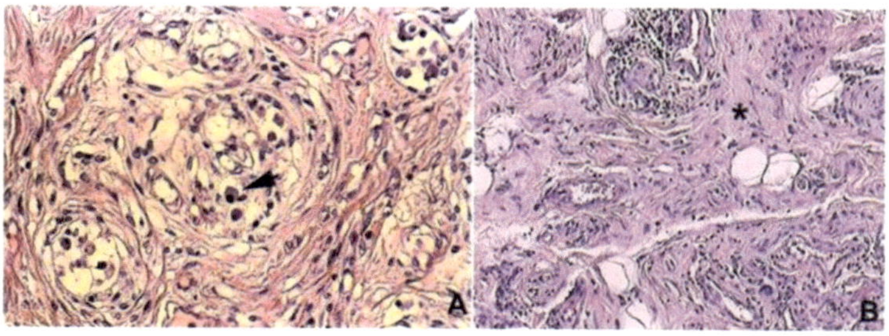

Figure 23. Carotid glomus. A Marked decrease in cells and moderate fibrosis. Typical rounded chief cells are shown in the centre of the section (arrowhead).Hematoxylin and eosin stain; ×400 objective lens. B Severe atrophy and, in some areas, absence of acinar structures with replacement by dense connective tissue with a so-called 'cirrhotic' appearance (asterisk). Hematoxylin and eosin stain; ×100 objective lens

There was a loss of the characteristic chief cells (more than 50%) and loss of their argyrophilic Grimelius-staining granules, suggesting a decrease in their catecholamine content. Fibrosis and glomic cell loss was assessed as 2.6±0.5. A focal reduction of glomus vascularization (more than 50%) was also observed in the areas of atrophy and fibrosis when capillaries were stained with anti-CD34, which was assessed as 2.76±0.6 (Figure 24) In a few cases, it was possible to observe autonomic ganglia showing moderate fibrosis, mild-to-moderate neuronal damage and lipofuscin deposits (Figure 25). Interestingly, the arterioles to the glomus showed severe fibrointimal proliferation and disruption of the internal elastic lamina, marked thickening of the media and luminal narrowing. Luminal thrombi were also observed, as well as focal areas of medial homogenization (Figure 26). At the outer media of the carotid sinus, corresponding to the deeper layers of the plaques, it was possible to identify damaged nerve endings that reacted specifically with S100 protein. No differences were found among groups for glomus area, number of type 1 cells, number of type 2 cells or the wall to lumen arteriole ratio. Also, no statistical differences could be demonstrated when complicated (intraplaque hemorrhage and/or rupture and/or thrombosis) and noncomplicated plaques were compared or when comparing age groups 1, 2 and 3. No correlation between morphometric data and age was found. Patients with stenosis of the extracranial carotid arteries constitute a multimorbid population that frequently shows several vascular risk factors, including hypertension and diabetes. Our study [179] demonstrated that, in patients who died from cerebral vascular disorders with critical carotid artery lesions, a strong involvement of the chemoreceptor structures and their supplying arterioles was found.

Accordingly, at the outer media of the carotid sinus, corresponding to the deeper fibrocalcified layers of the plaques and in periglomic areas, damaged nerve endings were observed as well as fibrotic autonomic ganglia. Therefore, a strong involvement of the baro-(carotid sinus) and chemoreceptor (carotid body or glomus) structures and their corresponding nerves and arterioles was observed in the group of elderly patients. These lesions were independent of patient age, as well as the presence of a complicated carotid plaque. Despite the observation that the connective tissue separating the glomic lobules increases with age, [166] the marked fibrotic involvement and the clear decrease in its rich vascularity, shown by the CD34 immunophenotyping, cannot be explained only in terms of aging. Several studies have found the grade of fibrosis to be dependent on age, [183] while others have demonstrated considerable differences, not only within comparable age groups but, in a few cases, between the right and left sides. [184]

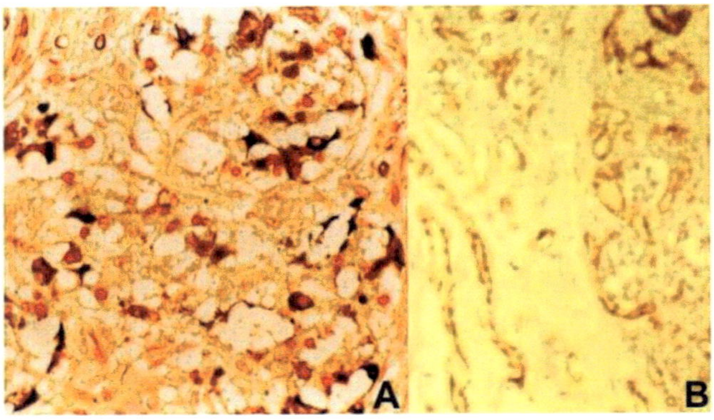

Figure 24. A :Acinar structure belonging to a carotid glomus showing a moderate-to-severe decrease in the number of chief cells, and loss of argyrophilic intracellular granules (shown in black). Grimelius stain; ×200 objective lens. B: Carotid glomus. A focal absence and global decrease of vascularization is shown in the areas of acinar atrophy and fibrosis. anti-CD34 stain; ×100 objective lens

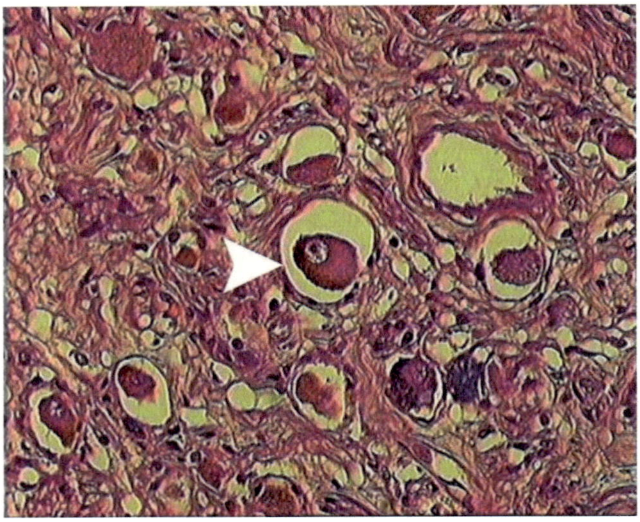

Figure 25. Autonomic ganglia showing moderate fibrosis and mild-to moderate neuronal damage with intracytoplasmic lipofuscin deposits (arrowhead).Hematoxylin and eosin stain; ×200 objective lens

On the other hand, examination of surgical specimens removed from patients older than 60 years of age showed that the organ almost had a 'cirrhotic' appearance. [181] This suggests an arteriolar involvement leading to fibrosis by a chronic hypoxic mechanism. Most of the autonomic parameters, including heart rate variability and baroreflex sensitivity, decline with

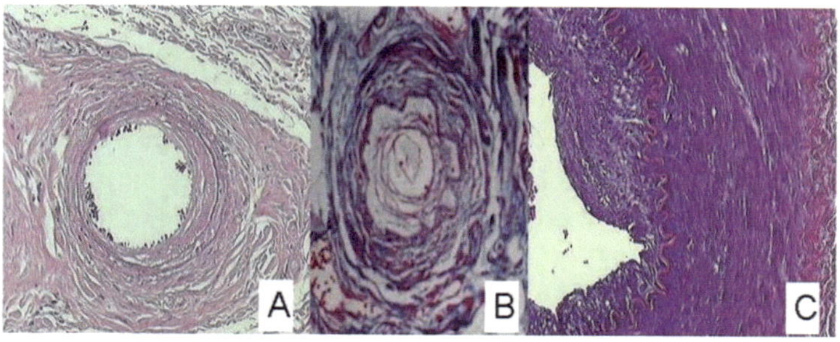

Figure 26. A::Glomic arteriole showing marked intimal fibrosis with moderate thickening of the media and focal areas of medial homogenization, and severe adventitial fibrosis. Hematoxylin and eosin stain; ×100 objective lens. B: Glomic arteriole with marked fibrointimal proliferation and thickening of the wall with luminal narrowing. Azan stain; ×100 objective lens. C: Small artery supplying the glomus. Marked fibrointimal fibrosis with reduction of the lumen and medial fibrosis. Azan stain; ×100 objective lens

age. [185] However, in the rat, aging of the cardiovascular system may not be associated with the attenuation of the baroreflex function. [184] Accordingly, the carotid baroreceptor reflex is well maintained in both young and old dogs, suggesting a lack of morphological involvement. [186] Nevertheless, the attenuation of the baroreflex is far less pronounced in patients in whom the possible effects of disease counteract the age effects. [187]

Therefore, it is possible that the age-related baroreflex attenuation observed in humans may not be due to aging *per se* but may instead reflect atherosclerotic and/or hypertensive processes. [188-189] There are few data concerning the dependency of the various kinds of chemoreflex sensitivity on age in healthy human subjects. A study [185] however, showed no significant correlation between chemoreflex sensitivity and age in patients with multiple organ dysfunction syndrome. The authors hypothesized that this lack of correlation can be interpreted as a confirmation that the effect of the disease prevails over aging in pathological conditions.

Early studies [187-189] speculated that a high systemic arterial pressure may deactivate the baroreceptor function by damaging the nerve endings in the arterial wall. An alternative explanation was issued by Heath and Smith, [190] who suggested that an increased stiffness of the arterial wall would splint the baroreceptor endings, reducing their sensitivity to changes in arterial pressure instead. These authors pointed out that, to some extent, atherosclerosis must depend on the orientation of the receptors in the arterial wall. If they are pulled circumferentially, an increased rigidity of the arterial wall should lead to a decreased baroreceptor response. In contrast, if the structure is compressed outwards from within, an increased rigidity of the vessel wall may not have such an effect. [191]

Baroreflex is aroused by changes in blood pressure that are collected by autonomic nerve 'sensors' that are distributed in the arterial tree and convey the stimuli elicited by mean pressure, rate of change in pressure (dP/dt), pulse pressure and heart rate. These mechanoreceptors, typically gathered in the outer tunica media of the carotid sinus, are found as nerve terminals and, occasionally, with the features of drumstick swellings. The smooth muscle layer is thinner there to allow for an increased vessel compliance favouring an enhanced mechanical stimulation. [192]

Adjustment of the respiration rate in response to changes in levels of oxygen, carbon dioxide and hydrogen ions in body fluids are mediated by a complex interplay between central and peripheral chemoreceptors. The peripheral arterial chemoreceptors, located in the carotid and aortic glomus, are responsible for the immediate ventilatory and arterial pressure increments during acute hypoxia. [165] Type 1 cells in the carotid and aortic glomus release neurotransmitters in response to hypoxia, causing depolarization of nearby afferent nerve endings. [191,192]

Unquestionably, permanent high blood pressure causes a deleterious effect in peripheral nervous structures. However, few studies deal with the findings reported in our papers [18,177,178] regarding the deleterious effect of arterial hypertension on carotid glomus and autonomic ganglia.

As said, our studies in SHRs has demonstrated a strong correlation between arterial hypertension and the development of lesions in the carotid glomus and autonomic ganglia characterized by extracellular matrix expansion, as well as a reduction in the number of ganglia neurons. [178]

Because lowering blood pressure is the first step in controlling the deleterious effects of arterial hypertension, we have evaluated the possible differences between the effects of the beta-blocker atenolol (AT) and the ACEI ramipril (RAM) regarding a protective role on these structures, as target organs in SHRs. [193] At the end of the experiment, SHRs receiving AT and SHRs receiving RAM (SHR-RAM) showed a similar control in blood pressure compared with untreated SHRs. However, SHR-RAM presented with a significant reduction in extracellular matrix expansion in the carotid glomus, autonomic ganglia and autonomic nerves. Moreover, the number of neurons was preserved with AT and even more with RAM compared with the untreated SHR group. TGF-β-1 and PAI-1 were increased in the carotid glomus and autonomic ganglia in SHRs and in SHRs receiving AT, whereas SHR-RAM showed a similar expression to the normotensive group (Wistar-Kyoto rats), indicating that RAM, but not AT, provided a significant protective role against structural changes in these structures caused by arterial hypertension in SHRs. This effect seems to be independent of blood pressure reduction. [194]

These structures were well preserved by an ACEI because permanent high blood pressure stimulates extracellular matrix expansion as a result of enhanced TGF-β-1 and PAI-1 production, through a mechanism regulated by the renin-angiotensin-aldosterone system. [193]

Previous studies have shown the existence of a local reninangiotensin-aldosterone system in the carotid glomus. [194] In agreement with this information, ACEIs could prevent fibrosis in barochemoreceptor structures observed in SHR by reducing local angiotensin II production. [194] The clinical importance of these data could be that the baroreflex attenuation in humans might be a consequence of atherosclerotic and/or hypertensive processes. [177,187,188]

Also the relationship between atherosclerosis and baroreflex sensitivity has been well documented in animal models. [55,63,194,195] Similar evidence in humans is both limited and indirect. [64] It is possible that the age-related baroreflex attenuation observed in humans may not be due to aging per se, but it may reflect atherosclerotic and/or hypertensive processes. [177,188,189]

Carotid barochemoreceptors are of utmost importance in the rapid adjustment of circulation and ventilation; the different degrees of involvement of these structures may explain various clinical responses. [196] These may encompass chronic hypertension, isolated systolic hypertension, blood pressure lability, postural lightheadedness and periodic orthostatic hypotension. [196] Elderly hypertensive patients with these relatively common conditions could be considered as a high-risk stroke group. [19,177]

Cooper et al [197] reported that the effect of both peripheral and central chemoreceptors on baroreflex function may contribute to promoting hypertension in patients with obstructive sleep apnea.Accordingly, Kario et al [196] investigated the clinical significance and mechanism of orthostatic blood pressure dysregulation in elderly hypertensive patients. They found that silent cerebrovascular disease is advanced in elderly patients with orthostatic hypertension.Elderly hypertensive patients with orthostatic hypertension or orthostatic hypotension may have an increased risk for developing cerebrovascular disease. In conclusion Severe carotid chemoreceptor damage exists in elderly patients who died from stroke and suffered from carotid atheromatosis, independently from aging and plaque type. The damage is plausibly related to a marked narrowing of their supplying arterioles as a consequence of hemodynamic (hypertension) and/or metabolic (diabetes, dyslipidemia) disturbances.

A high density of angiotensin II receptors was observed in the rat carotid body by in vitro autoradiography employing 125I- [SarÁ,IleÌ]-angiotensin II as radioligand. Displacement studies demonstrated that the receptors were of the AT1 subtype. [198]

As written above, the renin-angiotensin system has been shown to be responsible for ageing and hypertension which are the major risk factors for the development of cardiovascular and renal diseases.[197,199-202] We conducted an investigation [203] in which the the aim was to compare the effects of losartan, an angiotensin II type-1 receptor blocker, on systolic blood pressure, (SBP), and histopathologycal changes in the carotid body and autonomic lymphs in 14 spontaneously normotensive rats (WKY) They were divided into two groups, one of them treated with Losartan (n=7) and the other was a control group (n=7) not receving this drug. We also compared to spontaneously hypertensive rats (SHRs). As expected, at the end of the study the rats treated with losartan had a SBP of 105 ± 8.3 mm Hg, significantly less than controls (115 ± 8.1 mm Hg, $p = 0.0375$).The carotid body was found in the area fork or carotid bifurcation, formed by lobes compact traversed separated by connective tissue by numerous small blood vessels and nerve fibers blood (Figure 1). Parenchyma was formed by two cell types: primary cells or type I, large round nuclei and cells Hold or type II, elongated and located peripherally of the first (Figure 2). Lobes comprise the functional units of the structure they were best preserved in the group treated with losartan (Figure 3, A). Also, fibrous stroma was much more apparent in the control group, where the gap was increased with cell replacement and decreased in number (Figure 4, A). Clearly losartan treated rats showed glomus area more, a smaller thickness wall in the arterioles and a light periglómicas higher compared with the control group (Figures 3 and 4, A, B, C). All this made that the losartan group had a wall / lumen ratio significantly lower than controls in these vessels. These findings strongly suggest atrophy of the structures analyzed. Through the increasing age is mainly linked with decreased arterial blood supply them and that the inhibition of AT1 receptor would a prominent role in the prevention of such alterations.

In conclusion, a severe carotid chemoreceptor damage does exist in old patients who died from stroke and suffering from carotid atheromatosis. The damage involved the glomic structures and of note, a ''culprit'' narrowing of the arterioles belonging to those structures was also observed. The clinical implications of these findings related to the development and/or worsening of all types of blood pressure and ventilatory disturbances in elderly patients are obvious. Hypertension could play aa very important role in the development of carotid body lesions -Beta blockade or Ramipril or Losartan could prevent morphologic and functional abnormalities

7. Final conclusions

This chapter was based on our experience in the pathology of the carotid arteries and barroreceptor as well as what exists in the international literature. The importance of knowing the biological phenomena that produces the formation of carotid atheromatous plaque is clearly emphasized. We also mentioned different plaque types (stable, unstable and calcified) and its correlation with diagnostic techniques. Concepts approached in the chapter offer the reader elements to enhance decision making in patients suffering carotid atheromatous disease. Additionally we emphasized the need to report on the origin and hemodynamic behavior of the carotid dolichoarteriopathies. Finally, we have highlighted the functions and the various pathological processes that can be observed in the carotid glomus.

Acknowledgements

The authors wish to thank Dr. Gabriel Persi for his academic assistance.

Author details

Ricardo Luis Beigelman, Andrés María Izaguirre, Francisco Azzato and José Milei

*Address all correspondence to: ininca@fmed.uba.ar

Instituto de Investigaciones Cardiológicas ''Prof. Dr. Alberto C. Taquini'' School of Medicine, University of Buenos Aires–CONICET, Buenos Aires, Argentina

References

[1] Whitlow PL, Lylyk P; Londero H Mendiz, OA; Mathias K, Jaeger H, Parodi, J, Schönholz C, Milei, J. Carotid Artery Stenting Protected With an Emboli Containment System. Stroke. 2002;33:1308-1314.

[2] The global burden of disease: 2004 update. World Health Organization (WHO)Press; 2008. http://www.nhlbi.nih.gov/health/health-topics/topics/catd/ [Online]

[3] North American Symptomatic Carotid Endarterectomy Trial Collaborators. Beneficial effect of carotid endarterectomy in symptomatic patients with high-grade carotid stenosis. N Engl J Med. 1991;325: 445–453.

[4] European Carotid Surgery Trialists' Collaborative Group. MRC European Carotid Surgery Trial: interim results for symptomatic patients with severe (70–90%) or with mild (0–29%) carotid stenosis. Lancet. 1991;337:1235–1243.

[5] Mayberg MR, Wilson ES, Yatsu F, Weiss DG, Messina L, Hershey LA, Colling C, Eskridge J, Deykin D, Winn HR. Carotid endarterectomy and prevention of cerebral ischemia in symptomatic carotid stenosis. JAMA.1991;266:3289–94.

[6] Carotid artery stenting compared with endarterectomy in patients with symptomatic carotid stenosis (International Carotid Stenting Study): an interim analysis of a randomised controlled trial International. Carotid Stenting Study investigators - The Lancet, 2010;375 (9719): 985-97

[7] Brott TG, Hobson RWII, Howard G. Stenting versus Endarterectomy for Treatment of Carotid-Artery Stenosis" N Engl J Med 2010; 363:11-23

[8] Paraskevas KI, Mikhailidis DP, Moore WS, Veith FJ. Optimal contemporary management of symptomatic and asymptomatic carotid artery stenosis. Vascular. 2011;19(3): 117-20.

[9] Schneider PA, Naylor AR. Asymptomatic carotid artery stenosis—medical therapy alone versus medical therapy plus carotid endarterectomy or stenting. J Vasc Surg. 2010;52(2):499-507

[10] Inzitari D, Eliasziw M, Gates P, et al, North American Symptomatic Carotid Endarterectomy Trial Collaborators. The causes and risk of stroke in patients with asymptomatic internal-carotid-artery stenosis. New England Journal of Medicine 2000;342:1693e700.

[11] Golledge J, Greenhalgh RM, Davies AH. The symptomatic carotid plaque. Stroke 2000;31:774e81.

[12] Del Corso L, Moruzzo D, Conte B, et al. Tortuosity kinking and coiling of the carotid artery: Expression of atherosclerosis or aging? Angiology. 1998;49(5): 361-71.

[13] Togay-Işikay C, Kim J, Betterman K, Andrews C, Meads D, Tesh P, Tegeler C, Oztuna D. Carotid artery tortuosity, kinking, coiling: stroke risk factor, marker, or curiosity? Acta Neurol Belg. 2005 Jun;105(2):68-72.

[14] Ballotta E, Thiene G, Baracchini C, Ermani M, Militello C, Da Giau G, Barbon B, Angelini A.J Vasc Surg. 2005 ;42(5):838-46; Surgical vs medical treatment for isolated internal carotid artery elongation with coiling or kinking in symptomatic patients: a prospective randomized clinical study.

[15] Beigelman R, Izaguirre A, Robles M, Grana D, Ambrosio G, Milei J.inking of carotid arteries is not a mechanism of cerebral ischemia: a functional evaluation by Doppler echography. Int Angiol. 2011 Aug;30(4):342-8.

[16] Beigelman R, Izaguirre AM, Robles M, Grana DR, Ambrosio G, Milei J. Are kinking and coiling of carotid artery congenital or acquired? Angiology. 2010 Feb-Mar;61(1): 107-12.

[17] Beigelman R, Milei J, Barone A, Ale JJ, Grana D, Parodi JC- Does carotid ultrasound predict plaque morphology? Intercontinental Cardiology 2000;9 (3): 93-8

[18] Milei J.Kinking, Parodi JC, Fernandez Alonso G, Barone A, Grana D, Matturri L. Carotid rupture and intraplaque hemorrhage: immunophenotype and role of cells involved. Am Heart J 1998;136:1096-1105.

[19] Milei J.Kinking, Juan C. Parodi, MD,b Mariano Ferreira, MD,b Andrea Barrone, MD,b Daniel R. Grana, VMD,a and Luigi Matturri. Atherosclerotic plaque rupture and intraplaque hemorrhage do not correlate with symptoms in carotid artery stenosis J Vasc Surg 2003;38:1241-7.

[20] Peng Gao, PhD; Zuo-quan Chen, MS; Yu-hai Bao, MD; Li-qun Jiao, MD; Feng Ling, MD, PhD. Correlation Between Carotid Intraplaque Hemorrhage and Clinical Symptoms. Systematic Review of Observational Studies Stroke. 2007;38:2382-2390

[21] Lavezzi AM, Milei J, Grana DR, Flenda F, Basellini A, Matturri L. Expression of c-fos, p53 and PCNA in the unstable atherosclerotic carotid plaque. Int J Cardiol. 2003 Nov; 92(1):59-63.

[22] Watanabe Y, Nagayama M. MR plaque imaging of the carotid artery. Neuroradiology. 2010;52(4):253-74

[23] Takaya N, Yuan C, Chu B, Saam T, Underhill H, Cai J, Tran N, Polissar NL, Isaac C, Ferguson MS, Garden GA, Cramer SC, Maravilla KR, Hashimoto B, Hatsukami TS. Association between carotid plaque characteristics and subsequent ischemic. Stroke 2006;37:816-823

[24] Matturri L, Lavezzi AM, Silvestri F, Grana DR, Bussari R, Rossi L, Milei J. Severe carotid barochemoreceptor involvement in stroke. Int J Cardiol. 2005 Feb 28;98(3):439-45

[25] Lusby RJ, Ferrel LD, Ehrenfeld WK, Stoney J, Wylie EJ: Carotid plaque hemorrhage. Its role in the production of cerebral ischemia. Arch Surg 1982;117:1479-88.

[26] Disciascio G, Cowley M, Goudreau E, Vetrovec GW, Johnson DE: Histopathologic correlates of unstable ischemic syndromes in patients undergoing directional coronary atherectomy: In vivo evidence of thrombosis, ulceration and inflammation. Am Heart J 1994; 128: 419-26

[27] Falk E: Why do plaques rupture? Circulation 1992; 86 (Suppl III): 1130-42

[28] Burleigh MC, Briggs AD, Lendon CL, Davies MJ, Born GVR, Richardson PD: Collagen types I and III, collagen content, GAGs and mechanical strength of human atherosclerotic plaque caps: span-wise variations. Atherosclerosis 1992; 96: 71-81

[29] Van der Wal, Becker AE, van der Loos CM, Das PK: Site of intimal rupture or erosion of thrombosed coronary atherosclerotic plaques is characterized by an inflammatory process irrespective of the dominant plaque morphology. Circulation 1994; 89; 76-44

[30] Milei J, Parodi JC, Fernandez Alonso G, Barone A, Beigelman R, Ferreira LM, et al. Carotid atherosclerosis: immunocytochemical analysis of the vascular and cellular composition in endarterectomies. Cardiologia 1996;41:535-42

[31] Gown AM, Tsukada T, Ross R: Human atherosclerosis, II: immunocytochemical analysis of the cellular composition of human atherosclerotic lesion. Am J Pathol 1986; 125: 191-207

[32] Constantinides P: Plaque fissuring in human coronary thrombosis. Journal of Atherosclerosis Research 1966; 48: 19-44

[33] Friedman M, Van den Bovenkamp GJ: The pathogenesis of a coronary thrombus. Am.1 Pathol 1966; 48: 19-44

[34] Richardson PD, Davies AT, Born GVR: Influence of plaque configuration and stress distribution on fissuring of coronary atherosclerotic plaques. Lancet 1989; 2: 941-44

[35] Kishikawa H, Shimokama T, Watanabe T: Localization of T-lymphocytes and macrophages expressing IL-1, 1L-2 receptor, IL-6 and TNF in human aortic intima. Role of cell-mediated immunity in human atherogenesis. VirchowsArchiv A. Pathological Anatomy and Histopathology 1993; 423: 433-42

[36] Ross R: The pathogenesis of atherosclerosis: a perspective for the 1990s. Nature 1993; 362: 801-9

[37] Persson AV, Robichaux WT, Silverman M: The natural history of carotid plaque development. Arch Surg 1983; 118: 1048-52

[38] Coombs BD, Rapp JH, Ursell PC, Reilly LM, Saloner D. Structure of plaque at carotid bifurcation high-resolution MRI with histological correlation Stroke 2001;32:2516-21

[39] Kistler JP,Furie KL. Carotid endarterectomy revisited. N Engl J Med 2000;342:1743-5.

[40] Davies M, Bland J, Hangartner J,Angelini A,Thomas AC. Factors influencing the presence or absence of acute coronary thrombi in sudden ischaemic death. EurHeart J1989;10:203-8

[41] CL, Davis MJ, Born GVR, Richardson PD: Atherosclerotic plaque caps are locally weakened when macrophages density is increased. Atherosclerosis 1991; 87: 87-90

[42] Fisher CM,Ojemann RG. A clinicopathologic study of carotid endarterectomy plaques.RevNeurol1986;142:573-89

[43] Clinical advisory:carotid endarterectomy for patients with asymptomatic internal carotid artery stenosis.Stroke1994;25:2523-4

[44] Imparato AM,RilesTS, Mintzer, R,Baumann FG.The importance of hemorrhage intherelationship between gross morphologic characteristic sandcerebral symptoms in 376 carotid artery plaques. AnnSurg 1983;197:195-203

[45] Ammar AD, Wilson RL,Travers H, Lin JJ, Farha SJ, Chang FC. Intraplaque hemorrhage:its significance incerebrovascular disease. Am J Surg 1984;178:840-3

[46] Zukowski AJ, Nicolaides AN, LewisRT,Mansfield AO, Williams MA,HelmisE,e tal.Thecorrelation between carotid plaque ulceration and cerebra linfarction seen on CT scan. J Vasc Surg 1984;1:782-6.

[47] Fisher M,Blumenfeld AM, Smith TW. The importance of carotid artery plaque disruption and hemorrhage. Arch Neurol 1987;44:1086-9

[48] Sitzer M, Muller W, Siebler M,Hort W,Kniemeyer HW,Jancke L,etal. Plaque ulceration and lumen thrombus are the main sources of cerebra microemboli in high-grade internal carotid arterystenosis.Stroke1995;26:1231-3

[49] Sterpetti AV, Hunter WJ, Schultz RD. Importance of ulceration of carotid plaque in determining symptoms of cerebral ischemia. J Cardiovasc Surg (Torino). 1991;32(2): 154-8.

[50] Van Maravic C, Kessler C, van Maravic M. Clinical relevance of intraplaque hemorrhage in the internal carotid artery. EurJSurg1991;157:185-8

[51] Bornstein NM, Krajewski A, Lewis AJ, NorrisJW. Clinica lsignificance of carotid plaque hemorrhage. ArchNeurol1990;4:958-9.

[52] Carr S,Farb A,Pearce WH,Virmani R, Yao JST.Atherosclerotic plaque rupture in symptomatic carotid artery stenosis. J Vasc Surg 1996;23:755-66

[53] Reilly IM, Lusby RJ, Hughes L, Ferrell LD, Stoney RJ, Ehrenfeld WK. Carotid plaque histology using real-time ultrasonography: clinical and therapeutic implications Am J Surg 1983; 146:188-93

[54] Lenninhan L, Kupsky WJ, Mohr JP,Hauser WA, Correll JW, Quest DO.Lack of association between carotid plaque hematoma and ischemic cerebral symptoms. Stroke1987;18:879-81

[55] Bassiouny HS, Davis H, Massawa N,Gewertz BL, Glagov S,Zarins CK. Critical carotid stenoses: morphologic and chemical similarity between symptomatic and asymptomatic plaques.J VascSurg1989;9:202-12

[56] Torvik A, Svindland A,Lindboe CF. Pathogenesis of carotid thrombosis Stroke1989;20:1477-83.

[57] Fryer JA, Myers PC, Appleberg M. Carotid intraplaque hemorrhage: the significance of neovascularity.J Vasc Surg 1987;6:341-9.

[58] Montauban ADM, Elbers HRJ, Moll FL,de SetterJ, Ackerstaff RGA. Cerebral ischemic disease and morphometric analyses of carotidplaques. Ann Vasc Surg 1999;13: 468-74.

[59] Fisher M, Martin A, Cosgrove M, Norris JW. Stroke symptoms from carotid artery plaques [abstract]. Stroke 1994;25:272

[60] O'Donnell TF, Erdoes L, Mackey WC, McCullough J,Shepard A, Heggerick RVT et al. Correlation of B-mode ultrasound imaging and arteriography with pathologic findings at carotid endarterectomy.Arch Surg 1985;120:443-9

[61] Imparato AM, Riles TS, Gorstein F. The carotid bifurcation plaque:pathologic findings associated with cerebral ischemia.Stroke1979;10: 238-45.

[62] Van Damme,H, Vivario M, Boniver J, Limet R. Histologic characterization of carotid plaques. Cardiovasc Pathol 1994;3:9-17.

[63] Feeley TM, Leen EJ, Colgan MP, Moore DJ, Homihane DOB, Shanik GD.Histologic characteristics of carotid artery plaque. J Vasc Surg 1991;13:719-24

[64] Hatsukami TS, Ferguson MS, BeachK W, Gordon D, Detmer P, Burns D et al. Carotid plaque morphology and clinical events.Stroke1997; 28:95-100.

[65] Goldstein LB et al. Guidelines for the primary prevention of stroke: a guideline for healthcare professionals from the American Heart Association/ American Stroke Association. Stroke.2011;42(2):517-84.

[66] ParodiJC,Fustinoni Osvaldo.Siempre está indicado un tratamiento invasivo en la arteriopatía carotídea obstructiva asintomática? Rev ArgCardiol 2004,72(3): 209-11

[67] Brener BJ, Brief DK, Alpert J, Goldenkranz RJ, Parsonnet V. The risk of stroke in patients with asymptomatic carotid stenosis undergoing cardiac surgery: a follow-up study. J Vasc Surg1987;5:269-79.

[68] Hougaku H, Matsumoto M, Handa N, Maeda H, Itoh T, Tsukamoto Y, et al. Asymptomatic carotid lesions and silent cerebral infarction. Stroke 1994;25:566-70.

[69] Park AE, McCarthy WJ, Pearce WH, Matsumura JS, Yao JS. Carotid plaque morphology correlates with presenting symptomatology. J VascSurg 1998;27:872-8.

[70] Muluk SC, Muluk VS, Sugimoto H, Rhee RY, Trachtenberg J, Steed DL, et al. Progression of asymptomatic carotid stenosis:a natural history study in 1004 patients. J Vasc Surg 1999;29:208-14.

[71] Tegos TJ, Sabetai MM, Nicolaides AN, Robless P, Kalodiki E, Elatrozy TS, et al. Correlates of embolic events detected by means of transcranial Doppler in patients with carotid atheroma. J Vasc Surg 2001;33:131-8.

[72] Cheng SW, Ting AC, Ho P, Wu LL. Accelerated progression of carotid stenosis in patients with previous external neck irradiation. J VascSurg 2004;39:409-15.

[73] Consenso de estenosis carotídea Sociedad Argentina de Cardiología. Rev Arg Cardiol 2006;74:160-74.

[74] Aburahma AF, Thiele SP, Wulu JT Jr. Prospective controlled study of the natural history of asymptomatic 60% to 69% carotid stenosis according to ultrasonic plaque morphology. J Vasc Surg 2002;36:437-42.

[75] Executive Committee for the Asymptomatic Carotid Atherosclerosis Study. Endarterectomy for asymptomatic carotid stenosis. JAMA. 1995; 273:1421-8

[76] Cullen P, Baetta R, Bellosta S, Bernini F, Chinetti G, Cignarella A, vonEckardstein A, Exley A, Goddard M, Hofker M, Hurt-Camejo E, Kanters E, Kovanen P, Lorkowski S, McPheat W, Pentikäinen M, Rauterberg J, Ritchie A, Staels B, Weitkamp B, De Winther M. Ruptureof the atherosclerotic plaque: does a good animal model exist?.Arterioscler Thromb Vasc Biol. 2003; 23: 535-542

[77] Peter K, Chen YC, Bui AV, et al. A Novel Mouse Model of Atherosclerotic Plaque Instability for Drug Testing and Mechanistic / Therapeutic Discoveries Using Gene and microRNA Expression Profiling.Circ Res. 2013 Jun 7. [Epub ahead of print]

[78] Forte A, Grossi M, Turczynska KM et al.Local inhibition of ornithinedecarboxylase reduces vascular stenosis in a murine model of carotid injury. Int J Cardiol. 2013 May 13 Epub ahead of print

[79] Sirimarco G, Amarenco P, Labreuche J, Touboul PJ. Carotid atherosclerosis and risk of subsequent coronary event in outpatients with atherothrombosis. Stroke. 2013;44(2):373-9

[80] Greco G, Egorova NN, Moskowitz AJ et al A Model for Predicting the Risk of Carotid Artery Disease Ann Surg. 2013 Jan 17

[81] Geroulakos G, Ramaswami G, Nicolaides A. Characterization of symptomatic and asymptomatic carotid plaques using high-resolution real-time ultrasonography. Br J Surg 1993; 80: 1274-77

[82] Grant E et al. Carotid Artery Stenosis: Gray Scale and Doppler US.Diagnosis-Society of Radiologists in Ultrasound Consensus Conference Radiology 2003; 229-340-6

[83] Fustinoni O y col. Consenso de Estenosis Carotídea.Sociedad Argentina de Cardiología, Sociedad Neurológica Argentina Rev Arg Cardiol 2006; 74(2) 160-74

[84] Bluth El, Kay D, Merrit CRB. Sonographic characterization of carotid plaque: detection of hemorrhage. A J R 1986; 146: 1061-65.

[85] Seeger JM, Klingman N. The relationship between carotid plaque composition and neurological symptoms. J Surg Res 1987;43:78-85

[86] Johnson JM, Kennelly MM, Decesare D. Natural history of asymptomatic carotid plaque. Arch Surg 1985; 120: 1110-2.

[87] Hennerici M, Rautenberg W, Trockel U. Spontaneous progression and regression of small carotid atheroma. Lancet 1985; 1: 1415-9.

[88] Casanova study Group. Carotid surgery versus medical therapy in asymptomatic carotid stenosis. Stroke 1991; 22: 1229-35.

[89] Hobson RW, Weiss DG, Fields WS. Forthe Veterans Attair Cooperative Study Group.Etticacy ot carotid endarterectomy tor asymptomatic carotid stenosis. N EnglJ Med 1993;328: 221-7.

[90] O'Leary D, Nolen J, Ricotta J. Carotid bifurcation disease: prediction of ulceration with B-mode ultrasound. Radiology 1987;162:523-5

[91] Schenk EA, Bond MG, Aretz TH. Multicenter validation study of real time ultrasonography, arteriography and pathology: pathologic evaluation of carotid endarterectomy specimens. Stroke 1988;19:289-26.

[92] Colgan MP, Kingston W, Shanik GD. Asymptomatic carotid stenosis. Is prophylactic endarterectomy justifiable?. Br J Surg 1985; 72: 313-4.

[93] Pourcelot L. Continuous wave Doppler techniques in cerebral vascular disturbances, in Reneman RS, Hoeks APG (eds): Doppler Ultrasound in the Diagnosis of cerebrovascular Disease. Chichester, Research Studies Press, 1982: 103-28.

[94] Fell G, Phillips DJ, Chikos PM. Ultrasonic duplex scanning for disease of the carotid artery. Circulation 1981; 64:1191-95.

[95] Leahy A, McCollum PT, Grouden MC. Accuracy of duplex scanning in estimating carotid lumina' diameter. Br Med J 1987;80: 289.

[96] Roederer G, Langlois YE, Jager KA. The natural history of carotid arterial disease in asymptomatic patients with cervical bruits. Stroke 1984;15:605-13.

[97] Chamber BR, Norris JW. Outcome in patients with asymptomatic neck bruits. N Engl J Med 1986;315:860-5.

[98] Beigelman R, Milei J, Barone A, Ale JJ, Grana D, Parodi JC. "Does carotid ultrasond predict plaque mophology?" Intercont Cardiol 2000;9:93-98

[99] Lehay A, Mc Cohn.) P, Feeley MCh. Duplex Ultrasonography and selection of patients for carotid endarterectomy. Plaque morphology or luminal narrowing?. J Vasc Surg 1988; 8: 558-62.

[100] Goes E, Janssens W, Maillet B. Tissue characterization of atheromatous plaques: correlation between ultrasound image and histological findings. J Clin Ultrasound 1990;18 611-7.

[101] Thiele BL, Jones AM, Hobson RW, Standards in noninvasive cerebrovascular testing. Report from the Committee on Standards for Noninvasive Vascular Testing of the Joint Council of the Society for Vascular Surgery and the North American Chapter of the International Society for Cardiovascular Surgery. J Vasc Surg. 1992;15(3):495-503.

[102] Sitzer M, Muller W, Rademacher J. Color-Flow Doppler assisted duplex imaging tails to detect ulceration in high-grade internal carotid artery stenosis.J Vasc Surg 1996;23:461-5

[103] Hartmann A, Mbhr J, Thompson J. lnterrater reliability ot plaque morphology classification in patients with severe carotid stenosis. Acta Neurol Scand 1999; 99: 61-4.

[104] Julian OC, Dye WS, Javid H. Ulceration lesions of the carotid artery bifurcation. Arch Surg 1963; 86: 803-9.

[105] European carotid plaque study group. Carotid artery plaque composition. Relationship to clinical presentation and ultrasound B-mode imaging. EurJ Endovasc Surg 1995;10:23-30

[106] Noritomi T, Sigel B, Swami V. Carotid plaque typing by multiple- parameter ultrasonic tissue characterization. Ultrasound Med Biol 1997; 23: 643-50.

[107] Noritomi T, Sigel B, Gahtan V. ln vivo detection carotid plaque thrombus by ultrasonic tissue chraracterization.Carotid plaque typing by multiple-parameter ultrasonic tissue characterization. J Ultrasound Med 1997; 16: 107-11.

[108] Lee DJ, Sigel B, Swami VK. Determination of carotid plaque risk by ultrasonic tissue characterization. Ultrasound Med Biol 1998; 24: 1291-9

[109] Singh N, Moody AR, Gladstone DJ, et al. Moderate Carotid Artery Stenosis: MR Imaging–depicted Intraplaque Hemorrhage Predicts Risk of Cerebrovascular Ischemic Events in Asymptomatic Men. Radiology 2009; 252:((2) 502-8

[110] Cheung H, Moody A, Singh N et al. Late Stage Complicated Atheroma in Low-Grade Stenotic Carotid Disease: MR Imaging Depiction—Prevalence and Risk Factors. Radiology 2011:260 (3) 841-7

[111] Executive Committee for the Asymptomatic Carotid Atherosclerosis Study. Endarterectomy for asymptomatic carotid artery stenosis. JAMA. 1995;273(18):1421-28.

[112] Humes HD. Kelley's Essentials of Internal Medicine. 2nd Ed. Paris: Lavoiser Lib; 2001:2693.

[113] Weibel J, Fields WS. Tortuosity, kinking and coiling of the carotid artery. Neurology. 1965; 15:7-14.

[114] Verlato F, Camporese G, Rocco S, SalmistraroG,Signorini GP. Carotid kinks relationship to atherosclerosis and cerebral ischemia. J Vasc Surg. 2000; 32(2):293-98.

[115] Schechter DC. Dolichocarotid syndrome. Cerebral ischemia related to cervical carotid artery redundancy with kinking: Part I. NY State. J Med. 1979;79(9):1391-97.

[116] Macchi C, Gulisano M, Giannelli F, Catini C, Pratesi C, Pacini P. Kinking of the human internal carotid artery: A statistical study in 100 healthy subjects by echocolor Doppler. J Cardiovasc Surg. 1997; 38(6):629-37.

[117] Pellegrino L, Prencipe G, Vairo F. Dolicho-arteriopathies (kinking, coiling, tortuosity) of the carotid arteries: study by color Doppler ultrasonography. Minerva Cardioangiol 1998;46(3):69-76

[118] Pancera P, Ribul M, De Marchi S, Arosío E, Lechi A. Prevalence of morphological alterations in cervical vessels: A colour duplex ultrasonography study in a series of 3300 subjects. Int Angiol. 1998; 17(1):22-7.

[119] Mukherjee D, Inahara T. Management of the tortuous internal carotid artery. Am J Surg. 1985;149(5):651-5.

[120] Koskas F,Bahnin A, Waldern N,Kieffer E. Stenotic coiling and kinking of the internal carotid artery. Ann Vasc Surg. 1993;7(6):530-40

[121] Aleksic M, Schutz G, Gerth S, Mulch J. Surgical approach to kinking and coiling of the internal carotid artery. J CardiovascSurg (Torino). 2004;45(1):43-8.

[122] Togay-Isikay C, Kim J, Betterman K, et al. Carotid artery tortuosity, kinking, coiling: stroke risk factor, marker, or curiosity? ActaNeurol Belg. 2005;105(2):68-72

[123] Price RA, Vawter GF. Arterial fibromuscular dysplasia in infancy and childhood.Arch Pathol.1972;93(5):419-23.

[124] Ghilardi G, De Monti M, Trimarchi S, Bortolani E. Prevalenza del kinking carotideo in una popolazione residente. Minerva Cardioangiol.1993; 41(4):129-32.

[125] Ghilardi G, Longhi F, De Monti M, Bortolani E. Kinking Carotideo ed ipertensione arteriosa. Minerva Cardioangiol. 1993; 41(7-8):287-92.

[126] Quattlebaum J Jr, Upson E, Neville RL. Stroke associated with elongation and kinking of the internal carotid artery. Ann Surg. 1959;150:824-32.

[127] Pancera P, Ribul M, Presciuttini B, Lechi A. Prevalence of carotid artery kinking in 590 consecutive subjects evaluated by Echodoppler. Is there a correlation with arterial hypertension? J Intern Med. 2000; 248(1):7-12.

[128] Oliviero U, Scherillo G, Casaburi C, et al. Prospective evaluation of hypertensive patients with carotid kinking and coiling:an ultrasonographic 7-year study. Angiology. 2003;54(2):169-75.

[129] Kelly AB. Tortuosity of the internal carotid in relation to the pharynx. J Laring. 1925;40:15-20

[130] Harrison J, Dávalos P. Cerebral ischemia. Arch Surg.1962;84:109-12.

[131] Etheredge SN, Effeney DJ, Ehrenfeld WK. Symptomatic extrinsic compression of the cervical carotid artery. Arch Neurol. 1984;41(6):672-73.

[132] Del Corso L, Moruzzo D, Conte B, et al. Tortuosity, kinking and coiling of the carotid artery: Expression of atherosclerosis or aging? Angiology1998; 49(5):361-71.

[133] Sarkari NBS, Macdonald H, Bickerstaff E. Neurological manifestations associated with internal carotid loops and kinks in children. J Neurol Neurosurg Psychiatr. 1970;33(2):194-200

[134] Perdue GD, Barreca JP, Smith RB, King OW. The significance of elongation and angulation of the carotid artery: A negative view. Surgery 1975;77(1):45-52.

[135] Cairney J. Tortuosity of the cervical segment of the internal carotid artery. J Anat (Lond). 1924; 59 (pt 1):87-96.

[136] Ochsner JL, Hughes P, Leonard GL, Milis N. Elastic tissue dysplasia of the internal carotid artery. Ann Surg. 1997;185(6):684-91.

[137] Starr DS, Lawrie GM,Morris GC. Fibromuscular disease of carotid arteries: long results of graduated internal dilatation. Stroke.1981;12(2):196-99

[138] Mettinger KL, Ericson K. Fibromuscular dysplasia and the brain.Stroke.1982;13(1): 46-52.

[139] Danza R, Baldizán J, Navarro T. Surgery of carotid kinking and fibromuscular dysplasia. J Cardiovasc Surg.1983;24(6):628-33.

[140] Metz H, Murray-Leslie RM; Bannister RG, Bull JW, Marshall J. Kinking of the internal carotid artery. Lancet1961;1:424-6

[141] Vollmar J, Nadjafi AS, Stalker CG. Surgical treatment of kinked internal carotid arteries. Br J Surg.1976; 63:847-50

[142] Oliviero U, Scherillo G, Casaburi C, Di Martino M, Di Gianni A, Serpico R, Fazio S, Sacca L. Prospective evaluation of hypertensive patients with carotid kinking and coiling: an ultrasonographic 7-year study. Angiology 2003;54:169-75.

[143] Cioffi FA, Meduri M, Tomasello F, Bonavita V, Conforti P. Kinking and coiling of the intemal carotid artery: clínical-statistical observations and surgical perspectives J. Neurosurg Sci 1975;19: 15-22.

[144] Freeman TR, Uppitt WH. Carotid artery syndrome due to kinking: surgical treatment in forty-four cases. Am Surg 1962;28:745-8

[145] Kia-Noury M. Common carotid kinking and cerebral insufficiency. Int Surg 1973; 58: 646-7

[146] Stanton PE Jr, McClusky DA Jr, Lamis PA. Hemodynamic assessment and surgical correction of kinking of the internal carotid artery. Surgery 1978;84:793-802

[147] Stanton PE Jr, Rosenthal D, McClusky DA, Pano L. Hemodynamic assessment and surgical correction of the kinked intemal carotid artery. South Med J 1981; 74:1348-52.

[148] Mascoli F, Mari C, Uboni A, Virgili T, Marcello D, Mari F, Donini I. The elongation of the internal carotid artery. Diagnosis and surgical treatment. J Cardiovasc Surg (Torino) 1987; 28: 9-11

[149] Zanetti PP, Cremonesi V, Rollo S, lnzani E, Civardi C, Baratta V, Accordino R, Rosa G. La terapia chirurgica del Kinking della carotide interna.Minerva Quirurgica 1989;44:1561-7

[150] Koskas F, Kieffer E, Kieffer A, Bahnini A. Loops and folds of the carotid and vertebral arteries:indications for surgery.J Mal Vasc 1994;19 Suppl A: 51-4.

[151] Poulías GE, Skoutas B, Doundoulakis N, Haddad H, Karkanias G, Lyberiadis D. Kinking and coíling of intemal carotid artery with and without associated stenosis. Surgical considerations and long-term follow-up. Panminerva Med 1996;38:22-7.

[152] Ballotta E, Abbruzzese E, Thiene G, Bottio T, Dagiau G, Angelini A, Saladini M. The elongation of the intemal carotid artery: early and long-term results of patients having surgery compared with unoperated control. Ann VascSurg 1997;11:120-8

[153] Gugulakis AG, Matsagas MI, Vasdekis SN, Giannakakis SG, Lazaris AM, Sechas MN. Evolvíng techniques in the treatment of carotíd artery kinking: the use of resected redundant arterial segment.Am Surg 2001 Jan; 67:67-70

[154] Hines GL, Bilaniuk J, Cruz V. Management of carotid coils during routine carotid endarterectomy. J Cardiovasc Surg (Torino).2001;42:365-8

[155] Benes V, Mohapl M. Altemative surgery for the kinked intemal carotid artery. Acta Neurochir (Wien). 2001 Dec; 143:1267-71; discussion 1271-2.

[156] Grego F, Lepidi S, Cognolato D, Frigatti P, Morelli I, Deriu GP. Rationale of the surgical treatment of carotid kinking. J Cardiovasc Surg (Torino). 2003; 44:79-85.

[157] Illuminati G, Ricco JB, Caliò FG, D'Urso A, Ceccanei G, Vietri F. Results in a consecutive series of 83 surgical corrections of symptomatic stenotic kinking of the internal carotid artery.Surgery 2008;143:134-9.

[158] Gavrilenko AV, Abramian AV, Kuklin AV. Comparative analysis of the outcomes of surgical and conservative treatment of patients with pathological kinking of carotid arteries]. Angio lSosud Khir. 2012;18(4):93-9.

[159] Dadashov SA, Lavrentev AV, Frolov KB, Vinogradov OA, Dziundzia AN, Uljianov ND. Surgical treatment of pathological kinking of the internal carotid artery. Angio lSosud Khir. 2012;18(3):116-21.

[160] Osipenko DV, Marochkov AV.Analysis of postoperative quality of life and survival of patients after surgical interventions on carotid arteries. Angiol Sosud Khir. 2012;18(4):85-91

[161] Ballota E, Thiene G, Baraccini C, Ermani M, Militello C, Da Giau C, Barbon D, Angelini A. Surgical vs medical treatment for isolated internal carotid artery elongation with coiling or kinking in symptomatic patients: a prospective randomized clinical study. J Vasc Surg 2005; 42: 838-46

[162] Beigelman R, Izaguirre A, Robles M, Grana D, Ambrosio G, Milei Kinking of carotid arteries is not a mechanism of cerebral ischemia:a functional evaluation by Doppler echography.J.Int Angiol.2011;30(4):342-8.

[163] Cong TC, Duan X, Gao WH, Zhao EM, Yang XD, Wang H, Xiao SF, Qin Y. [Tortuosity and kinking of cervical segment of internal carotid artery: an analysis of 7 cases]. Zhonghua Er Bi Yan Hou Tou Jing Wai Ke Za Zhi. 2012; 47(11):913-7.

[164] Hering HE. Die Karotissinusreflexe auf Herz und Gefasse. Dresden:Steinkopff, 1927.

[165] Konig SA, Seller H. Historical development of current concepts on central chemosensitivity. Arch ItalBiol 1991;129:223-37

[166] Robertson D, Hollister AS, Biaggioni I, Netterville JL,Mosqueda Garcia R, Robertson RM. The diagnosis and treatment of of baroreflex failure. N Engl J Med 1993;329:1449-55

[167] Ejaz AA, Meschia JF. Thalamic hemorrhage following carotid endarterectomy-induced labile blood pressure: Controlling the liability with clonidine. A case report. Angiology 1999;50:327-30

[168] Rossi L. Bulbo-spinal pathology in neurocardiac sudden death of adults: A prognostic approach to a neglected problem. Int J Legal Med 1999;112:83-90.

[169] Timmers HJLM, Wieling W, Karemaker JM, Lenders WM.Denervation of carotid baro- and chemoreceptors in humans.J Physiol 2003;553:3-11.

[170] Timmers HJLM, Karemaker JM, Wieling W, Marres HAM, Folgering HTM, Lenders JWM. Baroreflex and chemoreflex function after bilateral carotid body tumor resection. J Hypertens 2003;21:591-9.

[171] Holton P, Wood JB. The effects of bilateral removal of the carotid bodies and degeneration of the carotid sinuses in two human subjects. J PhysiolLond 1965;181:365-78.

[172] Capps RB, de Takats G. The late effects of bilateral carotid sinus denervation in man. J Clin Invest 1938;17:385-9

[173] Smiley RH, Campbell GS, Thompson WM, et al. Successful treatment of a fulminant hypertensive crisis after bilateral carotid sinus denervation. Am J Surg 1967;114:784-7

[174] Smit AAJ, Timmers HLJM, Wieling W, et al. Long-term effects of carotid sinus denervation on arterial blood pressure in humans.Circulation 2002;105:1329-35.

[175] Hilz MJ, Stemper B, Neundorfer B. Physiology and methods for studying the baroreceptor stimuli. FortshcrNeurolPsychiatr2000;68:37-47

[176] Iturriaga R, Rey S, Del Río R. Cardiovascular and ventilator acclimatization induced by chronic intermittent hypoxia: A role for the carotid body in the pathophysiology of sleep apnea. Biol Res 2005;38:335-40

[177] Luigi Matturri, Anna Maria Lavezzia, Furio Silvestrib, Daniel R. Granac, Rossana Bussarib, Lino Rossia, Jose´ Milei,* Severe carotid barochemoreceptor involvement in stroke International Journal of Cardiology 98 (2005) 439– 445

[178] Milei J, Cao G, Grana DR, Toblli JE. Plasminogen activator inhibitor-1 and transforming growth factor-beta 1 in carotid glomus and autonomic ganglia from spontaneously hypertensive rats. J Hypertens 2004;22:1351-9.

[179] Milei J, Lavezzi a, Bruni A, Grana DR, Azzato F, Matturri L- Carotid barochemoreceptor pathological findings regarding carotid plaque status and aging-Can J Cardiol 2009; 25 (1) e6-e12

[180] Glenner GG, Grimley PM. Branchiomeric and intravagalparaganglia.In: Atlas of Tumor Pathology. Second series, fascicle 9. Tumors of the Extra-Adrenal Paraganglion System (Including Chemoreceptors). Washington: Armed Forces Institute of Pathology, 1974

[181] de Burgh Daly M. Peripheral Arterial Chemoreceptors and Respiratory-Cardiovascular Integratrion. Oxford: Clarendon Press, 1997:16-65.

[182] Adams WE. The comparative morphology of the carotid body and carotid sinus. Springfield: Charles C Thomas, 1958.

[183] Wei JY, Mendelowitz D, Anastasi N, Rowe JW. Maintenance of carotid baroreflex function in advanced age in the rat. Am J Physiol 1986;250:R1047-51.

[184] Schmidt H, Francis DP, Rauchhaus M, Werdan K, Piepoli MF.Chemo- and ergoreflexes in health, disease and ageing.Int J Cardiol 2005;98:369-78.

[185] Cox RH, Bagshaw RJ, Detweiler DK. Alterations in carotid sinus reflex control of arterial hemodynamics associated with experimental hyperlipemia in the racing greyhound. Circ Res 1980;46:237-44.

[186] Kleiger RE, Miller JP, Bigger JT Jr, Moss AJ. Decreased heart rate variability and its association with increased mortality after acute myocardial infarction. Am J Cardiol 1987;59:256-62.

[187] McGarry K, Laher M, Fitzgerald D, Horgan J, O'Brien E, O'Malley K.Baroreflex function in elderly hypertensives. Hypertension 1983;5:763-6

[188] Vlachakis ND, Mendlowitz M, Degusman D. Diminished baroreceptor sensitivity in elderly hypertensives: Possible role of atherosclerosis. Atherosclerosis 1976;24:243-9.

[189] Sleight P. What is hypertension? Recent studies on neurogenic hypertension. Br Heart J 1971;33(Suppl):109-12.

[190] Heath D, Smith P. The Pathology of the Carotid Body and Sinus. Caulfield East Victoria: Edward Arnold, 1985

[191] Rossi L. Structures of the human baroreflex arch in health and disease. Eur J Card Pacing Electrophysiol 1992;2:53-7.

[192] Prabhakar NR. Oxygen sensing by the carotid body chemoreceptors. J ApplPhysiol 2000;88:2287-95.

[193] Toblli JE, Grana D, Cao G, Milei J. Effects of ACE inhibition and β-blockade on Plasminogen Activator Inhibitor-1 and Transforming Growth Factor-β1 in carotid glomus and autonomic ganglia in hypertensive rats. Am J Hypertens 2007;20:326-34.

[194] Tamura K, Chen YE, Chen Q, et al. Expression of renin-angiotensin system and extracellular matrix genes in cardiovascular cells and its regulation through AT1 receptor. Mol Cell Biochem 2000;212:203-9.

[195] Van Damme H, Vivario M, Boniver J, Limet R. Histologic characterization of carotid plaques. CardiovascPathol 1994;3:9-17.

[196] Kario K, Eiguchi K, Hoshide S, et al. U-curve relationship between orthostatic blood pressure change and silent cerebrovascular disease in elderly hypertensives: Orthostatic hypertension as a new cardiovascular risk factor. J Am CollCardiol 2002;40:133-41

[197] Cooper VL, Pearson SB, Bowker CM, Elliott MW, Hainsworth R. Interaction of chemoreceptor and baroreceptor reflexes by hypoxia andhypercapnia – a mechanism for promoting hypertension in obstructive sleep apnoea. J Physiol 2005;568:677-87

[198] Angell-James JE. Arterial baroreceptor activity in rabbits with experimental atherosclerosis. Circ Res 1974;34:27-39

[199] Chapleau MW, Cunningham JT, Sullivan MJ, Wachtel RE, Abboud FM. Structural versus functional modulation of the arterial baroreflex. Hypertension 1995;26:341-7.

[200] Wilfert K, Drischel K, Unbehaun A, Guski H, Persson PB, Stauss HM. Vascular response to angiotensin II in atherosclerosis:Role of the baroreflex. Hypertension 2000;35:685-90.

[201] Mancia G, Ferrari A, Gregorini L, Ludbrook J, Zanchetti A.Baroreceptor control of the heart rate in human. In: Schwartz PJ,Brown AM, Malliani A, Zanchetti A, eds. Neural Mechanisms in Cardiac Arrhythmias. New York: Raven Press, 1978:323

[202] Allen AM. Angiotensin AT1 receptor-mediated excitation of rat carotid body chemoreceptor afferent activity. J Physiol. 1998 Aug 1;510 (Pt 3):773-81.

[203] Grana D, Cao G, Paglia N, Toblli J, Milei J.Efectos del losartán sobre el glomus carotídeo en ratas normotensas adultas Rev Arg Cardiol 2006: 74(5),384-8

Chapter 4

Carotid Plaque Morphology: Plaque Instability and Correlation with Development of Ischaemic Neurological Events

Reza Mofidi and Barnabas Rigden Green

Additional information is available at the end of the chapter

http://dx.doi.org/10.5772/57254

1. Introduction

Stroke is one of the major health care problems in the world today. It is the third leading cause of mortality in the western countries and the most common cause of mortality of any neurological disorder. Incidence of stroke is 160 per 100,000 population per year; 40 percent of victims require some type of special services and 10 percent require total care. [1, 2] Consequently, stroke rehabilitation places a large drain on national health care resources.

A significant proportion of strokes are ischemic in nature, one of leading causes for which is internal carotid artery (ICA) atherosclerosis. It is estimated that 20-25 percent of all strokes can be attributed directly to carotid bifurcation atherosclerosis. [1, 2]

Both internal carotid artery endarterectomy and carotid stenting in patients with preoperative ocular or cerebral embolic events are well established as procedures that reduce the risk of future ischaemic events. [3-7] In addition to the management of hypertension and commencement of antiplatelet and statin therapy, these interventions form the corner stone of stroke prevention policy in patients with significant ICA stenosis. As it is recognised that a significant proportion of patients have a disabling embolic stroke attributable to severe ICA stenosis without any prior symptoms, [8, 9] it would be advantageous if patients who are at highest risk of stroke from ICA stenosis could be identified and treated in advance of any ischaemic neurological events.

2. Atherosclerotic plaque morphology

Atherosclerotic plaques are not static lesions; they undergo dynamic changes in their size and morphological characteristics. These changes manifest themselves as changes in plaque volume and consistency, otherwise known as *plaque progression* and *regression*. These, together with adaptive responses of the arterial wall, determine the degree of stenosis in the diseased artery. [10-12] This degree of stenosis is the measurable clinical finding which, together with timing and nature of symptoms and co-morbidities, correlates with the risk of developing further neurological events. [13]

Over the last 20 years a lot has been learned about the morphological characteristics of an atherosclerotic plaque responsible for plaque progression and instability. [10-12] Morphological characteristics of atherosclerotic plaques can be discussed in the context of plaque surface characteristics and the composition of the atherosclerotic lesion.

3. Plaque surface characteristics

Julian *et al* in 1963 were the first to discuss the issue of carotid plaque ulceration. They reported 17 cases of macroscopic plaque ulceration with thrombosis in the ulcer crater and suggested this as a source for embolisation. [12] Ulceration has been described as an observable disruption of intima exposing the adjacent atheromatous plaque or media [13] (figure 1).

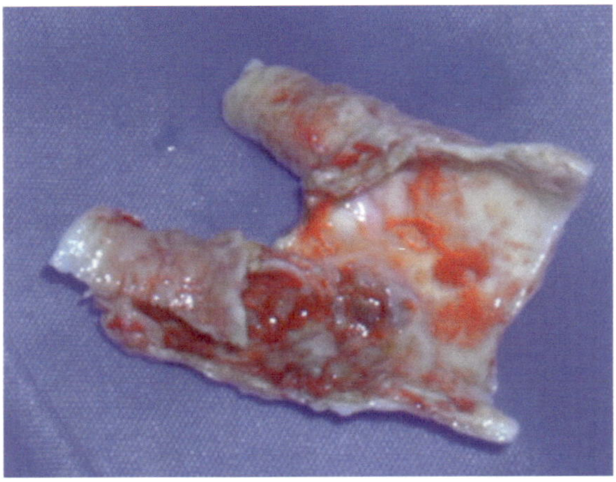

Figure 1. A carotid endarterectomy specimen containing a large ulcer which is associated with intra-plaque haemorrhage.

There has been conflicting evidence regarding the significance of plaque ulceration in the evolution of symptomatic disease. In a large study, Imparato *et al* did not find any significant difference in the incidence of ulceration between symptomatic and asymptomatic groups. [14-16]

Other researchers have found a definite increase in the incidence of plaque ulceration in patients with symptomatic carotid artery disease. Most notably, following review of 593 angiograms in the North American Symptomatic Carotid Endarterectomy Trial (NASCET), 34 percent of medically treated patients were found to have ulcerated plaques with reasonable certainty; this figure was 36 percent for those assigned to surgery. At 2 years, 30 percent of the medically treated group with ulceration had suffered a non-fatal stroke or vascular death compared to only 17 percent of those without plaque ulceration [17].

One reason for this difference may be the time interval between the duration of symptoms and surgery in some of the studies. Lusby *et al* reported re-endothelialisation of several plaques, and suggested that this is particularly likely when the time span between the onset of symptoms and endarterectomy exceeds 3 weeks. [18]

The strength of the evidence from the NASCET trial has meant that most clinicians recognise plaque cap ulceration as a risk factor for development of further carotid territory embolic neurological events. Preoperative evidence of plaque cap ulceration has been included in stroke risk calculators such as the Oxford Stroke Risk calculator. [19]

4. Composition of an atherosclerotic plaque

The raised lesion or fibro-lipid plaque is the archetypal lesion of atherosclerosis and complications of this lesion (fissure and ulceration) form the basis of the vast majority of cases of occlusive arterial disease. All atherosclerotic plaques share two basic morphological components:

Fibrous cap: a thick layer of fibrous connective tissue, which is significantly thicker and much less cellular than the normal intima and contains lipid-filled macrophages, collagen and smooth muscle cells;

Atheroma: A necrotic mass of lipid that forms the core of the lesion. Loss of continuity of the endothelium is the main step in the progression of a plaque and increases the permeability of the intima to lipoproteins, permits platelet-vessel wall interaction and release of growth factors leading to formation of thrombus on the vessel wall.

Leahy demonstrated that various elements of the plaque are available as potential emboli. [20] This includes the fibrous cap overlying complex plaques, the contents that include cholesterol crystals, the breakdown products of intra-plaque haemorrhage, and fibrous or cartilaginous material as well as calcified tissue. Hollenhorst showed the presence of cholesterol emboli in the retinal artery of patients suffering from amaurosis fugax, in the form of bright plaques that were seen in the extra-cranial carotid vessels. [21] Bock *et al* reported that soft plaques (lipid laden and haemorrhagic plaque) behave in an unstable way and tend to ulcerate, whilst fibrous or calcified plaques behave differently. [22]

Based on the natural history and pathological changes within the plaque the American Heart Association (AHA) has classified atherosclerotic lesions [23] (table 1). This classification that has been modified by Virmani and Naghavi *et al* divides the atheromatous lesions into non-atherosclerotic intimal lesions and progressive atherosclerotic plaques. [24, 25] The classification, although not particularly directed at the carotid atherosclerotic lesions, is however applicable when classifying carotid plaques. Progressive atherosclerotic plaques (AHA plaque types V and VI) are relevant in the setting of clinically significant carotid disease (figure-2).

Type I	Adaptive Lesion: Intimal Smooth Muscle Cells (SMC)
Type II	Fatty Streak, Foamy Macrophages and underlying SMCs
Type III	Pre Atheroma, Intimal Macrophages, deeper pools of extracellular lipid
Type IV	Atheroma (Fibrous Plaque), dense large extra cellular lipid core deep to intima, and close to media.
Type V	Fibroatheroma, multiple layers of lipid core encased in a fibrous cap
Type VI	Complicated plaque: VI a Disruption of the intimal surface VI b Intra Plaque Haemorrhage VI c Thrombosis related to the atherosclerotic plaque

Table 1. American Heart Association has classification of atherosclerotic lesions [23] (*Circulation* 1995;92: 1355-74)

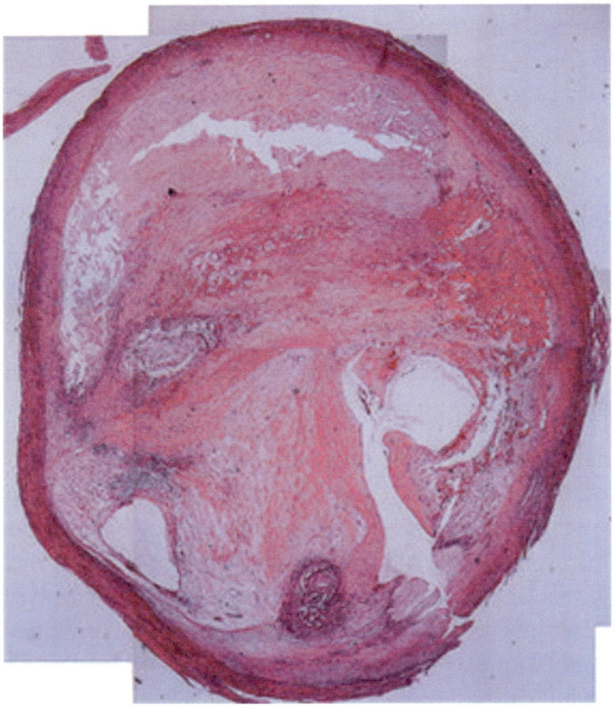

Figure 2. American Heart Association Type VI (Complicated atherosclerotic lesion) obtained from a carotid endarterectomy specimen. (*Br J Surg.* 2001;88:945–950.)

5. The concept of unstable atherosclerotic plaque

The concept that a sub-group of atherosclerotic plaques are prone to embolisation or thrombosis is not new. As early as 1926, Benson postulated that coronary thrombosis results from disruption of intima that exposes lipids to flowing blood. [26] Constantinides was the first to establish conclusively that plaque rupture was the immediate cause of coronary thrombosis. [27] In a series of subsequent studies Davies *et al* established the importance of plaque fissuring, ulceration and subsequent thrombosis in the development of acute coronary syndromes. [28-30] Further clinical and angiographic work has led to progression of this concept and introduction of thrombolytic therapy in the treatment of coronary artery atherosclerosis. [31-34]

Atherosclerotic plaques that are prone to rupture are known to have certain cellular, molecular and structural features. Notably these include an intense inflammatory process within the plaque, angiogenesis, and intra-plaque haemorrhage with gradual thinning of the fibrous cap, subsequent loss of plaque cap integrity and ulceration. [35] Burke *et al* defined a vulnerable plaque in the coronary arteries as a lesion with a cap thickness of less than 65 μM [36]. Gertz *et al* noted that the lipid cores were much larger in areas of atherosclerotic plaque disruption than in lesions with intact surfaces. [37-38] Inflammatory activity within the plaque is associated with plaque ulceration and has a role in pathogenesis of intimal damage. [39]

The evolution of atheroma is modulated by innate and adaptive immune responses which are recognized histologically as presence of an inflammatory infiltrate within the lesion [40]. These processes are responsible for replication and phenotypic change within the smooth muscle cell from contractile to secretory which results in formation of plaque cap and lesion growth. Intimal endothelial cell activation results in recruitment of macrophages and lymphocytes (predominantly CD4 positive T-cells) into evolving lesion. [40] Activation of Th-1 T-cells is known to initiate a potent inflammatory cascade which in turn leads to plaque instability [41]. Inflammatory cell infiltrate is a marker for plaque vulnerability. [42-47] Several factors such as oxidized lipoproteins, infectious agents or auto-antigens *(heat shock protein)* have been considered as the putative cause of the chronic inflammatory reaction in an atherosclerotic plaque. [40] This in turn results in weakening of the connective tissue framework of the plaque. [48, 49] Smooth muscles may help to counteract some of these effects by producing matrix protein, collagen and inhibitors of matrix degrading enzymes known as metalloproteinases. [50, 51] The net result of these two processes is thought to define whether or not the plaque ruptures or remains contained by the fibrous cap.

6. Angiogenesis in carotid atherosclerotic lesions

Normal human intima is devoid of blood vessels, [52] however newly formed blood vessels are often seen within atherosclerotic plaques [53-56] (figure-3). The presence and density of these new blood vessels in carotid atherosclerotic lesions has been associated with the histological features of plaque instability and intra-plaque haemorrhage as well as the

Structural:
Large Lipid rich core
Thin Fibrous Cap
Reduces Collagen content
Cellular:
Local Chronic inflammation
Increased macrophage density and activity
T Lymphocyte accumulation near site of rupture
Increased Neovascularity
Reduced Smooth muscle cell density
Increased number and activity of mast cells
Expression of markers of inflammatory activation
Molecular
Matrix Metalloproteinase Secretion
Increased Tissue Factor Expression

Table 2. Features of Rupture prone (Unstable) Plaques [40]

development and timing of ipsilateral ischaemic or ocular events and presence of ipsilateral cerebral infarction on computer tomography (CT) scanning. [57-62] Microarray gene chip analysis revealed that the presence of newly formed vessels is associated with increased angiogenic gene expression. [63, 64] These new blood vessels are weak and could be responsible for intraplaque haemorrhage. Moreover, the endothelial lining of these microvessels express high levels of E-Selectin, ICAM-1, and VCAM-1, which indicates that these endothelial cells are in an activated state. Activated endothelial cells act as local site of inflammatory cell recruitment into the atherosclerotic plaque, perpetuating the inflammatory process within the lesion and contribute to plaque destabilization. [65-69]

7. Plaque haemorrhage

Haemorrhage is a common feature of unstable carotid atherosclerotic lesions. [68-72] Intraplaque haemorrhage has been associated with the development and growth of the necrotic plaque core, rapid changes in plaque volume, development of plaque instability, and ischaemic neurological events. [73-76]

The origin of plaque haemorrhage is uncertain. It has been suggested that it may occur from fissures within the plaque cap. [76] Alternatively the new blood vessels within the atherosclerotic plaque may represent the first site of morphologic change that leads to intra-plaque haemorrhage; features such as microvessel density and perivascular inflammatory infiltrate have been associated with the presence and quantity of intra-plaque haemorrhage. [55, 77, 78]

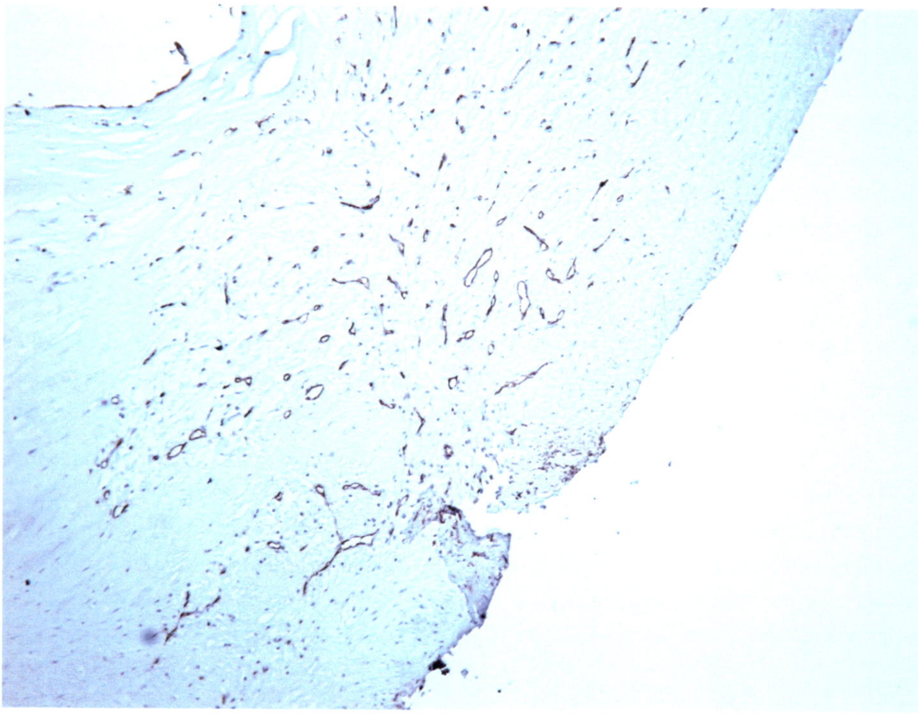

Figure 3. New blood vessels in a carotid atherosclerotic plaque. (*Ann Vasc Surg* 2008; 22(2): 266–272.)

There is ample clinical and histological evidence that carotid atherosclerotic plaques with large necrotic lipid core, thin plaque cap or ulceration, dense inflammatory infiltrate, intra-plaque haemorrhage and angiogenesis are vulnerable to rupture and development of ischaemic neurological and ocular events. In vivo identification of these changes within carotid atherosclerotic plaques gives these findings clinical significance in the context of patients with significant carotid atherosclerosis. For over two decades, non-invasive imaging modalities such as duplex ultrasound and magnetic resonance imaging have been in clinical use. They have been used for the measurement of internal carotid artery stenosis. [79-81] These imaging modalities can also be used to study morphological changes associated with plaque instability and development of ischaemic neurological events. [82-85]

8. Duplex ultrasound assessment of carotid plaque morphology

Duplex ultrasound is arguably the most important imaging modality for preoperative assessment of patients with carotid atherosclerotic disease. It is non-invasive, relatively inexpensive and very accurate at identification of significant ICA stenosis. [87-92] In measuring the degree of stenosis, the flow and velocity characteristics assessed by colour flow Doppler are utilized. Duplex devices also generate high resolution B-mode ultrasound images of the atherosclerotic lesion. These images do not contribute significantly to the assessment of carotid artery stenosis. However the B-mode ultrasound image can be used to assess morphologic characteristics of an atherosclerotic lesion. It has been known for some time that plaques that have low echogenicity (appear dark on Duplex ultrasound) or a high degree of heterogeneity are associated with histologic characteristics of plaque instability, ipsilateral neurological or ocular events, [93] CT evidence of carotid territory cerebral infarction or evidence of embolisation on trans-cranial ultrasound. [94] These ultrasound characteristics can be assessed subjectively and classified by a trained observer.

B-mode ultrasound assessment of atherosclerotic plaque morphology started some 30 years ago. Reilly *et al* recognised two distinct types of carotid atherosclerotic lesion. The first was termed homogenous and was defined as lesion with uniformly high or medium level echoes. Histologically, homogenous plaques are fibrous lesions. [95] The second type was termed heterogeneous and was defined as plaque with high, medium and low level echoes. [95]

Histologically heterogeneous plaques contain variable amounts of intra-plaque haemorrhage, lipids, cholesterol crystal and a loose stroma. A further refinement of subjective assessment of plaque morphology was the Gray-Wheal classification method (table-3). [96] In the Cardiovascular Health Study, which enrolled 5,201 individuals aged 65 years and over without prior cerebrovascular symptoms, and followed them for an average of 3.3 years demonstrated a significantly increased incidence of stroke in individuals who had echo-lucent plaques. [97]

Plaque Type	Ultrasound characteristics
Type-1	Predominantly echolucent with a thin echogenic cap
Type-2	Intermediate echolucent lesions with small areas of echogenicity
Type-3	Intermediate echogenic lesions with small areas of echolucency (<25%)
Type-4	Uniformly echogenic lesions (equivalent to homogenous).

Table 3. Gray-Wheal Classification of atherosclerotic plaques

Subjective observer dependent assessment of plaque morphology, whilst useful, is limited by high inter- and intra-observer variability, significantly limiting its clinical application. [98-99] Echogenicity and heterogeneity of an atherosclerotic plaque can be objectively assessed using image analysis techniques through the measurement of median grey scale (GS) value of the ultrasound image, percentage of echo-lucent pixels and entropy in GS characteristics of the lesion(figure-4). [99-103] In order to remove variability associated with acquisition of the ultrasound image, the US images are normalised using linear scaling so that the adventitia would have a grey scale median value of 185-195 and blood 0-5. Plaques with a low GS median were associated with a significantly higher annual risk of stroke. [99-104]

Interestingly, although characterisation of the internal structure of the plaque assessed by image analysis correlates closely with clinical symptoms, the correlation between computerised assessment of plaque morphology and histological features of the lesion is less strong. [94] This indicates that values such as GS median represent a median value of the whole atherosclerotic area and do not necessarily reflect the presence of particular regional components.

http://dx.doi.org/10.5772/57254

The use of stratified GS median measurements which create a profile of the regional GS median as a function of distance from plaque surface combined with colour mapping correlates better with the presence of various histopathological components and identify determinants of plaque instability with a high degree of accuracy. [94]

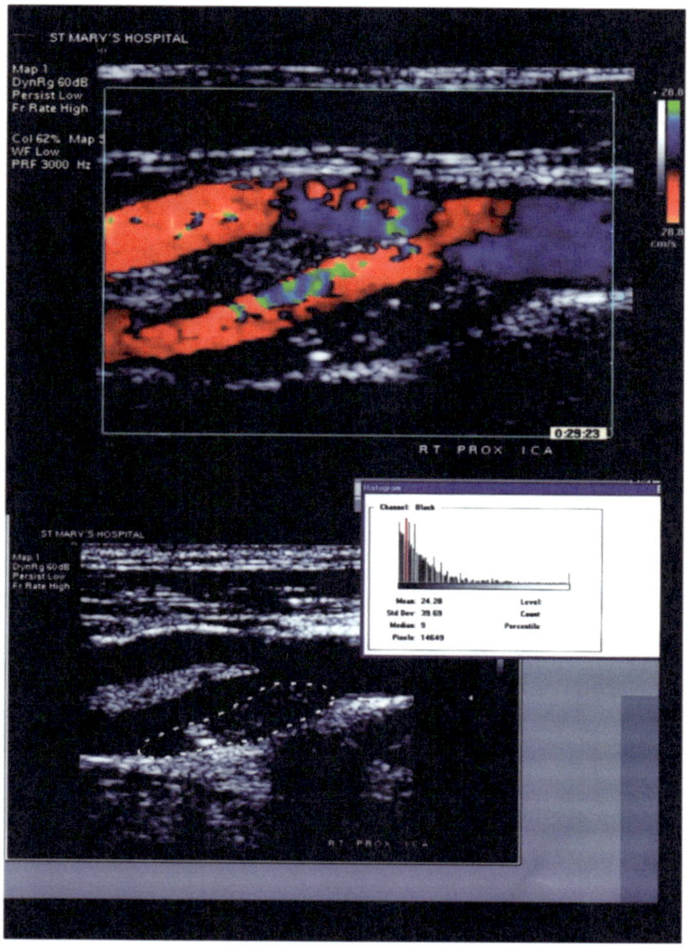

Figure 4. Calculation of Grey Scale Median of a hypo-echoic plaque. (*Swiss Med* 2005; 135:635–643.)

9. Magnetic resonance imaging assessment of plaque morphology

Magnetic resonance imaging (MRI) is a promising modality for characterisation of carotid plaque morphology and assessment of composition of atherosclerotic plaques. It can accurately identify the presence of ulcerated or thin plaque cap, [105-107] quantify intra-plaque haemorrhage [105-107], or the presence of a large necrotic plaque core [105-107]. Serial MRI examinations in asymptomatic patients with moderate (50-70-percent) ICA stenosis have revealed correlation between these plaque findings and development of subsequent ipsilateral ocular and ischaemic neurological events [108] (Figure-5).

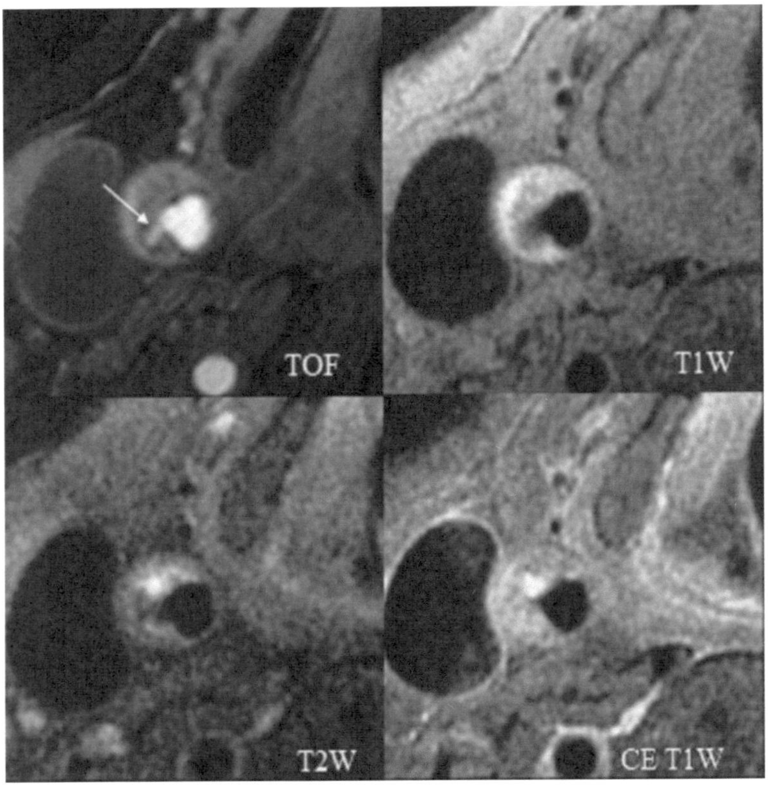

Figure 5. Identification of intra-plaque haemorrhage using high spatial resolution, multi-contrast MRI image. (*JACC Cardiovasc Imaging.* 2009; 2:883-96.)

One of the strengths of MRI is the availability of multi-contrast weighted protocols. The most common application of carotid MRI remains the acquisition of an angiogram which uses a bright blood sequence using a 3-dimensional time of flight sequence. This attenuates the signal from stationary (plaque) tissues. Black blood sequences eliminate the luminal signal and help to characterise plaque morphology. [105-109] Combining the information, multiple-contrast weightings can be used to identify all plaque components. [105-110] Plaque compositional characteristics can be assessed using automatic classifiers such as morphology enhanced probabilistic plaque segmentation (MEPPS) algorithms with a high degree of accuracy (Figure-6). [111, 112] Administration of gadolinium-DTPA together with T1-weighted sequences in addition to bright blood time of flight sequence can be used to create maximal intensity projection (MIP) images for measurement of the degree of ICA stenosis [105-107] and accurately measure the thickness of plaque cap in relation to the necrotic core volume. [105-107]

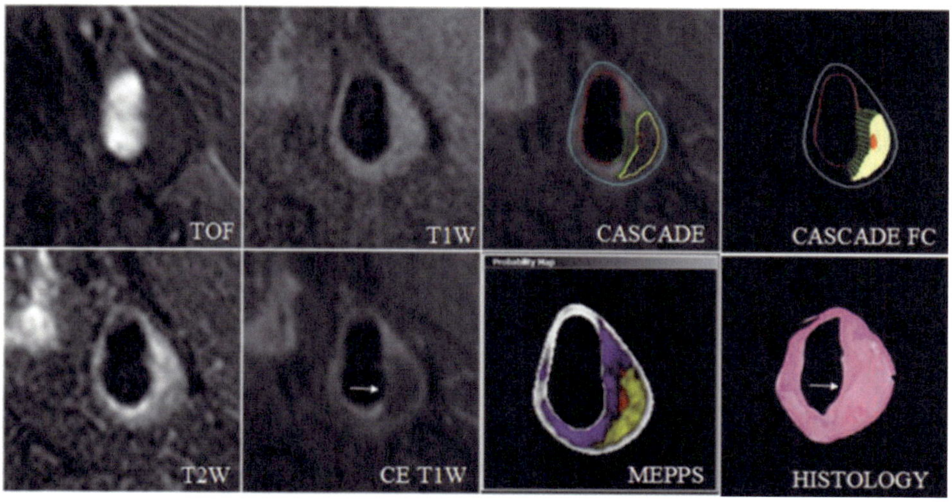

Figure 6. Automated segmentation of bright–and black-blood, high-spatial resolution, Multi-contrast in vivo MR images compared with histological characteristics of plaque. (*JACC Cardiovasc Imaging.* 2009; 2:883-96.)

High resolution MRI can identify and age intra-plaque haemorrhage. [113-115] Prospective serial MRI studies have demonstrated that haemorrhage in atherosclerotic plaques is associated with sudden increases in plaque volume, necrotic core, and progression of degree of stenosis. [115]

In addition to Duplex and MRI, other modalities such as fludeoxyglucose (FDG) positron emission tomography (PET) CT scanning has been used to assess the level of metabolic activity in carotid atherosclerotic plaque. This is used in turn as a surrogate marker of plaque instability.

PET CT scanning has shown some promise as a tool for assessment of plaque instability. [116] However it is unlikely to gain mainstream applicability due to its limited availability, expense, and the significant exposure to ionising radiation (meaning serial assessments are not possible) and availability of non-invasive accurate imaging modalities to assess plaque morphology.

10. Conclusion

Over the last 20 years the advances in technology have led to the evolution of non-invasive imaging modalities with high spatial resolution. The application of this technology in the assessment of carotid plaque morphology has advanced our understanding of the natural history of atherosclerotic lesions more than the assessment of histological characteristics of atherosclerotic plaques. Consequently for the first time, plaque morphology could be assessed against the two functions that ultimately matter the most: time and occurrence of future embolic ischaemic events.

New and continuing advances in MRI technology such as higher field strength, phased-array coils, and the application of 3-dimensional and contrast enhanced ultrasound will provide even more tools for assessment of carotid plaque morphology. Gradual application of these modalities in clinical practice will help clinicians select patients with significant ICA stenosis who are likely to benefit from carotid intervention prior to occurrence of ischaemic neurological events.

Author details

Reza Mofidi and Barnabas Rigden Green

James Cook University Hospital, Middlesbrough, United Kingdom

References

[1] Dennis M, Bamford J, Sandercock P, Warlow C. Prognosis of transient ischaemic attacks in the oxfordshire community stroke project. *Stroke* 1990; 21: 848-853

[2] Shah KH, Kleckner K, Edlow JA. Short term prognosis of patients diagnosed in the emergency department with a transient ischemic attack. *Ann Emerg Med* 2008; 51: 316-323.

[3] Barnet HJM, Taylor DW, M Eliasziw, Fox AJ. Benefit of Carotid endarterectomy in patients with Symptomatic moderate or severe stenosis. *N Engl J Med* 1998, 339: 1415-25

[4] North American Symptomatic Carotid Endarterctomy Trial collaborators. Beneficial effects of carotid endarterectomy for symptomatic patients with high grade stenosis. *N Engl J Med* 1991, 325: 445-83

[5] Medical Research Council European Carotid Surgery Trial. Interim results for symptomatic patients with severe (70-99%) or with mild (0-29%) carotid stenosis.*Lancet* 1991; 337: 1235-43

[6] European Carotid Surgery Trialists Collaborative Group.MRC. Risk of stroke in the distribution of asymptomatic carotid artery. *Lancet 1995 ;345: 209-12*

[7] European Carotid Surgery Trialists Collaborative Group.MRC. European Carotid Surgery Trial: Interim results for symptomatic patients with severe (70-99%) or with mild (0-29%) carotid stenosis. *Lancet; 337: 1235-43*

[8] Executive Committee for Asymptomatic Carotid Atherosclerosis Study. Endarterectomy for asymptomatic carotid artery stenosis *JAMA* 1995 273: 1421-8.

[9] Halliday A, Harrison M, Hayter E. Kong X, et al. 10-year stroke prevention after successful carotid endarterectomy for asymptomatic carotid stenosis (ACST-1): A randominsed trial. *Lancet* 2010; 376(9746):1074-1084.

[10] Virmani R, Farb A, Burke AP. Understanding the atherosclerotic plaque.*Progress in vascular surgery*. Yao JST, Pearce WH. *Appleton & Lange, USA. 1997; 3-19*

[11] Golledge J, Cuming R, Ellis M, Davies AH,Greenhalgh. Carotid Plaque characteristics and presenting symptoms. *British J Surg*. 1996, 84: 1697-1701.

[12] Lovett J, Walton J, Hands L, Gallagher P J, Rothwell PM. Histological correlates of angiographic carotid plaque ulceration. *Circulation* 2004; 110: 2190-97

[13] Rothwell PM, Eliasziw M, Gutnikov SA, Fox AJ, Taylor W, Mayberg MR, Warlow CP, Barnet HJM for the Carotid Endarterectomy Trialists' Collaboration. Pooled analysis of individual patient data from randomised controlled trials of endarterectomy for symptomatic carotid stenosis. *Lancet* 2003; 361: 107-16.

[14] Mofidi R, Powell TI, Brabazon A, Mehigan D, Sheehan SJ, MacErlaine DP, Keaveny TV. Prediction of the exact degree of internal carotid artery stenosis using an artificial neural network based on duplex velocity measurements. *Ann Vasc Surg*2005; 19(6): 829-37.

[15] Jahromi AS, Cina AS, LiuY, Clase CM. Sensitivity and specificity of color duplex ultrasound measurement in the estimation of internal carotid artery stenosis: a systematic review and meta-analysis. *J Vasc Surg* 2005; 41(6):962-72.

[16] Nederkoorn PJ, van der Graaf Y, Hunink MG. Duplex ultrasound and magnetic resonance angiography compared with digital subtraction angiography in carotid artery stenosis: a systematic review. *Stroke* 2003;34(5):1324-32.

[17] Makris GC, Lavida A, Griffin M, Geroulakos G, Nicolaides AN. Three-dimensional ultrasound imaging for the evaluation of carotid atherosclerosis.*Atherosclerosis* 2011; 219(2):377-83.

[18] Biasi GM, Froio A, Diethrich EB, Deleo G, Galimberti S, Mingazzini P, Nicolaides AN, Griffin M, Raithel D, Reid DB, Valsecchi MG. Carotid plaque echolucency increases the risk of stroke in carotid stenting: the Imaging in Carotid Angioplasty and Risk of Stroke (ICAROS) study. *Circulation* 2004 ; 110(6):756-62.

[19] Rothwell PM, Eliasziw M, Gutnikov SA, Fox AJ, et al. for the Carotid Endarterectomy Trialists' Collaboration. Pooled analysis of individual patient data from randomised controlled trials of endarterectomy for symptomatic carotid stenosis. *Lancet* 2003; 361: 107-16.

[20] Kawahara I, Morikawa M, Honda M, Kitagawa N.High-resolution magnetic resonance imaging using gadolinium-based contrast agent for atherosclerotic carotid plaque. *Surgical Neurology* 2007; 68(1):60-65.

[21] Watanabe Y, Nagayama M. MR plaque imaging of carotid artery.*Neuroradiology* 2010; 52: 253-274.

[22] Bock R Gray- Weale A C.Mock P. Natural history of asymptomatic carotid artery disease. *J Vasc Surg 1993*;17:160-71

[23] Stary HC, Chandler AS, Dinsmore RE, et Al. A definition of advanced type of Atherosclerosis, A report from the committee on vascular lesions of the council on atherosclerosis AHA. *Circulation* 1995;92: 1355-74

[24] Virmani R, Kolodgie FD, Burke AP, Farb A, Schwartz SM. Lessons from sudden coronary death: a comprehensive morphological classification scheme for atherosclerotic lesions. *Arterioscler Thromb Vasc Biol.* 2000;20(5):1262-75.

[25] Naghavi M, Libby P, Falk E, Ward-Casscells S et al. From Vulnerable Plaque to Vulnerable Patient. *Circulation* 2003; 108: 1664-1672.

[26] Benson RL. Present Status of Coronary Artery Disease. *Arch Pathol Lab Med* 1926;2:876-916

[27] Constantinides P. Plaque fissures in human Coronary thrombosis. *J Atherosclr Res* 1966;6:1-17

[28] Davies MJ Fulton WF, Robertson WB. Pathology of acute myocardial infarction with particular reference to occlusive coronary thrombi. *Br Heart J* 197638:659-64

[29] Davies MJ Thomas A. thrombosis and acute coronary artery lesions in sudden cardiac ischemic death.. *N Engl J Med* 1984;310:1137-40

[30] Davies MJ Thomas AC. Plaque fissuring-The cause of acute myocardial infarction, sudden ischemic death and cresendo angina..*Br Heart J* 1985;53:363-73

[31] DeWood MA, Spores J, Notske R, and Mouser LT et al. Prevalence of total coronary occlusion during the early hours of transmutable infarction. *N Engl J Med 1980*; 303:895-902

[32] Brown BG, Gallery CA, Badger RS, Kennedy JW et al. Incomplete lyses of thrombus in the moderate underlying atherosclerotic lesion during the intracoronary infusion of streptokinase for acute myocardial infarction: quantitative angiographic observations. *Circulation* 1986;73:653-61

[33] Little WC, Constantinescu M, Applegate RJ, Kutcher MA et al. Can coronary angiography predict the site of subsequent myocardial infraction in patients with mild-to-moderate coronary artery disease? *Circulation* 1988;78:1157-66

[34] Kullo I, Edwards WD, Schwartz RS. Vulnerable Plaque: Pathobiology and Clinical Implications. *Ann. Intern. Med.* 1998; 129:150-60

[35] Virmani R, Burke AP, Farb A, Kolodgie FD. Pathology of the vulnerable plaque. *J Am Coll Cardiol.* 2006; 47: (8 Suppl):C13-8.

[36] Burke AP, Farb A, Malcom GT, Liang YH, Smialek J et al. Coronary risk factors and plaque morphology in men with coronary disease who died suddenly. *New Engl J Med* 1997; 336 (18): 1276-82.

[37] Gertz SD, Roberts WC Heamodynamic Shear force in rupture of coronary arterial atherosclerotic plaque. *Am J Cardiology* 1990;66:1368-72

[38] Loree HM, Tobias BJ, Gibson LJ, Kamm RD et al. Mechanical properties of model atherosclerotic lesion lipid pools. *Arterioscler Thrmb* 1994;14:230-4

[39] Spagnoli LG, Bonanno E, Sangiorgi G, Mauriello A. Role of inflammation in atherosclerosis. *J Nucl Med* 2007; 48:1800-1815.

[40] Hansson GK, Jonasson L, Lojsthed B, Stemme S, et al. Localisation of T Lymphocytes and macrophages in fibrous and complicated human atherosclerotic plaques *Arteriosclerosis* 1988;72: 135-41.

[41] Benagiano M, Azzurri A, Ciervo A, et al. T helper type 1 lymphocytes drive inflammation in human atherosclerotic lesions. *Proc Natl Acad Sci* 2003;100: 6658–6663.

[42] Annovazzi A, Bonanno E, Arca M, et al. 99mTc-Interleukin-2 scintigraphy for the in vivo imaging of vulnerable atherosclerotic plaques. *Eur J Nucl Med Mol Imaging.* 2006;33:117–126.

[43] Benagiano M, D'Elios MM, Amedei A, et al. Human 60-kDa heat shock protein is a target autoantigen of T cells derived from atherosclerotic plaques. *J Immunol.* 2005;174:6509–6517.

[44] Mauriello A, Sangiorgi G, Fratoni S, et al. Diffuse and active inflammation occurs in both vulnerable and stable plaques of the entire coronary tree a histopathologic study of patients dying of acute myocardial infarction. *J Am Coll Cardiol.* 2005;45:1585–1593.

[45] Libby P. Molecular basis of the acute coronary syndrome. *Circulation* 1995; 91:, 2844-50.

[46] Fustor V, Badimon J, Chesebro JH, Mechanisms of disease I: the pathogenesis of coronary artery disease and the acute coronary syndromes. *N Engl J Med.* 1992; 326:242-50

[47] Falk E. Why do plaques rupture? *Circulation* 1992; 86(Suppl III): 36-42

[48] Amento EP, Ehsani N, Palmer H, Libby P. Cytokines positively and negatively regulate interstitial collagen gene expression in human vascular smooth muscle cells. *Arteriosclerosis Throm.* 1991; 11: 1223-30.

[49] Moreno PR, Purushothaman KR, Fuster V, O'Connor WN. Intimomedial interface damage and adventitial inflammation is increased beneath disrupted atherosclerosis in the aorta: implications for plaque vulnerability. *Circulation.*2002; 105:2504–2511.

[50] Uemura S, Matsushita H, Li W, et al. Diabetes mellitus enhances vascular matrix metalloproteinase activity: role of oxidative stress. *Circ Res.*2001;88:1291–1298.

[51] Garcia-Touchard A, Henry TD, Sangiorgi G, et al. Extracellular proteases in atherosclerosis and restenosis. *Arterioscler Thromb Vasc Biol.*2005;25:1119–1127.

[52] Geiringer E. Intimal vascularisation and atherosclerosis. Histologic characteristics of carotid atherosclerotic plaque. *J Path. Bacteriol.* 1951 63: 201-11

[53] Barger AC, Beewikes R, Lainey LL, Silverman KJ. Hypothesis: Vasa vasarum and neo-vascularization of the human coronary arteries. *N Engl J Med* 1984, 310: 175-77

[54] O'Brien ER, Garvin RD, Stewart DK, Hinohara T et al. Angiogenesis in human coronary atherosclerotic plaques. *Am. J. Pathology* 1994,145 (4): 833-94.

[55] Jeziorska M, Woolley DE. Local Neovascularisation and cellular composition within vulnerable regions of atherosclerotic plaques of human carotid arteries. *J. Pathology* 1999; 188,189-96.

[56] Jeziorska M, Woolley DE. Neovascularization in early atherosclerotic lesions of human carotid arteries: its potential contribution to plaque development. *Hum. Pathol.* 1999; 30(8): 919-25.

[57] McCarthy MJ, Loftus IM, Thompson MM, Jones L, et al. Angiogenesis and the atherosclerotic carotid plaque: an association between symptomatology and plaque morphology. *J Vasc Surg.* 1999; 30(2): 261-8.

[58] Mofidi R, Crotty TB, McCarthy P, Sheehan SJ, Mehigan D, Keaveny TV. Association between plaque instability, angiogenesis and symptomatic carotid occlusive disease. *Br J Surg.* 2001;88:945–950.

[59] Mofidi R, Powell TI, Crotty TB, McCarthy P, et al. Angiogenesis in Carotid Atherosclerotic Lesions Is Associated with Timing of Ischemic Neurological Events and Presence of Computed Tomographic Cerebral Infarction in the Ipsilateral Cerebral Hemisphere. *Ann Vasc Surg* 2008; 22(2): 266–272.

[60] Dunmore BJ, McCarthy MJ, Naylor AR, Brindle NP. Carotid plaque instability and ischemic symptoms are linked to immaturity of microvessels within plaques *J Vasc Surg.* 2007; 45(1): 155-159.

[61] Post S, Peeters W, Busser E, Lamers D, et al. Balance between Angiopoietin-1 and Angiopoietin-2 Is in Favor of Angiopoietin-2 in Atherosclerotic Plaques with High Microvessel Density. *J Vasc Res* 2008; 45: 244–250.

[62] Virmani R, Ladich ER, Burke AP, Kolodgie FD et al. Histopathology of carotid atherosclerotic disease. *Neurosurgery* 2006; 59(S3): 219-227.

[63] Virmani R, Kolodgie F, Burke AP, Finn AV et al. Atherosclerotic Plaque Progression and Vulnerability to Rupture Angiogenesis as a Source of Intraplaque Hemorrhage. *Arterioscler Thromb Vasc Biol.*2005;25: 2054-61.

[64] Davies MJ, Gordon JL, Gearing AJ, Pigott R, et al. The expression of Adhesion Molecules ICAM-1, VCAM-1, PECAM, and E Selectin in Human Atherosclerosis. *J Pathol* 1993; 171(3): 223-9.

[65] Mofidi R, Crotty T, McCarthy P, Mehigan D et al. Neovascular endothelial-cell activation: the link between angiogenesis, intimal leukocyte content, and development of symptomatic carotid occlusive disease. *Int J Angiology* 2004; 13(1):15-21.

[66] O'Brien KD, McDonald TO, Chait A, Allen MD, Alpers CE. Neovascular expression of E-selectin, intercellular adhesion molecule-1, and vascular cell adhesion molecule-1 in human atherosclerosis and their relation to intimal leukocyte content. *Circulation* 1996; 93(4): 672-82.

[67] Galkina E, Ley K. Vascular Adhesion Molecules in Atherosclerosis. *Arterioscler Thromb Vasc Biol.*2007; 27: 2292–2301.

[68] Paterson JC. Capillary rupture of with intimal haemorrhage as the causative factor in coronary thrombosis. *Arch Pathol.* 1938; 25: 474-87.

[69] Imparato AM, Riles TS, Mintzer R, Baumann FG The importance of hemorrhage in the relationship between gross morphologic characteristics and cerebral symptoms in 376 carotid artery plaques. Ann. Surg. 1983; 197(2):195-203

[70] Lusby RJ, Ferrell LD, Ehrenfeld WK, Stoney RJ, Wylie EJ. Carotid plaque hemorrhage. Its role in production of cerebral ischemia. *Arch Surg* 1982; 117(11): 1479-88.

[71] Milei J, Parodi JC, Alonso GF, Barone A, et al. Carotid rupture and intraplaque hemorrhage: immunophenotype and role of cells involved. *Am. Heart J.* 1998; 136(6): 1096-105.

[72] Fryer JA, Myers PC, Appleberg M. Carotid intraplaque haemorrhage: The significance of neovascularity. *J. Vasc. Surg.* 1987; 6 (4): 341-9

[73] von Maravic C, Kesler C, von Maravic M, Hohlbach G, Kompf D. Clinical relevance of intraplaque hemorrhage in the internal carotid artery. *Eur J Surg* 1991; 157(3): 185-8.

[74] Feely TM, Leen EJ, Colgan MP, Moore JD, et al. Histologic Characteristics of carotid artery plaque. *J Vasc Surg* 1991, 13:719-24.

[75] Mofidi R, Powell TI, Crotty TB, Sheehan SJ, et al. Increased Internal Carotid Artery Peak Systolic Velocity Is Associated with Presence of Significant Atherosclerotic Plaque Instability Independent of Degree of ICA Stenosis. *Int J Angiology* 2005; 14(2): 74-80.

[76] Davies MJ, Thomas AC. Plaque fissuring: the cause of acute myocardial infarction, sudden ischaemic death, and crescendo angina. *Br Heart J.*1985; 53:363–373.

[77] Moreno PR, Purushothaman KR, Sirol M, Levy AP, Fuster V. Neovascularization in human atherosclerosis. *Circulation* 2006; 113: 2245–2252.

[78] Türeyen K, Vemuganti R, Salamat MS, Shahriar M, Dempsey RJ. Increased Angiogenesis and Angiogenic Gene Expression in Carotid Artery Plaques from Symptomatic Stroke Patients. *Neurosurgery* 2006; 59: 971-977.

[79] Mofidi R, Powell TI, Brabazon A, Mehigan D, Sheehan SJ, MacErlaine DP, Keaveny TV. Prediction of the exact degree of internal carotid artery stenosis using an artificial neural network based on duplex velocity measurements. *Ann Vasc Surg* 2005; 19(6): 829-37.

[80] Jahromi AS, Cina AS, LiuY, Clase CM. Sensitivity and specificity of color duplex ultrasound measurement in the estimation of internal carotid artery stenosis: a systematic review and meta-analysis. *J Vasc Surg* 2005; 41(6):962-72.

[81] Nederkoorn PJ, van der Graaf Y, Hunink MG. Duplex ultrasound and magnetic resonance angiography compared with digital subtraction angiography in carotid artery stenosis: a systematic review. *Stroke* 2003;34(5):1324-32.

[82] Makris GC, Lavida A, Griffin M, Geroulakos G, Nicolaides AN. Three-dimensional ultrasound imaging for the evaluation of carotid atherosclerosis. *Atherosclerosis* 2011; 219(2):377-83.

[83] Biasi GM, Froio A, Diethrich EB, Deleo G, et al. Carotid plaque echolucency increases the risk of stroke in carotid stenting: the Imaging in Carotid Angioplasty and Risk of Stroke (ICAROS) study. *Circulation* 2004 ; 110(6):756-62.

[84] Kawahara I, Morikawa M, Honda M, Kitagawa N.High-resolution magnetic resonance imaging using gadolinium-based contrast agent for atherosclerotic carotid plaque. *Surgical Neurology* 2007; 68(1):60-65.

[85] Watanabe Y, Nagayama M. MR plaque imaging of carotid artery. *Neuroradiology* 2010; 52: 253-274.

[86] Perkins JM, Galland RB, Simmons MJ, Magee TR. Carotid duplex imaging: variation and validation. *Br J Surg* 2000; 87: 320-322.

[87] Padayachee TS, Cox TC, Modaresi KB, Colchester AC, Taylor PR. The measurement of internal carotid artery stenosis: comparison of duplex with digital subtraction angiography. *Eur J Vasc Endovasc Surg* 1997; 13: 180-185.

[88] Chen JC, Salvian AJ, Taylor DC, Teal PA, Marotta TR, Hsiang YN. Predictive ability of duplex ultrasonography for internal carotid artery stenosis of 70%-99%: a comparative study. *Ann Vasc Surg* 1998; 12: 244-247.

[89] Hood DB, Mattos MA, Mansour A, et al. Prospective evaluation of new duplex criteria to identify 70% internal carotid artery stenosis. *J Vasc Surg* 1996;23:254-261.

[90] Moneta GL, Edwards JM, Papanicolaou G, et al. Correlation of North American Symptomatic Carotid Endarterectomy Trial (NASCET) angiographic definition of

70-99% internal carotid artery stenosis with duplex scanning. *J Vasc Surg* 1993; 17: 152-159.

[91] Geroulakos G, Hobson W, Nicolaides A. Ultrasonographic carotid plaque morphology in predicting stroke risk. *Br J Surg.* 1996; 83:582-87.

[92] TJ Tegos, MM Sabetai, AN Nicolaides, Robless P. et al. Correlates of embolic events detected by means of transcranial Doppler in patients with carotidatheroma *J Vasc Surg* 2001; 33(2): 131-138.

[93] Golledge J, Cuming R, Ellis M, Davies AH, Greenelgh. Carotid Plaque Characteristics and presenting symptoms. *Br J Surg.* 1996; 84:1697-1701.

[94] Sztajzel S. Ultrasonographic assessment of the morphological characteristics of the carotid plaque. *Swiss Med* 2005; 135:635–643.

[95] Reilly LM, LusbyRJ, Hughes L, Ferrell LD, StoneyRJ, Ehrenfeld WK.. Carotid plaque histology using real-time ultrasonography. *Am J Surg* 1983, 146:188-193.

[96] Gray-Weale AC, Graham JC, Burnett JR, Byrne K, Lusby RJ. Carotid artery atheroma: Comparison of preoperative B Mode ultrasound appearance with carotid endarterectomy specimen pathology. *J Cardiovascular Surg.* 1988; 29:676-81

[97] Polak JI, Shemanskil, O'Leary D, Lefkowitz D, Price TR, Savage P et al. Hypoechoic plaque at US of the carotid artery: An independent risk factor for individual stroke in adults aged 65 years or older. *Radiology* 1998, 208:649-654.

[98] Sabetai MM, Tegos TJ, Nicolaides AN, Dhanjil S, et al. Reproducibility of Computer-Quantified Carotid Plaque Echogenicity Can We Overcome the Subjectivity? *Stroke* 2000;31: 2189-2196.

[99] Arnold JAC, Modaresi KB, Thomas N, Taylor PR, Padayachee TS. Carotid plaque characterization *Vascular* by duplex scanning: observer error may undermine current clinical trials. *Stroke.* 1999; 30:61–65.

[100] Sabetai MM, Tegos TJ, Nicolaides AN, El-Atrozy T, et al. Hemispheric symptoms and carotid plaque echomorphology. *J Vasc Surg* 2000; 31(1): 39–49.

[101] El Atrozy T, Nicolaides A, Tegos T, Griffin M. Objective Characterization of Carotid Plaque Features. *Eur J Vasv Endovasc Surg.* 1998; 16:223-30.

[102] Tegos TJ, Sabetai MM, Nicolaides AN, El-Atrozy T, et al. Patterns of brain computed tomography infarction and carotid plaque echogenicity. *J Vasc Surg* 2001; 33(2): 334-339.

[103] Nicolaides AN, Kakkos SK, Griffin M, Sabetai M et al. Effect of Image Normalization on Carotid Plaque Classification and the Risk of Ipsilateral Hemispheric Ischemic Events: Results from the Asymptomatic Carotid Stenosis and Risk of Stroke Study. *Vascular* 2005;13: 211-221.

[104] Kakkos SK, Stevens JM, Nicolaides AN, et al. Texture analysis of ultrasonic images of symptomatic carotid plaques can identify those plaques associated with ipsilateral embolic brain infarction. *Eur J Vasc Endovasc Surg* 2007;33; 422-429.

[105] Kerwin WS, Hatsukami T, Yuan C, Zhao XQ. MRI of Carotid Atherosclerosis. Am J Roentgenology 2013; 200(3): 304-313.

[106] Wasserman BA. Advanced Contrast-Enhanced MRI for Looking Beyond the Lumen to Predict Stroke Building a Risk Profile for Carotid Plaque. *Stroke* 2010;41: 512-516.

[107] Chu B, Ferguson MS, Chen H, Hippe DS, et al. Magnetic resonance imaging features of the disruption-prone and the disrupted carotid plaque. *JACC Cardiovasc Imaging.* 2009; 2(7):883-96.

[108] Sievers M. Detection of unstable carotid artery stenosis using MRI. *J Neurol* 2007; 254: 1714-1722.

[109] Altaf N, Akwei S, Auer DP, MacSweeney ST, et al. MR detected carotid plaque hemorrhage is associated with inflammatory features in symptomatic carotid plaques. *Ann Vasc Surg* 2013;27(5): 655–661.

[110] Kawahara I, Morikawa M, Honda M, Kitagawa N, et al. High-resolution magnetic resonance imaging using gadolinium-based contrast agent for atheroscleroticcarotid plaque. *Surgical Neurology* 2007;68(1):60-65.

[111] Kerwin W, Xu D, Liu F, Saam T, Underhill H, et al. Magnetic resonance imaging of carotid atherosclerosis: plaque analysis. *Top Magn Reson Imaging.* 2007;18: 371–378.

[112] Liu F, Xu D, Ferguson MS, Chu B, et al. Automated in vivo segmentation of carotid plaque MRI with Morphology-Enhanced probability maps. *Magn Reson Med.* 2006; 55:659–668.

[113] Chu B, Kampschulte A, Ferguson MS, Kerwin WS et al. Hemorrhage in the Atherosclerotic Carotid Plaque: A High-Resolution MRI Study *Stroke* 2004;34: 1079-1084.

[114] Honda M, Kitagawa N, Tsutsumi K, Nagata I, et al. High-Resolution Magnetic Resonance Imaging for Detection of Carotid Plaques. *Neurosurgery* 2006; 58: 338-346.

[115] Takaya N, Yuan C, Chu BC, Saam T, Polissar NL, et al. Presence of Intraplaque Hemorrhage Stimulates Progression of Carotid Atherosclerotic Plaques: A High-Resolution MRI study. *Circulation* 2005; 111: 2768–2775.

[116] Sakalihasan N, Michel JB. Functional Imaging of Atherosclerosis to Advance Vascular Biology. *Eur J Vasc Endovasc Surg* 2009; 728-734.

Chapter 5

Update on Carotid Revascularization: Evidence from Large Clinical Trials

Hussien Heshmat Kassem, Foad Abd-Allah and Mohammad Wasay

Additional information is available at the end of the chapter

http://dx.doi.org/10.5772/57153

1. Introduction

In the era of evidence-based medicine, doctors rely on clinical trials to guide their decisions. The best method of treating carotid stenosis is still debatable after six decades from the first carotid surgical revascularization performed. Despite the conduct and publication of dozens of trials on carotid revascularization, the truth remains shaggy. The interpretation of these trials is influenced by the design, inclusion criteria, credentialing of the operators and even their specialties. We will try to discuss the trials of carotid endarterectomy and carotid artery stenting trying to reach a conclusion of where is the truth regarding carotid revascularization. We will discuss the trials of CEA versus medical therapy, then the initials registries of CAS, then the trials that compared CEA against CAS, we will elaborate on the two techniques in peculiar situations and finally we will give a short notice about ongoing trials and future directions.

2. Carotid endarterectomy

Carotid endarterectomy (CEA) started in the early 1950s and is now the most commonly performed peripheral arterial surgery in the USA. The aim of CEA is to remove the entire atherosclerotic plaque from the carotid bifurcation en bloc leaving a rough surface to be endothelialized over the following weeks. Most procedures are performed under general anesthesia. However, local anesthesia and mild intravenous sedation are sometimes successful and can allow monitoring of neurologic functions during surgery. Local anesthesia also should be considered in the hemodynamically unstable patient or in situations where general anesthesia may be too risky.

3. The early years of carotid endarterectomy

Early attempts at reconstruction of the carotid artery at the bifurcation were carried out by Carrea, Molins, and Murphy in 1951 and subsequently by Eastcott, Pickering, and Robb in 1954. In 1965 DeBakey reported that he performed the first CEA in 1953. Although not published, there is controversy about this claim.[1] Subsequently, a group of neurologists, vascular surgeons, and neurological surgeons performed a study on the "new technique" comparing it with medical therapy. Interestingly, the surgical mortality was surgical mortality of 4.5% in 2400 operations. This early study the study delineated careful methods of measuring common carotid and internal carotid and vertebral artery stenosis. The study also determined the upper level of ready surgical accessibility as well as the contraindications to the operation.[2] Additionally, myocardial infarction was identified as the principal cause of late mortality in those patients undergoing successful surgical treatment. Providing the patients survived the surgical therapy, the occurrence of new stroke was 4% in the surgical group. However, the superiority of surgery over medical therapy was not definitive. Despite criticism, CEA became extremely popular. It became the most commonly performed peripheral arterial procedure in the United States, reaching a peak of 107,000 operations in nonveteran hospitals in the United States in 1985.[1] At that time, however, neurologists were skeptical. Their fears were supported by reports that the rates of death or stroke from CEA were 10%. Endarterectomy turned from a great procedure to an operation "that has escaped critical analysis to be let loose on an unsuspecting public"![3] These concerns stressed the need to perform well-designed randomized trials under independent neurological audit. Those trials established the role of CEA versus medical treatment for stroke prevention.

4. The landmark trials of CEA versus medical therapy; NASCET, ACAS and ECST

The role of CEA in prevention of stroke was established based on large randomized trials performed mostly in the early 1990s.

This meta-analysis of ECST and NASCET trials showed that surgery increased the 5-year risk of ipsilateral ischemic stroke in patients with <30% stenosis (absolute risk reduction of –2.2%, P = 0.05), had no effect in patients with 30-49% stenosis (absolute risk reduction of 3.2%, P = 0.6), was of marginal benefit in those with 50% to 69% stenosis (absolute risk reduction of 4.6%, P =0.04), and was highly beneficial in those with ≥70% stenosis without near-occlusion (absolute risk reduction of 16.0%, P < 0.001). There was a trend toward benefit from surgery in patients with near occlusion at 2 years' follow up (absolute risk

http://dx.doi.org/10.5772/57153

	No of patients in specified trial	Medical risk (%) at 2 years	Surgical risk (%) at 2 years	Risk difference (%)	Relative risk reduction (%)	No need to treat*	Perioperative stroke and death rate (%)
Symptomatic patients							
70-99% NASCET	659	21.4	8.6	12.8	60	8	5.8
70-99%ECST**	501	19.9	7.0	12.9	65	8	5.6
50-69% NASCET	858	14.2	9.2	5.0	35	20	7.1
50-69% ECST**	684	9.7	11.1	-1.4	-14	-	9.8
<50%NASCET	1368	11.6	10.1	1.5	13	67	6.5
<50% ECST**	1882	4.3	9.5	-5.2	-109	-	6.1
Asymptomatic patients							
≥50%, VA, men only	444	7.7†	5.6†	2.1	27	48	4.4
ACAS	1662	5.0	3.8‡ (actual)	1.2	24	83	2.6
ACE	2848	5.0§ **(assumed)**	5.8	-0.8	-	-	4.6

ACE=aspirin and carotid endarterectomy trial.

*NNT = Number needed to treat by CEA to prevent one stroke in 2 years after the procedure, compared with medical treatment alone.

**By NASCET measurement.

†Extrapolated from results.

‡Assigning a perioperative risk of 2.6% based on 724 of 825 patients who actually received endarterectomy in the surgical arm of ACAS, and utilizing the 0.6% risk of stroke in each of the two years after endarterectomy. The same

1.2% risk is assumed for the ACE patients and VA patients.

§No medical arm—assumed from ACAS data.

Table 1. Number needed to treat by endarterectomy to prevent one stroke in 2 years in patients with carotid stenosis

reduction of 5.6%, P = 0.19), but no benefit at 5 years (absolute risk reduction of –1.7%, P =0.9). Both ACST and ACAS studies showed benefit from CEA in >60% asymptomatic stenosis. However, neither showed increasing benefit from surgery with increasing degree of stenosis. This observation was assumed to be attributable to a lack of statistical power of the trials. The benefit from CEA relates to the complication rates. Reported benefits were predicated on operative risks of stroke or death of 7.5% in the ECST and 6.5% in the NASCET. If the disabling stroke and death rates exceed this by as little as 2%, the benefit from CEA disappears.[4]

5. The spread of CEA among vascular surgeons worldwide

There have been a dramatic fall and a rise in the rates of carotid endarterectomy in both the United States and Canada, which correlate with the publication of first unfavorable and then favorable clinical studies. The absence of selective referral of patients to centers with the lowest mortality rates raises questions about whether the benefits of carotid endarterectomy in the general population are similar to those demonstrated in the clinical trials. Rates of carotid endarterectomy fell in all three regions from 1984 to 1989 (from 126 to 66 per 100,000 adults 40 years of age or older in California, from 65 to 40 per 100,000 in New York, and from 40 to 15 per 100,000 in Ontario), after the publication of studies demonstrating that the rates of complications of carotid endarterectomy were unacceptably high. However, the clinical trials of the 1990s, which showed benefit from carotid endarterectomy, were associated with a dramatic resurgence in the rates of the procedure from 1989 to 1995 (from 66 to 99 per 100,000 in California, from 40 to 96 per 100,000 in New York, and from 15 to 38 per 100,000 in Ontario). These increased rates were not associated with proportionally greater numbers of referrals of patients to hospitals with low mortality rates.[5]

6. The limitations of carotid endarterectomy

This NASCE, ACAS and ESCT trial as well as the spread of carotid endarterectomy worldwide unveiled the problems and limitations inherent to the procedure. It became clear that the coexistence of cardiac co-morbidity is a powerful predictor of mortality and that myocardial infarction can be the most dreaded complication, even more than stroke. This was evident, despite the fact that patients with myocardial infarction in the prior six months, congestive heart failure and patients scheduled for coronary revascularization were excluded from the large CEA trials.[6] Other limitations of the procedure were more located to the local environment in the neck as prior endarterectomy, prior neck dissection or radiation, cranial nerve palsies and inaccessible high/low carotid bifurcations. The presence of contra-lateral carotid occlusion also posed a problem during cross clamping that increased the risk of CEA.

7. Carotid angioplasty

While carotid endarterectomy was growing to maturity, anther contender was born. After the fundamental work in endovascular therapy by Charles Dotter and Andreas Grüntzig, it was inconceivable at the end of the 1970s to apply their work to arteries supplying the brain. Klaus Mathias chose to ignore this strict limit and was able to successfully perform angioplasty of atherosclerotic stenoses at the carotid bifurcation in 1980.[7] The technique evolved slowly from simple balloon dilatation to involve stenting, used first by Théron in 1990 and then widespread use of cerebral protection devices.

8. The initial case-series and registries of carotid stenting

Author	No of Patients	No of stents	Asymptomatic stenosis (%)	Technical success rates (%)	30-day Morbidity or Mortality (%)	No of Deaths/ Mortality Rate	Major Stroke Rate (%)	Minor Stroke Rate (%)	Restenosis rate
Roubin	146	210	37	99	NS	1 / 0.65	1.3	4.6	6 mo, ,5%; 12 mo, ID
Theron	69	69	NS	100	NS	...	...	...	4% (time not specified)
Diethrich	110	129	72	99.1	7.3	2 / 1.8%	2	4.5	6 mo, NS; 12 mo, NS
Yadav	107	189	36	100	7.9	1 / 0.9%	1.9	6.5	6 mo, 4.9%; 12 mo, NS
Vozzi	22	19	55	96	NS	1 / 4.5%	4.5	4.5	6 mo, NS; 12 mo, ID
Criado	33	NS	27	100	NS	0	0	0	3% (mean 8-mo follow-up)
Wholey	108	NS	44	95	NS	2/ 1.9%	1.8	1.8	1% (mean 6-mo follow-up)
Henry	163	178	35	99.4	NS	0/ ..	1.8	1.2	6 mo, 2.3%; 12 mo, ID
Teitelbaum	22	31	32	96.2	27.3	1 / 4.5%	13.6	9.0	6 mo, 14.3%; 12 mo, NS
Waigand	50	56	72	100	2	1 / 2%	2	2	8.7% (mean 8-mo follow-up
Bergeron	99	99	42	97	2.0	0/...	0	1	4.2% (mean 13-mo follow-up)

Table 2. Carotid Stent Series [8]

9. Results of multicenter registries

The Global Carotid Artery Stent Registry: In 1998, Wholey et al collected data from major interventional centers worldwide as well as from peer-reviewed journals. The total number of procedures that have been performed till that date included 2,048 cases, with a technical success of 98.6%. The stroke rate was 3.08%. The 30-day post-procedure mortality rate was 1.37%. The registry was updated in 2003. The total number of stent procedures performed then became 12392 with a technical success rate of 98.9%. Overall, there was TIA rate of 3.07%, minor strokes of 2.14%, major strokes of 1.20%, and procedure-related deaths of 0.64%. There were 6753 cases done without protection and which incurred a 5.29% rate of strokes and procedure-related deaths. In the 4221 cases with cerebral protection, there was a 2.23% rate of strokes and procedure-related deaths. The rate of neurologic events was 1.2%, 1.3%, and 1.7% at 1, 2, and 3 years, respectively.[9]

In the following years, several registries that were supported by the device industry were reported. These registries included patients who are considered high risk for CEA because one or more of the following features:

1. Class-III/IV congestive heart failure
2. Left ventricular ejection fraction<30%
3. Open heart surgery within 6 weeks
4. Recent myocardial infarction (>24 h <30 d)
5. Unstable angina: class III/IV
6. Concurrent requirement for coronary revascularization
7. Severe pulmonary disease
8. Contralateral carotid occlusion
9. Previous radiation to head/neck
10. Previous CEA
11. Age >80 y
12. Surgically inaccessible lesions

Acronym	Sponsor	Stent	Protection device	Result; 30-day death/ stroke/MI rate
BEACH	Boston Scientific	WallStent	Ex filter	5.4%
CABERNET	Boston Scientific/ Endotex	Nex Stent	EPI Filter	3.9%
ARCHER	Guidant	AccuLink	AccuNet	7.8%
MAVErIC	Medtronic	Exponent	PercuSurge	4%
PASCAL	Medtronic	Exponent	Any approved	8%
SECuRITY	Abott	Xact	Emboshield	7.2%

Table 3. Carotid stent industry-supported high-risk registries

10. Comparisons of stenting versus endarterectomy

Markus et al studied the effect of carotid PTA compared to CEA on cerebral hemodynamics of symptomatic stenoses as reflected by CO_2 reactivity. After PTA there was a significant improvement in ipsilateral hypercapnic reactivity. There was a similar improvement in ipsilateral hypercapnic reactivity after CEA.[10]

Golledge et al performed a systematic comparison of the 30-day outcome of angioplasty with or without stenting and CEA for symptomatic carotid disease reported in single-center studies, published between 1990 and 1999. All the results were in favor of CEA. Mortality within 30 days of angioplasty was 0.8% compared with 1.2% after CEA (P=0.6). The stroke rate was 7.1% for angioplasty and 3.3% for CEA (P<0.001).[11]

11. The UK Leicester halted trial

The most outstanding negative trial of carotid angioplasty was form Leicester Royal Infirmary. The study consisted of 23 patients with focal carotid territory symptoms and severe ICA stenosis (>70%) who were randomized to either CEA or CAS. However, only 17 had received their allocated treatment before trial suspension. All 10 CEA operations proceeded without complication, but 5 of the 7 (71.4%) patients who underwent CAS had a stroke, 3 of which were disabling at 30 days. The Data Monitoring Committee invoked the stopping rule and the trial was suspended. The investigators and the Ethics Committee subsequently decided that the trial should not be restarted even in an amended format because of problems with informed consent.[12, 13]

The CAVATAS (Carotid and Vertebral Artery Transluminal Angioplasty Study), was the first randomized trial of CEA versus CAS. 504 patients were randomized from 22 centers in between 1992 and 1997. The majority of patients had recently symptomatic lesions. Only 26% of the angioplasty patients received a stent. The rates of major outcome events within 30 days of first treatment did not differ significantly between endovascular treatment and surgery (6.4% vs. 5.9%, respectively, for disabling stroke or death; 10.0% vs. 9.9% for any stroke lasting more than 7 days, or death). (Figure 21) At 1 year after treatment, restenosis was more usual after endovascular treatment (14%vs. 4%, p<0.001). Complications of cranial nerve injury and myocardial ischemia were only reported in the surgical group. The trial described rates of death and disabling stroke after 3 years of 14.3% in the endovascular group and 14.2% in the surgical group.[14]

Crawley et al compared cerebral hemodynamics and microembolization during CAS versus CEA using TCD. The period during which the ICA was occluded by PTA balloon or by clamp during CEA was timed. Ischemic time was defined as the period during which mean MCA velocity fell to a third or less of baseline. CEA resulted in significantly longer occlusion time and ischemic time than PTA. There were significantly more microembolic signals during PTA than during CEA. There was no correlation between any of the parameters measured and periprocedural stroke.[15]

The SAPPHIRE trial (Stenting and Angioplasty with Protection in Patients at High Risk for Endarterectomy) randomized patients with co-morbid conditions that represented exclusion criteria from the previous major randomized trials of CEA. The rationale was that patients with these co-morbid conditions appear to represent the majority of patients undergoing CEA, and concerns have been raised about the generalizability of the CEA trial results in view of the exclusion of those patients in major CEA trials. SAPPHIRE was designed to test "non-inferiority" of CAS versus CEA in the high-risk population with >50% symptomatic or >80% asymptomatic stenosis.[16, 17]

All carotid stenting procedures were done with the Angioguard protection device. The trial was conducted at 29 US centers which all had mean complication rate less than 3% for CEA and 4% for CAS. All patients were seen by a team made up of a neurologist, a surgeon, and an interventionist. If the surgeon felt that he or she could not operate, and the interventionist felt that intervention was possible, the patient was entered into a stent registry. Conversely, if the interventionist did not feel that he or she could perform the intervention, and the surgeon felt that surgery was possible, the patient was entered into a surgical registry. 723 patients were enrolled initially. Consensus was achieved in 307 patients who were randomized to either stenting (n = 156) or CEA (n = 151). The stent registry consisted of 409 patients, and the surgical registry included seven. Individual endpoints of death, stroke, and MI at 30 days were lower in patients randomized to stenting. The combined endpoint of death/stroke/MI was statistically significantly lower in patients randomized to stenting vs. CEA. The death, stroke or myocardial infarction rate was 11.9% in the CAS group and 19.9 % in the CEA group after 1-year. The SAPPHIRE results indicated that CAS has become a promising alternative to CEA, at least "not inferior".

12. SAPPHIRE long-term results

At 3 years, data were available for 260 patients (77.8%), including 85.6% of patients in the stenting group and 70.1% of those in the endarterectomy group. There was no significant difference could be shown in long-term outcomes between patients who underwent carotid artery stenting with an emboli-protection device and those who underwent endarterectomy The prespecified major secondary end point occurred in 41 patients in the stenting group (cumulative incidence, 24.6%; Kaplan–Meier estimate, 26.2%) and 45 patients in the endarterectomy group (cumulative incidence, 26.9%; Kaplan–Meier estimate, 30.3%) (absolute difference in cumulative incidence for the stenting group, −2.3%; 95% confidence interval, −11.8 to 7.0). There were 15 strokes in each of the two groups, of which 11 in the stenting group and 9 in the endarterectomy group were ipsilateral.[18]

The SAPPHIRE data are specific to patients who are at high surgical risk, and they provide no insight into outcomes of treatment of a carotid artery stenosis in patients at low-to-moderate risk. On the basis of the similar long-term outcomes among high-risk patients in the two treatment groups, it may be tempting to infer that endarterectomy is preferable for lower-risk patients.

13. The CARESS trial

Carotid REvascularization with Stenting Systems was a prospective, multicenter non-randomized industry-sponsored trial compared standard CEA to carotid stenting in patients with symptomatic (≥50%) and asymptomatic (≥75%) carotid stenosis. There was no significant difference in the 30-day combined all-cause mortality and stroke rate between CEA (2%) and CAS (2%). There was no significant difference in the secondary endpoint of combined 30-day all-cause mortality, stroke, and myocardial infarction between CEA and CAS.[19]

Following the publication of the SAPPHIRE and the CARESS trials, carotid artery stenting rocketed. There was a general felling that carotid artery stenting will prevail and become the preferred choice for carotid revascularization. However, the following randomized trials did not come in favor of carotid stenting.

14. SPACE

Stent-protected angioplasty versus carotid endarterectomy in symptomatic patients included 1183 patients with symptomatic carotid-artery stenosis. Patients were randomly assigned within 180 days of transient ischemic attack or moderate stroke (modified Rankin scale score of < or =3) to carotid-artery stenting (n=605) or carotid endarterectomy (n=595). The primary endpoint of this hospital-based study was ipsilateral ischemic stroke or death from time of randomization to 30 days after the procedure. The non-inferiority margin was defined as less than 2.5% on the basis of an expected event rate of 5%. Analyses were on an intention-to-treat basis. The rate of death or ipsilateral ischemic stroke from randomization to 30 days after the procedure was 6.84% with carotid-artery stenting and 6.34% with carotid endarterectomy (absolute difference 0.51%, 90% CI -1.89% to 2.91%). The one-sided p value for non-inferiority is 0.09. SPACE failed to prove non-inferiority of carotid-artery stenting compared with carotid endarterectomy for the periprocedural complication rate.[20]

Lon term data showed that in both the intention-to-treat and per-protocol analyses the Kaplan-Meier estimates of ipsilateral ischemic strokes up to 2 years after the procedure and any periprocedural stroke or death do not differ between the carotid artery stenting and the carotid endarterectomy groups (intention to treat 9 5% vs. 8 8%; hazard ratio (HR) 1 10, 95%CI 0 75 to 1 61; log-rank p=0 62; per protocol 9 4% vs. 7 8%; HR 1 23, 95%CI 0 82 to 1 83; log-rank p=0 31). In both the intention-to-treat and per-protocol populations, recurrent stenosis of 70% or more is significantly more frequent in the carotid artery stenting group compared with the carotid endarterectomy group, with a life-table estimate of 10 7% versus 4 6% (p=0 0009) and 11 1% versus 4 6% (p=0 0007), respectively.[21]

15. EVA-3S

262 patients were randomly assigned to endarterectomy and 265 to stenting. The cumulative probability of periprocedural stroke or death and non-procedural ipsilateral stroke after 4

years of follow-up was higher with stenting than with endarterectomy (11 1% vs. 6 2%, hazard ratio [HR] 1 97, 95% CI 1 06–3 67; p=0 03). The HR for periprocedural disabling stroke or death and non-procedural fatal or disabling ipsilateral stroke was 2 00 (0 75–5 33; p=0 17). A hazard function analysis showed the 4-year differences in the cumulative probabilities of outcomes between stenting and endarterectomy were largely accounted for by the higher periprocedural (within 30 days of the procedure) risk of stenting compared with endarterectomy. After the periprocedural period, the risk of ipsilateral stroke was low and similar in both treatment groups. For any stroke or periprocedural death, the HR was 1 77 (1 03–3 02; p=0 04). For any stroke or death, the HR was 1 39 (0 96–2 00; p=0 08). The results of this study suggest that carotid stenting is as effective as carotid endarterectomy for middle-term prevention of ipsilateral stroke, but the safety of carotid stenting needs to be improved before it can be used as an alternative to carotid endarterectomy in patients with symptomatic carotid stenosis.[22]

In the same study, the rate of carotid restenosis of ≥50% or occlusion was significantly higher after CAS (12.5%) than after CEA (5.0%; time ratio, 0.16; 95% CI, 0.03–0.76; *P*=0.02). The rates of severe restenosis of ≥70% or occlusion were low and did not differ significantly between the 2 groups (3-year rates are 3.3% in the CAS group and 2.8% in the CEA group). Age at baseline was the only vascular risk factor significantly associated with carotid restenosis. Our study could not detect any effect of carotid restenosis on ipsilateral stroke.[23]

It was notable that the risk of ipsilateral stroke or death increased significantly with age in the CAS group (p=0 001) but not in the CEA group (p=0 534). Classification and regression tree analysis showed that the age that gave the greatest separation between high-risk and low-risk populations who had CAS was 68 years: the rate of primary outcome events was 2 7% (8/293) in patients who were 68 years old or younger and 10 8% (34/314) in older patients.[24]

In the first 120 days after randomization (ITT analysis), the primary outcome event occurred in 153/1725 patients in the CAS group (8.9%) compared with 99/1708 patients in the CEA group (5.8%, risk ratio [RR] 1.53, 95% confidence interval [CI] 1.20–1.95, p = 0.0006; absolute risk difference 3.2, 95% CI 1.4–4.9). Age was the only subgroup variable which significantly modified the treatment effect: in patients <70 years old (the median age), the 120-day stroke or death risk was 5.8% in CAS and 5.7% in CEA (RR 1.00, 0.68–1.47); in patients 70 years or older, there was an estimated two-fold increase in risk with CAS over CEA (12.0% vs. 5.9%, RR 2.04, 1.48–2.82, interaction p = 0.0053).[25]

Endarterectomy was safer in the short-term than stenting, because of an increased risk of stroke associated with stenting in patients over the age of 70 years. Stenting should be avoided in older patients, but may be as safe as endarterectomy in younger patients. Determination of the efficacy and ultimate balance between the two procedures requires further data on long-term stroke recurrence.[25]

16. ICSS study

The incidence of stroke, death, or procedural myocardial infarction was 8.5% in the stenting group compared with 5.2% in the endarterectomy group (72 vs. 44 events; HR 1.69, 1.16-2.45, p=0.006), Risks of any stroke (65 vs. 35 events; HR 1.92, 1.27-2.89) and all-cause death (19 vs. seven events; HR 2.76, 1.16-6.56) were higher in the stenting group than in the endarterectomy group. Three procedural myocardial infarctions were recorded in the stenting group, all of which were fatal, compared with four, all non-fatal, in the endarterectomy group.[26]

At 1 month, there were changes on fluid-attenuated inversion recovery sequences in 28 (33%) of 86 patients in the stenting group and six (8%) of 75 in the endarterectomy group (adjusted OR 5 93, 95% CI 2 25–15 62; p=0 0003). In patients treated at a center with a policy of using cerebral protection devices, 37 (73%) of 51 in the stenting group and eight (17%) of 46 in the endarterectomy group had at least one new DWI lesion on post-treatment scans (adjusted OR 12 20, 95% CI 4 53–32 84), whereas in those treated at a center with a policy of unprotected stenting, 25 (34%) of 73 patients in the stenting group and ten (16%) of 61 in the endarterectomy group had new lesions on DWI (adjusted OR 2 70, 1 16–6 24; interaction p=0 019).[27]

These discordant results may be explained by the fact that the EVA-3S and SPACE studies differ from ours in numerous ways, including in the selection criteria (e.g., the EVA-3S and SPACE trials included neither patients with a high surgical risk nor asymptomatic patients), the rate of use of specific emboli-protection devices (in 92% of cases in the EVA-3S trial and 27% in the SPACE trial), and the experience level of the physician who placed the stent (in the EVA-3S trial, stents could be placed by physicians who had performed as few as five previous carotid-stent procedures or, if working under the direction of a tutor, no previous procedures).[18]

The results of the previous studies were a major setback for stenting. They created a general belief among practicing physicians and neurologists that carotid artery stenting has only a limited role in the prevention of stroke. This set the stage ready for a more comprehensive larger trial trying to reach the truth.

17. CREST trial

The CREST (Carotid Revascularization Endarterectomy vs. Stent Trial) was a multicenter trial supported by the National institute of health. The study includes symptomatic (>50% stenosis) and asymptomatic (>70% stenosis) patients. The CREST was probably the largest study on carotid revascularization and had the best design. Centers were required to have a team consisting of a neurologist, an interventionist, a surgeon, and a research coordinator. Patients could not be randomly assigned to a treatment group until the operators performing carotid artery stenting and carotid endarterectomy had been certified. Certification was achieved by 477 surgeons, whose clinical results were audited by means of a validated selection process documenting that they performed more than 12 procedures per year and that the rates of complications and death were less than 3% among asymptomatic patients and less than 5% among symptomatic patients. The 224 interventionists were certified after satisfactory evaluation of their endovascular experience, carotid-stenting results, participation in hands-on training, and participation in a lead-in phase of training.[28]

There was no differential treatment effect with regard to the primary end point according to symptomatic status (P = 0.84) or sex (P = 0.34). The 4-year rate of stroke or death was 6.4% with stenting and 4.7% with endarterectomy (hazard ratio, 1.50; P = 0.03); the rates among symptomatic patients were 8.0% and 6.4% (hazard ratio, 1.37; P = 0.14), and the rates among asymptomatic patients were 4.5% and 2.7% (hazard ratio, 1.86; P = 0.07), respectively. Periprocedural rates of individual components of the end points differed between the stenting group and the endarterectomy group: for death (0.7% vs. 0.3%, P = 0.18), for stroke (4.1% vs. 2.3%, P = 0.01), and for myocardial infarction (1.1% vs. 2.3%, P = 0.03). After this period, the incidences of ipsilateral stroke with stenting and with endarterectomy were similarly low (2.0% and 2.4%, respectively; P = 0.85).[28]

The results of the CREST were "satisfying" for both surgeons and interventionists. Surgeons were glad to prove that CEA resulted in lower stroke rates in the short term and the long term. Interventionists were reassured that the primary end-point was similar in the two methods.

Restenosis and occlusion were infrequent and rates were similar up to 2 years after carotid endarterectomy and carotid artery stenting. Subsets of patients could benefit from early and frequent monitoring after revascularization.[29]

CAS was associated with better health-related quality of life HRQOL during the early recovery period as compared with CEA-particularly with regard to physical limitations and pain-but these differences diminish over time and are not evident after 1 year. Although CAS and CEA are associated with similar overall quality of life at 1 year, event-specific analyses confirm that stroke has a greater and more sustained impact on HRQOL than MI.[30]

The MI rates were slightly lower after CAS (1.3% vs. 2.6%; P =.24). In performing CAS, vascular surgeons had outcomes for the periprocedural primary end point comparable to the outcomes of all interventionists (HR, 0.99; 95% CI, 0.50-2.00) after adjusting for age, sex, and symptomatic status. Vascular surgeons also had similar results after CEA for the periprocedural primary end point compared with other surgeons (HR, 0.73; 95% CI, 0.42-1.27).[31]

18. Carotid endarterectomy and stenting in specific situations

18.1. Restenosis after carotid stenting

The restenosis rate after carotid stenting is remarkably low at 2.3-10% compared to other endovascular interventions. Although self-expanding carotid stents generate considerable neointimal hyperplasia, the process is balanced by marked late stent enlargement. Small stent dimensions immediately post-procedure were associated with a higher risk of restenosis.[32] In the 2003 global carotid stent registry, restenosis rates have been 2.7%, 2.6%, and 2.4% at 1, 2, and 3 years, respectively.[9] A retrospective, single-center review was conducted of 399 carotid stent procedures in 363 patients over 9 years, with a mean follow-up of 24 months (range 6-99 months). Overall, restenosis occurred in 15 patients (3.8%). However, the restenosis occurred in 7 of 35 (20%) patients who had previous neck radiation, 6 of 57 (10.5%) patients who had previous CEA, and 2 of 9 (22%) patients who previously had both CEA and neck

http://dx.doi.org/10.5772/57153

radiation. The only analyzed variables that were significantly associated with an increased risk of restenosis were previous CEA (OR 4.28, P = 0.008) or XRT (OR 11.3, P <or=<or= 0.0001).[33] In another study, among 215 CAS procedures that had clinical and serial carotid duplex ultrasound investigations, restenosis was detected in 6.1% of patients. Contralateral carotid occlusion (OR 10.11, 95% CI 2.06-49.63, p = 0.004), carotid endarterectomy (CEA) restenosis (OR 8.87, 95% CI 1.68-46.84, p = 0.010) and postprocedural carotid duplex ultrasound with a PSV >/=120 cm/s (OR 6.33, 95% CI 1.27-31.44, p = 0.024) were independent predictors of stent restenosis.[34] Most restenoses occur within 6 to 12 months after the intervention. Usually they are located either in the mid or at the distal end of the stent. Restenoses are often overestimated by ultrasound compared to angiography. Most of restenoses can be treated by balloon angioplasty. Drug-eluting balloons can be a promising modality[35] and only rarely, stent removal and eversion endarterectomy will be required.[36]

18.2. Restenosis after carotid endarterectomy

The incidence ranges from 1.2% to 23.9% depending on the operative technique. The highest rates of restenosis, 21.4%, after CEA came with direct suture and the lowest rate 3.9% were after patch angioplasty only Long-term risk of recurrence is about 1% per year. The risk is highest in the first few years after CEA and is very low later.[37]. Most of restenoses are asymptomatic and only 1.2-3.6% require re-intervention.[38]

The type of operative technique for reoperations depends on the cause of the recurrent disease. Myointimal hyperplasia has a smooth luminal surface and appears to be associated with a low potential for embolization therefore simple patching may be all that is necessary. By contrast, the soft nature of the plaque in recurrent atherosclerosis, which appears later, has a greater potential for embolization therefore repeat CEA with carotid patch angioplasty is preferable. AbuRahma et al showed the 30-day perioperative stroke and transient ischemic attack rates for reoperation and primary CEA were 4.8% versus 0.8% (P=0.015) and 4% versus 1.1%, respectively. There was an increase in the number of transient cranial nerve injuries in the reoperation group compared with the primary CEA group (15.3% versus 4.9%).[39]

CAS for restenosis after CEA has a complication rate lower than primary CAS. The time interval between CEA and CAS did not influence micro embolic load.[40] Statistical analysis demonstrated that post-CEA restenosis was the most important predictive factor for the development of in-stent restenosis after CAS. This review of our 10-year experience confirms that patients who develop restenosis after CEA are also prone to developing in-stent restenosis after CAS.[41]

18.3. Carotid stenosis in patients requiring bypass cardiac surgery

Patients who have concomitant severe carotid and coronary artery disease pose a serious dilemma. Stroke remains a major non-cardiac complication after CABG and myocardial infarction is the major non-neurological cause of early and late morbidity after CEA. The risk of stroke after CABG ranges from 0.7-5.2%[42]

Hemodynamically significant carotid stenoses are associated with 30% of early post-CABG strokes. The perioperative stroke risk is <2% when carotid stenoses are <50%, 10% when stenoses are 50% to 80%, 11% to 18.8% in patients with stenoses >80%. The risk shoots to 20% with untreated, bilateral, high-grade stenoses or an occluded carotid artery and contralateral high-grade stenosis.[43]

The majority of strokes happen after the first 24 hours post CABG. This suggests that majority of strokes cannot be simply be ascribed to an adverse intra-operative event (low flow, hypotension and carotid embolism). The overall case fatality following post-CABG stroke as 23.1%. [43]In real life, it is not possible to state how often carotid stenosis of any degree of severity contributes to the incidence of ischemic stroke after CABG. Naylor et al concluded that primary carotid thromboembolic disease alone was not responsible for up to 59% of post CABG strokes. A significant proportion of post-operative strokes was in the vertebro-basilar territory or located contralateral to the severely stenosed carotid or ipsilateral to an insignificant stenosis. Aortic arch atherosclerosis embolization may be an important cause of stroke in the majority of cases.[43]

19. Approaches to treatment

1. Staged approach: Advocates of a staged procedure perform CEA several days prior to CABG or several weeks following cardiac surgery. The rationale of the staged procedure is to decrease the risk of stroke in the cardiac procedure and eliminate the need for longer and more stressful combined procedure. Increased cardiac morbidity and mortality resulting from CEA may offset potential benefits of this approach.[42]

In those with a history of TIA or stroke who have a significant carotid artery stenosis (50% to 99% in men or 70% to 99% in women), the likelihood of a post-CABG stroke is high; as a result, they are likely to benefit from carotid revascularization. Conversely, CABG alone can be performed safely in patients with asymptomatic unilateral carotid stenoses, because a carotid revascularization procedure offers no discernible reduction in the incidence of stroke or death in these individuals. Men with asymptomatic bilateral severe carotid stenoses (50% to 99%) or a unilateral severe stenosis in conjunction with a contralateral carotid artery occlusion may be considered for carotid revascularization in conjunction with CABG. Little evidence exists to suggest that women with asymptomatic carotid artery disease benefit from carotid revascularization in conjunction with CABG. Whether the carotid and coronary revascularization procedures are performed simultaneously or in a staged, sequential fashion is usually dictated by the presence or absence of certain clinical variables. In general, synchronous combined procedures are performed only in those with both cerebrovascular symptoms and ACS.[44]

2. Combined approach: performing CEA and CABG in the same setting: If the combined approach can be done safely, a second surgical procedure and hospital stay may be eliminated, with significant cost reduction. Long-term stroke free survival may also be significantly improved.[42] The problem with this approach is that the stroke rate is exceedingly high.

http://dx.doi.org/10.5772/57153

3. Ignoring the carotid disease initially and addressing it weeks to months later after the CABG procedure may be another approach. This idea is supported by a retrospective review of 94 patients with asymptomatic high-grade carotid stenosis undergoing CABG. There was one perioperative stroke and no deaths in this group of patients. These data combined with findings of Naylor et al that prophylactic CEA could barely prevent < 40% of post-CABG strokes [43] would support this approach in asymptomatic carotid stenoses. In the absence of clear guidelines, the decision is better individualized dealing with the more symptomatic vascular bed first. The simultaneous performance of CABG and CEA carries a high risk but is warranted in patients with recent symptoms of both severe coronary disease (unstable angina) and severe carotid stenosis.

Carotid stenting can be an alternative in endarterectomy in this subset of patients.[45, 46] A recent Comparison of Early and Late Outcomes with Three Approaches to Carotid Revascularization and Open Heart Surgery showed that Staged CAS-OHS and combined CEA-OHS are associated with similar risk of death, stroke or MI in the short term, with both being better than staged CEA-OHS. However, the outcomes are significantly in favor of staged CAS-OHS after the first year.[47]

20. CEA in the presence of contralateral occlusion

Patients with contralateral carotid occlusion have higher surgical risk for CEA due to multiple reasons; reduced collateral circulation during carotid clamping, cerebral hemorrhage secondary to hyperperfusion syndrome, and the overall advanced status of the vascular disease. Surgical mortality was extremely high in patients with a contralateral carotid occlusion and only 34% of the surgically treated patients were alive at 66 months in contrast to 63% of medically treated patients.(88) Results from the NASCET study demonstrated that medically treated patients with a contralateral occluded carotid were more than twice as likely to have a stroke compared to patients with a patent contralateral artery. However, when compared with medically treated patients, the overall risk of stroke contralateral to an occluded carotid artery was significantly reduced in the surgical patients. The risk of stroke in medically treated patients was 69% at 2 years versus 22% in patients treated surgically. (2) Thus, CEA with contralateral occlusion is a risky procedure but its risk may be justified considering the natural history of the disease.

21. CEA vs. CAS in the real world

21.1. The limitations of published trials comparing CEA and CAS

The influence of the industry is strong, where all the industry-sponsored registries had lower rates of complications compared to randomized trials. The levels of expertise of operators vary significantly among trials as well as the obligatory use of protection devices. The percentage of symptomatic and asymptomatic patients also varies rendering interpretation of results and generalizing them to the general practice an intriguing issue. There also seems a publication bias in reporting the trial results. Vascular surgery periodicals tend to note better results with CEA while cardiology journals tend to report superiority or non-inferiority of CAS.

22. Ongoing trials and future directions

The modern medical treatment and optimized medical therapy (OMT) were not available at the time of some landmark trials like NASCET and ECST. There is a growing enthusiasm to test if OMT renders intervention unnecessary or only restricted to high risk patients. A new set of trials called "Trials 2" are now developing and ongoing:

- **European Carotid Surgery Trial-2 (ECST-2):** The trial will include patients with symptomatic or asymptomatic moderate or severe carotid stenosis at low or intermediate risk of future stroke. The trial compares the risks and benefits of treatment by modern optimized medical management alone versus the addition of immediate carotid surgery (or stenting) to optimize medical management.
- **Asymptomatic Carotid Surgery Trial-2 (ACST-2):** To compare carotid endarterectomy with carotid artery stenting in the prevention of stroke in patients with asymptomatic carotid stenosis.
- **Stent-protected angioplasty in asymptomatic carotid artery stenosis vs. endarterectomy Trial-2 (SPACE-2):** A three-arm randomized-controlled clinical trial. The trial based on German speaking countries. The trial initially randomized patients with asymptomatic stenosis between carotid artery stenting vs. Carotid endarterectomy and recently the trial modified to include third arm with optimized medical therapy (OMT) only.
- **Carotid Revascularization Endarterectomy versus Stenting Trial-2(CREST-2):** North American trial testing revascularization vs. contemporary medical management alone.

23. Conclusion

What we can infer from these trials that CEA has a lower stroke rate than CAS but CAS has a lower MI rate than CEA. If mortality, stroke and MI are mingled together as a single end-point, then both strategies are equivalent on the long-term. Advancing age is strongly against selecting CAS as the initial choice of revascularization. The results of either technique are critically dependent on the skills of the performing physician. Restenosis after CAS may be slightly more than restenosis after CEA but the severe, clinically significant restenosis is uncommon. In patients with concomitant coronary and carotid disease, stenting may have an advantage over CEA.

There remains a need for more trials assessing the future roles of medical management, carotid stenting, and carotid endarterectomy. Future trials should be designed with the assumption that some patients will be best managed medically, some with medical therapy plus stenting, and some with medical therapy plus endarterectomy. These treatments are complementary and not competing. Varying treatment algorithms including more or less liberal use of each modality can be designed, patients randomly assigned to one of the algorithms, and their results compared.[48]

Author details

Hussien Heshmat Kassem[1*], Foad Abd-Allah[2] and Mohammad Wasay[3]

*Address all correspondence to: hheshmat@kasralainy.edu.eg

1 Department of Cardiovascular Medicine, Faculty of Medicine, Cairo University, Egypt

2 Department of Neurology, Faculty of Medicine, Cairo University, Egypt

3 Department of Neurology, Aga Khan University, Pakistan

References

[1] Robertson, J.T., Carotid Endarterectomy: A Saga of Clinical Science, Personalities, and Evolving Technology: The Willis Lecture. Stroke, 1998. 29(11): p. 2435-2441.

[2] Blaisdell, W.F., et al., Joint study of extracranial arterial occlusion. IV. A review of surgical considerations. JAMA, 1969. 209(12): p. 1889-95.

[3] Remarks, W.C., carotid endarterectomy, in Cerebrovascular Diseases, Plum F and P. W., Editors. 1985, Raven Press Publishers: New York, NY.

[4] Barnett, H.J.M., M. Eliasziw, and H.E. Meldrum, Prevention of ischaemic stroke. BMJ, 1999. 318: p. 1539-43.

[5] Tu, J.V., et al., The Fall and Rise of Carotid Endarterectomy in the United States and Canada. New England Journal of Medicine, 1998. 339(20): p. 1441-1447.

[6] Beneficial effect of carotid endarterectomy in symptomatic patients with high-grade carotid stenosis. North American Symptomatic Carotid Endarterectomy Trial Collaborators. N Engl J Med, 1991. 325(7): p. 445-53.

[7] Theron, J., My history of carotid angioplasty and stenting. J Invasive Cardiol, 2008. 20(4): p. E102-8.

[8] Phatouros, C.C., et al., Carotid Artery Stent Placement for Atherosclerotic Disease: Rationale, Technique, and Current Status1. Radiology, 2000. 217(1): p. 26-41.

[9] Wholey, M.H., N. Al-Mubarek, and M.H. Wholey, Updated review of the global carotid artery stent registry. Catheter Cardiovasc Interv, 2003. 60(2): p. 259-66.

[10] Markus, H.S., et al., Improvement in cerebral hemodynamics after carotid angioplasty. Stroke, 1996. 27(4): p. 612-6.

[11] Golledge, J., et al., Systematic comparison of the early outcome of angioplasty and endarterectomy for symptomatic carotid artery disease. Stroke, 2000. 31(6): p. 1439-43.

[12] Naylor, A.R., Randomized study of carotid angioplasty and stenting versus carotid endarterectomy: a stopped trial. Journal of Vascular Surgery, 1998. 28(2): p. 326-334.

[13] Hobson, R.W., 2nd, Regarding "Randomized study of carotid angioplasty and stenting versus carotid endarterectomy: a stopped trial". J Vasc Surg, 2000. 31(3): p. 622-4.

[14] Endovascular versus surgical treatment in patients with carotid stenosis in the Carotid and Vertebral Artery Transluminal Angioplasty Study (CAVATAS): a randomised trial. Lancet, 2001. 357(9270): p. 1729-37.

[15] Crawley, F., et al., Comparison of hemodynamic cerebral ischemia and microembolic signals detected during carotid endarterectomy and carotid angioplasty. Stroke, 1997. 28(12): p. 2460-4.

[16] Mozes, G., et al., Carotid endarterectomy in sapphire-eligible high-risk patients: implications for selecting patients for carotid angioplasty and stenting. Journal of Vascular Surgery, 2004. 39(5): p. 958-965.

[17] Yadav, J.S., et al., Protected Carotid-Artery Stenting versus Endarterectomy in High-Risk Patients. New England Journal of Medicine, 2004. 351(15): p. 1493-1501.

[18] Gurm, H.S., et al., Long-Term Results of Carotid Stenting versus Endarterectomy in High-Risk Patients. New England Journal of Medicine, 2008. 358(15): p. 1572-1579.

[19] Carotid Revascularization Using Endarterectomy or Stenting Systems (CaRESS) phase I clinical trial: 1-year results. Journal of Vascular Surgery, 2005. 42(2): p. 213-219.

[20] null, et al., 30 day results from the SPACE trial of stent-protected angioplasty versus carotid endarterectomy in symptomatic patients: a randomised non-inferiority trial. Lancet, 2006. 368(9543): p. 1239-1247.

[21] Eckstein, H.-H., et al., Results of the Stent-Protected Angioplasty versus Carotid Endarterectomy (SPACE) study to treat symptomatic stenoses at 2 years: a multinational, prospective, randomised trial. The Lancet Neurology, 2008. 7(10): p. 893-902.

[22] Mas, J.-L., et al., Endarterectomy Versus Angioplasty in Patients with Symptomatic Severe Carotid Stenosis (EVA-3S) trial: results up to 4 years from a randomised, multicentre trial. The Lancet Neurology, 2008. 7(10): p. 885-892.

[23] Arquizan, C., et al., Restenosis Is More Frequent After Carotid Stenting Than After Endarterectomy: The EVA-3S Study. Stroke, 2011. 42(4): p. 1015-1020.

[24] Stingele, R., et al., Clinical and angiographic risk factors for stroke and death within 30 days after carotid endarterectomy and stent-protected angioplasty: a subanalysis of the SPACE study. The Lancet Neurology, 2008. 7(3): p. 216-222.

[25] Bonati, L.H. and G. Fraedrich, Age Modifies the Relative Risk of Stenting versus Endarterectomy for Symptomatic Carotid Stenosis – A Pooled Analysis of EVA-3S, SPACE and ICSS. European Journal of Vascular and Endovascular Surgery, 2011. 41(2): p. 153-158.

[26] Ederle, J., et al., Carotid artery stenting compared with endarterectomy in patients with symptomatic carotid stenosis (International Carotid Stenting Study): an interim analysis of a randomised controlled trial. 2010.

[27] Bonati, L.H., et al., New ischaemic brain lesions on MRI after stenting or endarterectomy for symptomatic carotid stenosis: a substudy of the International Carotid Stenting Study (ICSS). The Lancet Neurology, 2010. 9(4): p. 353-362.

[28] Brott, T.G., et al., Stenting versus Endarterectomy for Treatment of Carotid-Artery Stenosis. New England Journal of Medicine, 2010. 363(1): p. 11-23.

[29] Lal, B.K., et al., Restenosis after carotid artery stenting and endarterectomy: a secondary analysis of CREST, a randomised controlled trial. Lancet Neurol, 2012. 11(9): p. 755-63.

[30] Cohen, D.J., et al., Health-related quality of life after carotid stenting versus carotid endarterectomy: results from CREST (Carotid Revascularization Endarterectomy Versus Stenting Trial). J Am Coll Cardiol, 2011. 58(15): p. 1557-65.

[31] Timaran, C.H., et al., Differential outcomes of carotid stenting and endarterectomy performed exclusively by vascular surgeons in the Carotid Revascularization Endarterectomy versus Stenting Trial (CREST). J Vasc Surg, 2013. 57(2): p. 303-8.

[32] Clark, D.J., et al., Mechanisms and predictors of carotid artery stent restenosis: a serial intravascular ultrasound study. J Am Coll Cardiol, 2006. 47(12): p. 2390-6.

[33] Younis, G.A., et al., Predictors of carotid stent restenosis. Catheter Cardiovasc Interv, 2007. 69(5): p. 673-82.

[34] Wasser, K., et al., Clinical impact and predictors of carotid artery in-stent restenosis. J Neurol, 2012. 259(9): p. 1896-902.

[35] Sangiorgi, G., E. Romagnoli, and G. Biondi-Zoccai, Commentary: drug-eluting balloons for carotid in-stent restenosis: can this technology deliver the goods? J Endovasc Ther, 2012. 19(6): p. 743-8.

[36] Jost, D., et al., Surgical treatment of carotid in-stent-restenosis: novel strategy and current management. Thorac Cardiovasc Surg, 2012. 60(8): p. 517-24.

[37] Raithel, D., Recurrent carotid disease: optimum technique for redo surgery. J Endovasc Surg, 1996. 3(1): p. 69-75.

[38] Frericks, H., et al., Carotid recurrent stenosis and risk of ipsilateral stroke: a systematic review of the literature. Stroke, 1998. 29(1): p. 244-50.

[39] AbuRahma, A.F., et al., Redo carotid endarterectomy versus primary carotid endarterectomy. Stroke, 2001. 32(12): p. 2787-92.

[40] Vos, J.A., et al., Carotid angioplasty and stenting: Treatment of postcarotid endarterectomy restenosis is at least as safe as primary stenosis treatment. Journal of Vascular Surgery, 2009. 50(4): p. 755-761.e1.

[41] Setacci, F., et al., Carotid restenosis after endarterectomy and stenting: a critical issue? Ann Vasc Surg, 2013. 27(7): p. 888-93.

[42] Safa, T.K., et al., Management of coexisting coronary artery and asymptomatic carotid artery disease: report of a series of patients treated with coronary bypass alone. Eur J Vasc Endovasc Surg, 1999. 17(3): p. 249-52.

[43] Naylor, A.R., et al., Reprinted article "Carotid artery disease and stroke during coronary artery bypass: a critical review of the literature". Eur J Vasc Endovasc Surg, 2011. 42 Suppl 1: p. S73-83.

[44] Eagle, K.A., et al., ACC/AHA 2004 guideline update for coronary artery bypass graft surgery: a report of the American College of Cardiology/American Heart Association Task Force on Practice Guidelines (Committee to Update the 1999 Guidelines for Coronary Artery Bypass Graft Surgery). Circulation, 2004. 110(14): p. e340-437.

[45] Chiariello, L., et al., Simultaneous hybrid revascularization by carotid stenting and coronary artery bypass grafting. Ann Thorac Surg, 2006. 81(5): p. 1883-5.

[46] Versaci, F., et al., Simultaneous hybrid revascularization by carotid stenting and coronary artery bypass grafting: the SHARP study. JACC Cardiovasc Interv, 2009. 2(5): p. 393-401.

[47] Shishehbor, M.H., et al., A Direct Comparison of Early and Late Outcomes with Three Approaches to Carotid Revascularization and Open Heart Surgery. J Am Coll Cardiol, 2013.

[48] Mackey, W.C., Clinical studies of carotid artery stenting: Why don't they tell us what we need to know? Journal of vascular surgery : official publication, the Society for Vascular Surgery [and] International Society for Cardiovascular Surgery, North American Chapter, 2008. 47(2): p. 470-475.

Chapter 6

Oxidised Low Density Lipoprotein (LDL) Modification with Statin Therapy is Associated with Reduction in Carotid Stenosis

Elias Skopelitis, Dimitrios Levisianou,
Helen Lydataki and Sofoklis Kougialis

Additional information is available at the end of the chapter

http://dx.doi.org/10.5772/57188

1. Introduction

1.1. Carotid stenosis and atheromatous process

Carotid artery stenosis due to atherosclerosis is a major complication of hyperlipidemia, diabetes mellitus and hypertension. Moreover, the extent of carotid intima media thickness is a measure of atheromatosis and therefore of cardiovascular disease (CVD).

The effect of cholesterol in the process of atheromatosis is now well established. High levels of total cholesterol, as well as of low-density lipoprotein (LDL), very low-density lipoprotein (VLDL), intermediate-density lipoprotein (IDL), lipoprotein a (Lp-α), and triglycerides, coupled with decreased levels of high-density lipoprotein (HDL) are responsible for the creation of atheromatous plaques [1-3]. Of the above factors, LDL cholesterol, and especially the oxidized LDL is considered as the most important contributor of atheromatosis [4].

The atheromatous process is completed in the following three stages:

1. In the first stage, LDL cholesterol enters the vessel wall, binds to gluxosaminoglucanes, which are part of the extracellulat matrix of the intima. This binding is facilitated by apolipoprotein B-100 (ApoB–100). The accumulation of LDL in the vessel wall contributes to the formation of fatty strikes. Following LDL adhesion in the vessel wall, it undergoes oxidation by free radicals produced locally, the molecule is altered and chemokines are produced by adjacent vessel wall cells, such as MCP – 1, together with growth factors, which are responsible for the accumulation of monocytes and macrophages. The latter,

cause further oxidation of LDL, resulting in negative charge, recognition by scavenger receptors on macrophage membrane and increased uptake of LDL inside the macrophages, as these receptors are not inhibited by increased intracellular concentration of cholesterol. The final result is an enormous accumulation of LDL in the macrophages, which are transformed to foamy cells. These cells represent the first step in the atheromatous process [5] (figure 1).

2. During the second stage, the atheromatous plaque is formed. Foamy cells produce growth factors and together with oxidized LDL result to the attraction of smooth muscle cells. The latter, are then differentiated to fibroblasts and start producing collagen. This collagen covers foamy cells, which either are destroyed or are forced to apoptosis. The final result is the formation of a pool of extracellular cholesterol trapped under a fibrous capsid (figure 2). The part which is close to the yet intact vessel wall is the active one of the plaque, where the foamy cells are produced. As the plaque extents to the inner layers of the vessel wall, the point of foamy cell formation becomes instable and may cause rapture of the plaque [5] (figure 3).

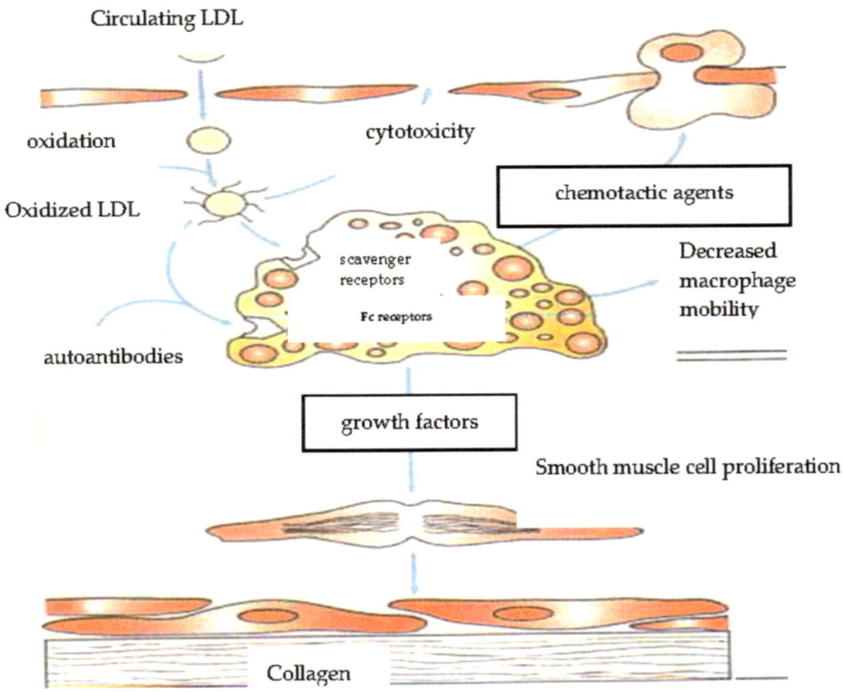

Figure 1. Atherogenesis. Fatty strikes are characterized by macrophages containing an excess of lipids (foamy cells). Foamy cells are derived by blood monocytes which are attracted to vessel intima and start phagocytosing lipoproteins, such as oxidized LDL. The convertion of fatty strike to atheroma depends on proliferation and differentiation of smooth muscle cells to fibroblasts. The latter produce collagen resulting in intima thickening. As the lesion extents further, foamy cells are destroyed releasing large amounts of cholesterol trapped in a fibrous capsid. The active site of atheroma is the point which is adjacent to normal endothelium, where foamy cells are formed (adopted from Durrington & Sinderman, 2002).

http://dx.doi.org/10.5772/57188

3. In the third stage, that of the complicated lesion, the rapture of the fibrous capsid of the atheromatous plaque leads to massive evacuation of the cholesterol reservoir. The artery may occult due to the accumulation of platelets and clotting, leading to infarction (figure 4). If not so, then the plaque will be further enlarged [5].

Avoiding the formation and the instability of the atheromatous plaque is top priority for patients at risk for cardiovascular events. Statins may contribute towards this direction [6,7]

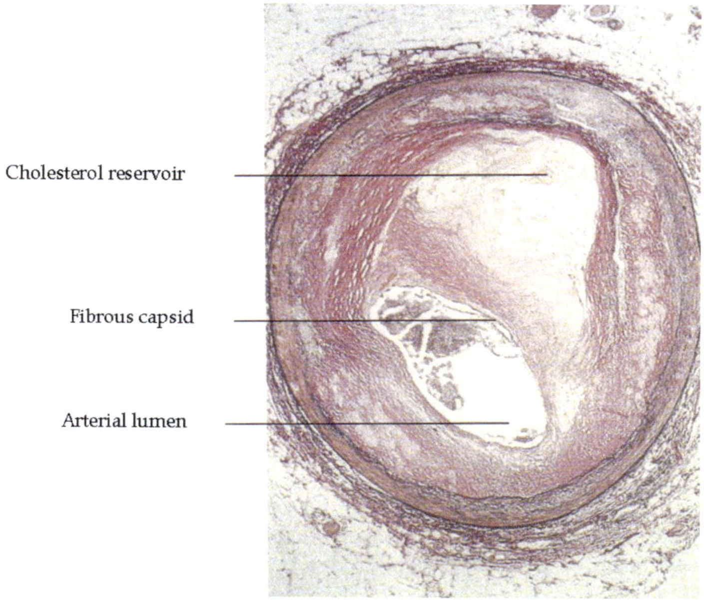

Figure 2. Advanced atheromatous plaque causing arterial lumen occlusion of 70% (adopted from Durrington & Sinderman, 2002).

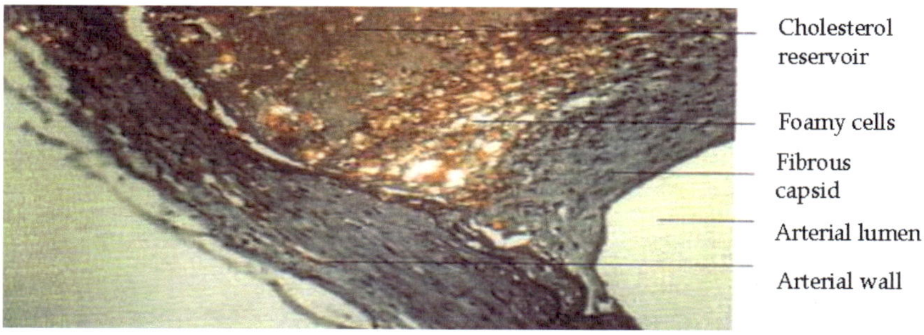

Figure 3. The point of the atheromatous plaque which active enlargement is occurring. Formation of new foamy cells, increased cholesterol uptake and increased instability of the plaque (adopted from Durrington & Sinderman, 2002).

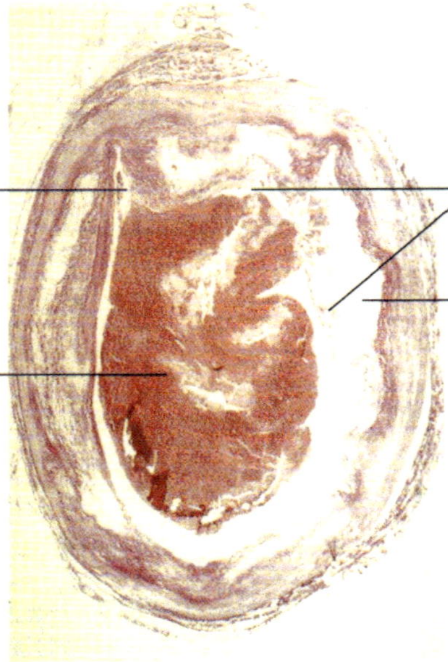

Figure 4. A raptured ahteromatous plaque, in which the cholesterol reservoir has evacuated itself under the fibrous capsid. A clot has in the endothelial surface at the site of rapture is completely occulting the lumen (adopted from Durrington & Sinderman, 2002).

1.2. Oxidised LDL

Oxidized low density lipoprotein LDL (oxLDL) cholesterol in humans is found mainly in two types:

a. conjugated form, attached to the atheromatous plaque and

b. circulating form found in serum.

Oxidized LDL is produced following oxidation of LDL by free radicals and other oxidadive factors, a procedure called oxidative stress. The circulating oxidized LDL is the measurable fraction of oxidized LDL in plasma. Oxidised LDL is a key element of the pathway leading to the formation of the atheromatous plaque and has been extensively studied both as a marker of atheromatosis and as a possible target of therapeutic intervention. Circulating oxLDL is considered a risk marker for atherosclerosis [8] and coronary heart disease (CHD) [8-10]. Increased oxLDL levels in circulation and the vessel wall are associated with endothelial dysfunction [11] in such patients [9,10,12], contributing to atheromatous plaque instability [9].

Oxidative modification of LDL leads to rapid focal accumulation in macrophages [13], which is the first step in atheromatous process. The increased retention time of LDL in the intima offers enhanced probability to be oxidized by free radicals produced by endothelium, smooth muscle cells or macrophages [14]. Oxidized LDL then acts chemotactic for monocytes and smooth muscle cells through binding to scavenger receptors [15], leading to the formation of foam cells. Oxidized LDL is also capable to elicit endothelial dysfunction by altering the secretory activity of endothelial cells [15], inhibiting the nitric oxide-mediated vasodilatation through reduction of the expression of endothelial nitric-oxide synthase (eNOS), inducing the expression of adhesion molecules on the endothelium thus mediating the adhesion of monocytes to intima [15], and inducing the expression of inflammatory cytokines [16]. Indeed, oxLDL is a potent inducer of inflammation [17], contributing to the chronic inflammatory process which results to atherosclerosis [18].

1.3. Statins

The 3-hydroxy-3-methylglutaryl-coenzyme A reductase inhibitors, or statins, reduce total cholesterol (TC), LDL cholesterol, apolipoprotein B (apoB), and, to a lesser degree, triglycerides and lipoprotein a (Lp-a). Statins also have pleiotropic effects [19], such as the modulation of inflammatory molecules and monocyte maturation and differentiation [19], the suppression of smooth muscle-cells migration and proliferation [19], the reduction of the monocyte adhesion to the endothelium [20], the restoration of the impaired endothelium-dependent vessel wall relaxation [21], and the modification of cell-mediated LDL oxidation [22,23]. All of the above mechanisms contribute to the reversion of atheromatosis. Undeniably, statins reduce the incidence of coronary events and are a cornerstone in the primary and secondary prevention of CHD [24]. Previous studies have detected some efficacy in reducing the circulating oxLDL levels, but whether this effect is due to the reduction of LDL or is an independent, pleiotropic phenomenon remains a matter of controversy [25,26]. Furthermore, little is known about the definite clinical benefit of such oxidative marker reduction.

The aim of the present study was to evaluate the efficacy of atorvastatin in reducing stenosis, to investigate the effect on oxLDL and to search for possible associations of oxLDL modification with changes of stenosis in patients managed conservatively and in pre-treated with percutaneous catheter interventional procedures patients with carotid atheromatosis. We hypothesise that atorvastatin therapy will confer remission of oxLDL levels in vivo and this will be associated with significant reduction of carotid artery stenosis.

2. Patients and methods

Between January 2005 and February 2008 a total of 100 patients were randomly selected from the lipid clinic and the carotid angioplasty clinic of a large tertiary hospital in Athens for inclusion in the study. Informed consent was obtained from each patient at recruitment according to our institutional policies. Eligible were patients with carotid artery stenosis from various causes and with a range of predisposing factors. Exclusion criteria included: acute cardiovascular disease, severe or unstable angina pectoris, clinically evident cardiac failure, severe arrhythmias, recent surgical procedures, inflammatory diseases, active liver disease or liver impairment, excessive alcohol consumption (>4 units/day) or history of alcohol abuse, known allergic reaction to statins, poorly controlled diabetes mellitus as defined by a haemoglobin A1c (HbA1c) level of >7mg/dl, uncontrolled hypertension indicated by systolic blood pressure (SBP) >140mmHg and/or diastolic pressure >85mmHg, history of deep vein thrombosis, bleeding tendency, serum triglycerides >350mg/dl, evidence of thyroid dysfunction, use of systemic steroids or other anabolics, pernicious anaemia, impaired vitamin B12 or folate acid levels, abnormal serum urate at baseline, serum creatinine phosphokinase elevation of >1.5fold at baseline, pregnancy or lactation, and end-stage renal disease or dialysis.

Patients were allocated into two groups according to the degree of carotid artery stenosis: those with arterial lumen occlusion of >70% in at least one common or internal carotid vessel consisted group A; those with stenosis <70% comprised group B. Patients in both groups were naive to statin therapy or if otherwise, a 6-month washout period was allowed before enrolment in the study. Group A underwent percutaneous transluminal carotid angioplasty with stenting by the same interventional cardiologist, prior to the initiation of statin therapy. Those patients were additionally administered clopidrogrel and salicylate. Both groups had to follow an American Heart Association step II diet and were encouraged to exercise.

All patients were placed on atorvastatin once daily at bedtime in individualised doses, tittered to achieve and maintain serum LDL cholesterol levels of <100mg/dl (and ideally <70mg/dl, if hypertension, renal impairment, smoking, hyperlipidemia, symptomatic peripheral arterial obstructive disease, or diabetes mellitus were present). The most common doses used to achieve the above levels of LDL ranged between 10 to 40mg, while seldom it was required to administer higher doses such as 60mg (median atorvastatin dose for the total population = 20mg, range 10 – 60mg). The use of other drugs known to act synergistically with statins causing rhabdomyolysis was prohibited during the study. Adverse events were assessed in every visit in a non-specific manner: every newly reported symptom was documented as possible adverse reaction due to statin therapy and subsequently evaluated by an expert in clinical biochemistry. Adherence to the medication regimen was assessed indirectly by the low LDL levels compared with baseline.

Medical anamnesis, anthropometrics, smoking habits, blood pressure, and laboratory investigations comprising of complete blood count, fasting glucose, HbA1c, liver and kidney biochemistry, detailed lipid profile (TC, LDL cholesterol, high density lipoprotein [HDL] cholesterol, serum triglycerides [TG], apoB, and apolipoprotein A), urate, B12 and folate, thyroid function tests, homocysteine, Lp-a, and oxLDL were obtained at baseline and during follow-up visits, which were arranged at baseline, one, three, and six months; the final assessment was carried out in 12 months. Blood samples were collected after an at least 12-hour fast and a light, low-fat meal the night before sample collection was advised. Venous blood samples were collected in standard biochemistry vacutainer tubes. For the analysis of homocysteine and whole blood count, ethylenediaminetetraacetic acid (EDTA) vacutainer was used. Serum for biochemistry analysis was obtained by centrifugation (4000g) at 4°C for 7 min and was immediately tested.

Lipid profiles (TC, HDL, TG) were determined using commercially available enzymatic colourimetric methods (Dade Behring, Newark, USA) with a Dade Behring analyser. LDL was calculated with the use of Friedewald's formula as all had TG <350mg/dl [27]. For the measurement of circulating oxLDL, a commercially available kit (Mercodia, Uppsala, Sweden), based on a double antibody (4E6 and mouse monoclonal antiapoB) [28] capture ELISA test, was used. This method primarily detects malondialdehyde LDL (MDA-LDL). The normative range (reference range) in our lab was 31-61mU/l. Apolipoprotein A, B and Lp-a were measured using immuno-nephelometry with rabbit antisera (Dade Behring, Newark, USA) in a Dade Behring analyser.

The evaluation of stenosis was conducted by Triplex ultrasonography using an Apogee 800 plus scanner with a 7.5 MHz transducer (ATL Inc., Bothell WA, USA) at baseline and 12 months. The stenosis was calculated in three sections in each common and internal carotid artery, and the final measure was the mean value of the three. The value of stenosis in the most occluded vessel was used in the statistical analysis. Specifically, the internal carotid artery (ICA) and common carotid artery (CCA) bilaterally were evaluated for each patient using coloured and grey Doppler ultrasonography. An effort was made to completely visualize the vessels. Additionally, the pulse wave was estimated with Doppler phasmatometry as well as the blood flow velocity of the two vessels. Results were recorded in a validated form. Stenosis was defined as the presence of visual plaque in coloured or grey Doppler. The degree of stenosis was calculated by measuring the decrease of the lumen diameter and the maximum systolic blood flow velocity. In difficult cases, other parameters were taken into account, such as ICA/CCA max blood flow velocity ratio and the ICA end-diastolic velocity. A degree of stenosis >70% was considered as sever and angioplasty was advised. A degree of stenosis between 60 – 70% was defined as high, between 50 – 60% as moderate and <50% as mild. High, moderate and mild stenoses were treated conservatively. The intima media thickness (IMT) and plaque morphology were not studied due to specific lab requirements, not readily available in our institution.

2.1. Statistical analysis

Continuous variables were presented as mean values ± standard deviation, while qualitative variables were presented as absolute and relative frequencies. Normality tests were applied using the Kolmogorov-Smirnov criterion as well as Shapiro-Wilk test. Univariate analysis was initially applied to test the associations of oxLDL with carotid stenosis for each patient group as well as to identify first order correlations with various clinical parameters. Correlations between skewed continuous or discrete variables were evaluated using Spearman's p-coefficient, whereas correlations of normally distributed variables were evaluated by calculating the Pearson's r-coefficient. Comparisons between normally distributed, continuous variables and categorical variables were made using the Student t-test. Analysis of categorical data was carried out with the [chi]2 test or Fischer's exact test when appropriate.

The association of oxLDL with carotid stenosis was also tested through multiple Cox proportional hazard model. The results obtained were presented as Hazard Ratios (HR) and the 95% Confidence Intervals (CI). A backward elimination procedure was applied to all multivariate models (using P<5% as the threshold for removing a variable from the models). All models were adjusted for age, gender, SBP and TC. Kaplan-Meier curves concerning stenosis over the study period were plotted and Log rank test was performed. All reported P-values were based on two-sided tests and compared to a significance level of 5%. STATA 8.0 software (Stata Corporation, 2003, Texas, USA) was used for the analysis.

3. Results

3.1. Patients' characteristics

A total of 612 patients were evaluated, of which 123 fulfilled the eligibility criteria; finally, 100 had complete data to enter the analysis, 76 males and 24 females, median age 68 years (range 45-81). Diabetes mellitus was recorded in 26 of the 100 patients and hypertension in 66. Twenty patients had metabolic syndrome according to the national cholesterol education programme-adult treatment panel III (NCEP-ATP III) criteria [29]. Active smoking (defined as current of discontinued as far back as 5 years) was reported by 58 patients. Mean atorvastatin dose at baseline was 24.31±11.49 mg for group A and 20.62±10.39 mg for group B (p=0.1). By the end of the study period, the respective mean values were significantly increased to 30.45±16.27 mg for group A (p=0.044) and 28.75±17.57 mg for group B (p=0.007).

Each of the study group (A and B) comprised 50 patients. The two groups were comparable with regard of their baseline characteristics (table 1).

3.2. Lipid profile and oxidised LDL

Mean serum TC, LDL-cholesterol, TG, Lp-a, homocysteine, HDL-cholesterol, and oxLDL were significantly reduced at 12 months compared to baseline (table 2). Specifically, mean oxLDL dropped from 62.26±22.03 mU/l to 44.49±21.75 (p<0.001). A marked decrease was noticed during the first 6 months and a plateau thereafter (Figure 5).

Characteristic	Total	Group A	Group B	p value
males / females	72 / 28	36 / 14	36 / 14	
mean age in years ± SD	67.57±7.15	68.46±5.71	66.68±8.31	0.21
number of pts with DM (percentage)	37 (37%)	18 (36%)	19 (38%)	0.83
number of pts with HTN (percentage)	67 (67%)	36 (72%)	31 (62%)	0.29
number of smokers (percentage)	54 (54%)	29 (54%)	25 (46%)	0.33
number of pts with CAD (percentage)	51 (51%)	24 (47%)	27 (53%)	0.55
mean ± SD total cholesterol (mg/dl)	232.23±47.8	235.24±49.2	229.22±46.7	0.53
mean ± SD LDL cholesterol (mg/dl)	151.27±41.7	154.16±42.8	148.84±40.9	0.52
mean ± SD HDL cholesterol (mg/dl)	51.97±12.7	52.12±12.1	51.82±13.4	0.9
mean ± SD triglycerides (mg/dl)	145.59±73.1	146.04±73.2	145.14±73.7	0.95
mean ± SD oxidized LDL (mU/l)	64.66±24.8	65.8±25.3	63.53±24.5	0.65
mean ± SD homocysteine (mU/l)	13.99±4.8	13.5±4.6	14.47±5.1	0.32

Pts: patients, DM: diabetes mellitus, HTN: arterial hypertension, MS: metabolic syndrome, SD: standard deviation, LDL: low density lipoprotein, HDL: high density lipoprotein, CAD: coronary artery disease

Table 1. Study population baseline characteristics

A significant correlation between LDL and oxLDL levels was detected (Pearson's correlation coefficient r=0.7, p<0.01) (Figure 6). Similar correlation was found between oxLDL and apoB levels (r=0.65, p<0.001), while no significant correlation was shown with Lp-a.

Between smokers mean oxidized LDL was reduced from 60.68±24.09 mU/l at baseline to 45.84±24.89 mU/l at the end of study period (difference 14.84 mU/l, p = 0.0036). Similarly, between non-smokers it was reduced from 69.33±25.11 to 40.36±5.6 (difference 28.97, p<0.001). Non-smokers had approximately double decline of oxidized LDL levels compared to smokers. Carotid artery stenosis was reduced between smokers from 29.68±25.59% at baseline to 23.06±21.71% at 12 months (p = 0.002). Non-smokers also presented significant reduction of stenosis during the study period 24.67±26.22% vs 20±21.45%, p = 0.004). Non-smokers and smokers had similar decline of carotid stenosis in 12 months (6.61% vs 4.67%, Table 3).

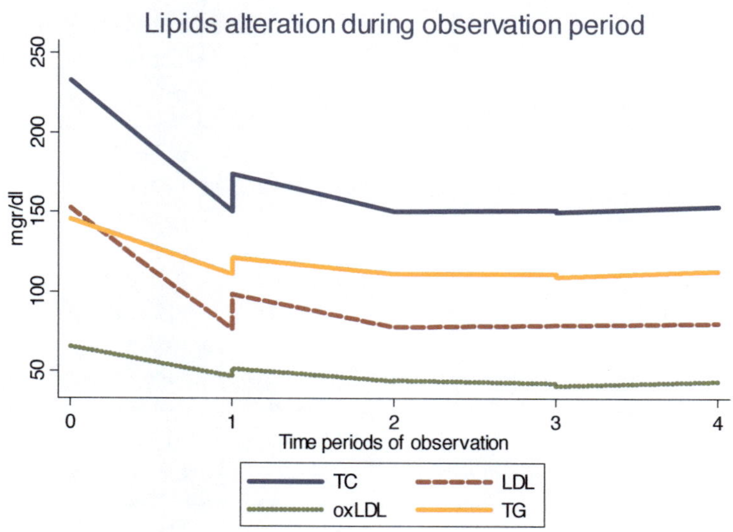

TC: total cholesterol, LDL: low density lipoprotein cholesterol, oxLDL: oxidised LDL, TG: triglycerides, 0=baseline, 1=one month, 2=three months, 3=six months, 4=twelve months.

Figure 5. Time curve of change of total cholesterol, LDL cholesterol, triglycerides and oxidised LDL levels during the observation period.

In further analysis, the group of smokers was subdivided to mild (≤5 cigarettes/day), moderate (5 – 15 cigarettes/day) and heavy (≥15 cigarettes/day) smokers. The statistical significant reduction of oxidized LDL levels and degree of carotid stenosis was apparent in the subgroup of mild smokers (oxidized LDL at baseline 48.24±8.74 mU/l vs 41.54±9 mU/l at 12 months, p = 0.027 and stenosis at baseline 27.63±25.68% vs 23.42±21.74% at 12 months, p = 0.009), while it was not apparent in the subgroups of moderate and heavy smokers (oxidized LDL at baseline 86.82±37.7 mU/l vs 42.92±10.77 mU/l at 12 months, p = 0.077 and stenosis at baseline 34±31.9% vs 22±24.9% at 12 months, p = 0.186, for moderate smokers; respective values for oxidized LDL were 66.29±15.88 mU/l vs 34.81±5.48 mU/l, p = 0.06 and for stenosis 32.14±24.13% vs

22.86±22.8%, p = 0.174, for heavy smokers). The above described effect of smoking was taken into consideration during Cox-regression analysis.

Investigations	Total	Group A	Group B
total cholesterol (mg/dl) baseline	232.23 ± 47.8	235.24±49.1	229.22±46.7
total cholesterol (mg/dl) 12months	153.36±17.2	154.24±16.9	152.48±17.7
p value	<0.0001	<0.0001	<0.0001
LDL cholesterol (mg/dl) baseline	151.5±41.7	154.16±42.8	148.84±40.9
LDL cholesterol (mg/dl) 12months	79.75±12.7	79.54±13.2	79.96±12.3
p value	<0.0001	<0.0001	<0.0001
triglycerides (mg/dl) baseline	145.59 ± 73.1	146.04±73.2	145.14±73.7
triglycerides (mg/dl) 12months	111±53.1	112.1±54.7	109.9±51.96
p value	0.0002	0.01	0.0069
oxidized LDL (mU/l) baseline	64.67±24.8	65.8±25.3	63.53±24.6
oxidized LDL (mU/l) 12months	43.38±18.9	42.16±17.6	44.65±26.1
p value	<0.0001	<0.0001	0.0007
HDL cholesterol (mg/dl) baseline	51.97±12.7	52.12±12.1	51.82±13.4
HDL cholesterol (mg/dl) 12months	51.32±15.5	52.22±16.3	50.42±14.8
p value	0.74	0.97	0.62
homocysteine (mg/dl) baseline	13.99±4.8	13.5±4.6	14.48±5.1
homocysteine (mg/dl) 12months	11.89±3.5	11.88±3.8	11.9±3.4
p value	0.0006	0.057	0.0036
apolipoprotein A (mg/dl) baseline	156.57±26.7	156.46±27.3	156.68±26.4
apolipoprotein A (mg/dl) 12months	160.35±25.3	162.02±23.7	158.68±27.1
p value	0.3	0.28	0.7
apolipoprotein B (mg/dl) baseline	129.95±31.3	131.84±31.4	128.05±31.4
apolipoprotein B (mg/dl) 12months	77.1±11.8	77.58±13.1	76.62±10.47
p value	<0.0001	<0.0001	<0.0001
lipoprotein a [Lp(a)] (mg/dl) baseline	25.08±23.8	25.67±24.1	24.47±23.8
lipoprotein a [Lp(a)] (mg/dl) 12months	27.72±29.1	29.42±29.8	26.01±28.7
p value	0.48	0.49	0.77

LDL: low density lipoprotein, HDL: high density lipoprotein

Table 2. Comparison of mean ± standard deviation and respective p values of measured laboratory investigations at baseline and 12 months, in the total population, and the two groups.

http://dx.doi.org/10.5772/57188

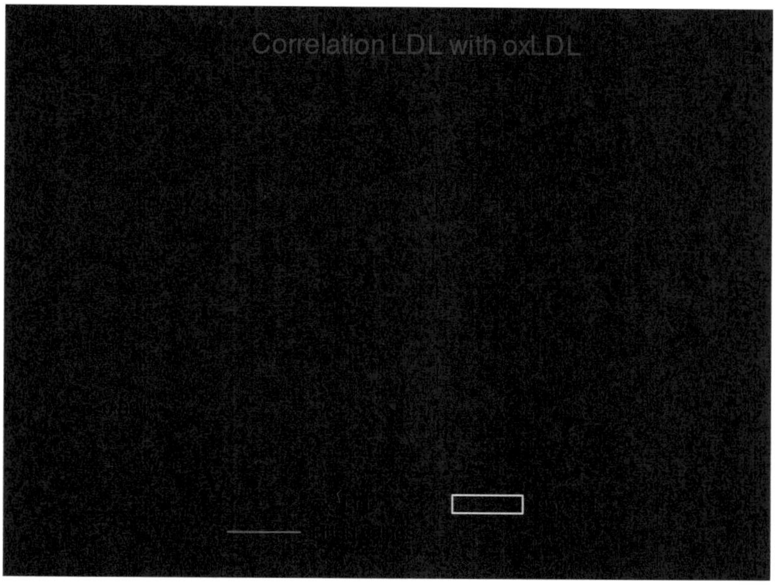

LDL: low density lipoprotein cholesterol, oxLDL: oxidised LDL, CI: confidence intervals.

Figure 6. Correlation of low density lipoprotein (LDL) with oxidised LDL (oxLDL) levels at baseline (Pearson's correlation coefficient r=0.7, p<0.001)

	Smokers	P value	Non Smokers	P value
ox LDL (mg/dl) baseline 12 months difference	60.68±24.09 45.48±24.89 14.84	0.0036	69.33±25.11 40.36±5.6 28.97	0.001
stenosis (%) baseline 12 months difference	29.68±25.59 23.06±21.71 6.61	0.002	24.67±26.22 20±21.45 4.67	0.004
Correlation of oxLDL change with stenosis change in 12 months	Pearson's r = 0.412	0.021	Pearson's r = 0.198	0.03

Table 3. Comparison of mean oxidized LDL values and degree of carotid stenosis change during the 1 year follow-up period, between smokers and non-smokers.

Within group B, the subgroup of patients with high degree of stenosis (>60%) had oxLDL 63.47±19.18 mU/l at baseline, while those with moderate and mild degree of stenosis (<60%) had 40.32±20.72 mU/l (p<0.001). Corresponding values at 12-months were 33.18±17.78 and

38.81±29.02, representing a marked decline for patients with >60% initial stenosis and a far less decline for patients with <60% initial stenosis; yet the differences were not significant (table 4).

	Stenosis >60<70%	Stenosis <60%	P value
Baseline Mean oxidized LDL	63.47±19.18 mU/l	40.32±20.72 mU/l	< 0.001
12 months Mean oxidized LDL	33.18±17.78 mU/l	38.81±29.02 mU/l	NS

Table 4. Comparison of mean oxidized LDL levels at baseline and 12 months within patients of group B (n = 50), according to degree of stenosis at enrollment.

3.3. Anthropometrics

Body mass index (BMI), weight, waist circumference and waist:hip ratio did not change significantly during the study period.

3.4. Carotid stenosis

Patients in group A had null stenosis at recruitment due to prior angioplasty with stenting. At the end of the 12-month statin therapy, no case of clinically important restenosis (>70%) was reported in this group (as restenosis was defined any increase of the carotid lumen diameter >5%). Patients in group B had mean percentage of stenosis at baseline 47.6±13.2%, which was significantly reduced following 12-month statin therapy (37.7±15.7%, p<0.001) (Table 5).

	baseline	12 months	p value
Mean % carotid stenosis ± standard deviation	47,6 ± 13,2	37,7 ± 15,7	0,001

Table 5. Change of the percentage of carotid artery stenosis between baseline and 12months for patients in group B.

3.5. Association of stenosis with oxidised LDL

Group B patients in the highest quartile of oxLDL values had a 12-month risk ratio for restenosis of 1.025, 95%CI=1.006-1.044, p=0.0083 (figure 7). After adjusting for gender, age, smoking, SBP, TC, and LDL levels, these patients demonstrated a HR for restenosis of 4.319 compared with those in the lowest quartile (p<0.001, figure 7). This means that an increase of oxidized LDL by one unit increases the degree of carotid stenosis by 2.5%, for patients in group B. A weak but significant correlation was detected between oxLDL levels and the degree of carotid artery stenosis (r=0.17, p=0.018). Similar correlation was found between LDL cholesterol levels and carotid stenosis (r=0.18, p=0.0085). The strength of Pearson's correlation of mean oxidised LDL change with degree of carotid stenosis change during the 12-month period was greater for smokers compared to non-smokers (table 3).

3.6. The effect of LDL levels

Patients in group B who achieved LDL levels <70mg/dl during the observation period had a greater (28.08±28% vs 22.31±22.7%, difference 5.77%, p =0.06) reduction of carotid stenosis compared to those with LDL levels between 70 and 100 mg/dl (26.98±25.3% vs 21.35±21.3%, difference 5.63%, p < 0.001), but this difference was not statistically significant. Thus, in conservatively treated group B, further reduction of LDL than the limit of 100mg/dl was not associated with additional improvement of stenosis.

4. Discussion

This study demonstrates that atorvastatin administered in indivudualised doses, tittered to maintain serum LDL cholesterol levels <100mg/dl, significantly decreased lipid profile and oxLDL, reduced carotid artery stenosis in patients managed conservatively and prevented restenosis in patients with prior angioplasty. Oxidised LDL in this study correlated positively with the degree of carotid artery stenosis; it was also shown by multivariate analysis that oxLDL represented an independent risk factor for restenosis. To our knowledge this is the first prospective study with a long observation period of 12 months to report such a clear, significant reduction of oxLDL levels following atorvastatin therapy for carotid atheromatosis of various causes and to report an association of the degree of oxLDL reduction with remission of carotid stenosis. It is also of major importance that this robust, long-standing decline of oxLDL was achieved with doses of atorvastatin used in everyday clinical practice. Interestingly, this beneficial effect was completed in the first six months, while practically no further reduction was noticed past this time point.

The mechanism by which statins modulate oxLDL levels has been controversial in the literature. Moreover, the association of oxLDL level modification with improvement of carotid atheromatosis and clinical outcome is not unequivocally established by large, double-blinded, randomised trials. Under this perspective, the present observational study provides reasonable evidence that reducing oxLDL may independently improve carotid stenosis.

Carotid intima media thickness (IMT) is a validated measure of carotid atherosclerosis. It is well established that carotid atherosclerosis, serves as an independent surrogate marker for CHD [30] and CVD [31]. Nevertheless, in the present study it was preferred to estimate the degree of carotid stenosis with a more direct approach, because this is more readily available in most hospital settings and because there is an obvious relation with clinical symptoms and signs. Besides, it represents a reliable method with sufficient reproducibility and it is practically the method of choice when evaluated patients candidate for endarterectomy or angioplasty. Evaluating carotid stenosis in turn, is an established method for estimating coronary risk [30] and cardiovascular risk [31]. Other parameters of vessel wall function, such as IMT and plaque morphology, even if clearly associated with cardiovascular risk in the literature, require well equipped laboratory and are not readily available in our hospital. Future research on the field should, ideally, comprise such measurements.

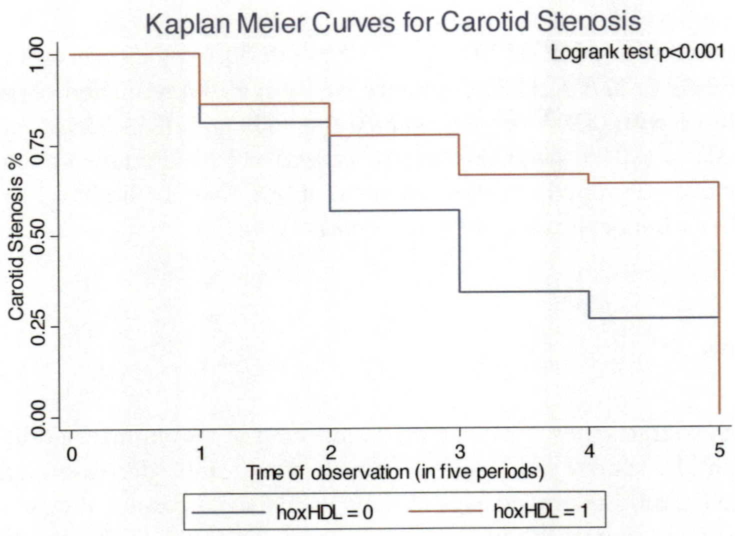

hoxLDL=0: low quartile of oxidised LDL levels, hoxLDL=1: high quartile of oxidised LDL levels, 0=baseline, 1=one month, 2=three months, 3=six months, 4=twelve months.

Figure 7. Kaplan Meier survival analysis for the estimation of the risk ratio for restenosis according to the levels of oxidised LDL (oxLDL). With red line those with oxLDL levels in the highest quartile of the values. With blue line those with oxLDL levels in the lowest quartile of the measurements (risk ratio 1.025, logrank test $p<0.001$).

Oxidised LDL has long been recognized as a risk factor for carotid atherosclerosis in asymptomatic men [32] and has also been linked with CVD [33]. Oxidized LDL levels [34], autoantibodies against epitopes of oxLDL [34] and oxLDL:LDL ratio [30] are independently associated with increased risk for coronary atheromatosis and ischemic heart disease. Increased levels of oxLDL [9] and MDA-LDL [10] in such cases are related to plaque instability. On the other hand, it has been reported that oxLDL is weakly associated with carotid IMT, but not with carotid plaque occurrence [35]. Oxidised LDL impairs endothelium relaxation [36] by inhibition of the expression of eNOS and of the transport pathways of nitric oxide (NO) from the endothelial cell, reduces the responsiveness of smooth muscle cell to NO [37], inhibits the NO-mediated vasodilation [16,36,38], induces the expression of adhesion molecules [39], acts directly chemotactic to circulating monocytes [16], stimulates endothelial cells to produce monocyte chemoattractant protein-1 (MCP-1) [40], facilitates monocyte adhesion to intima [41], exhibits cytotoxic properties against endothelial cells [16], and induces the expression of inflammatory molecules [16]. All of the above contribute directly to dysfunction of the endothelium [13] and foam cell formation, which is the first step in the development of fatty streaks [18], the first visible step of atherosclerosis. These effects are mediated by preferential binding of oxLDL with type A scavenger receptors (SRA, SRA-II and CD36) on subendothelial resident macrophages and smooth muscle cells [42] and lectin-like oxLDL receptor-1 (LOX-1) on endothelial cells [43] rather than the typical LDL receptor, resulting in an unrestricted uptake of cholesterol.

Statins reduce the incidence of cardiovascular events, an effect attributable to their hypocholesterolemic properties [44]. However, the extent of clinical benefit and accumulating laboratory evidence suggest additional mechanisms of action, the so-called pleiotropic effects [19]. The most important among such effects are the suppression of smooth muscle cell migration and proliferation [45], the reduction of monocyte adhesion to the vascular endothelium [20], the improvement of endothelial function [21], the inhibition of cell-mediated LDL oxidation [22,23], the immuno-modulation of monocyte maturation and differentiation, and the modification of production of inflammatory cytokines [46].

Atorvastatin suppresses cellular uptake of oxLDL from differentiating monocytes by reducing the expression of LOX-1 and scavenger receptors [47] and accelerates the LDL-receptor-mediated removal of the non oxidized LDL particles [48]. Hydroxymetabolites of atorvastatin protect the LDL against oxidation [31]. The antioxidant potency of atorvastatin metabolites has been confirmed by the reduction of IgG antibodies against LDL, a marker well-associated with CHD [23]. It has even been reported that these active atorvastatin metabolites may have greater anti-atherosclerotic effects than other statin molecules [49].

In acute coronary syndromes, atorvastatin therapy was linked to modulation of short- and long-term immune response towards LDL due to inhibition of lipoprotein-associated phospholipase A2 (Lp-LPA2) enzyme [34]. The apparent benefit from statin therapy after acute coronary events may also be attributed to the stabilization of the plaque and removal of oxLDL from the vessel wall [50]. Increased mobilization of oxidized phospholipids from the vessel wall, transient binding with apoB-100 particles and clearance from the circulation may be the possible underlying mechanism. Under this perspective the increase in oxLDL:apoB ratio detected with atorvastatin therapy might represent a marker of oxLDL efflux from the vessel wall. Removal of oxLDL contributes to improved endothelial function as oxLDL is highly immunogenic and vasoconstrictive. In our study there was no significant change in oxLDL:apoB ratio. Atorvastatin also inhibits the oxLDL-mediated LOX-1 expression by endothelial cells, the uptake of oxLDL in endothelium and the oxLDL-mediated reduction of protein kinase B (PKB) phosphorylation [24]. The activation of PKB is critical for the expression of eNOS, which promotes vessel relaxation. However, a meta-analysis provided no clear evidence that statin therapy have a favourable effect on oxLDL [51].

In STAT trial [52] the antibodies against oxLDL were equally decreased with both aggressive and conventional lipid-lowering therapy. This indicates that the statin-related reduction of oxLDL is not a dose-dependent phenomenon, a finding which is in agreement with our results. It might therefore represent a pleiotropic effect, independent -at least partially- from the hypocholesterolemic action. A study by Orem et al detected a significant decrease of autoantibodies against oxLDL with low doses of atorvastatin (10mg) [53], similar to doses used in our study. In statin exposed patients, intensification of the regimen offers no additional benefit and only those with LDL>125mg/dl benefited from a more aggressive statin therapy [52]. Statins have a dose-related response with regard to clinical outcome, but this dose-related response has not been confirmed with regard to oxidative stress [54]. This might alternatively be explained by the hypothesis that statins achieve their uttermost benefit on oxLDL after a certain time point [52], after which further continuation of treatment serves only the purpose of maintenance.

Atorvastatin has been shown to reduce small dense LDL subfractions, remnant-like particles cholesterol and oxLDL, and improve endothelial function, after just few weeks of therapy [55,56]. Such time-related effect has not been fully elucidated, but may possibly account for our finding that in the first six months there was an accelerated decline of oxLDL levels followed by a milder reduction rate thereafter.

Additional pleiotropic effects of statins have been reported in the literature and might account for the observed beneficial effects in the current study. Lysophosphatidylcholine is elevated during LDL oxidation and is responsible for some of the biological effects of oxLDL. Atorvastatin alters the ability of oxLDL to impair the endothelium relaxation, by modulating the hydrolysis of phosphatidylcholine to lysophosphatidylcholine when LDL is being oxidized [57]. Statins remove predominately "aged LDL" from plasma, which is more prone to oxidation [53], through stimulation of hepatic LDL receptor activity and inhibition of very-low density lipoprotein (VLDL) and LDL production by the liver cells [53]. Statins also reduce oxygen species generation [54]. Atorvastatin promotes adipocyte uptake of oxLDL in rabbits by increasing the expression of CD36 and peroxisome proliferators-activated receptor γ (PPARγ) in adipocytes [58]. The increased expression of such receptors by adipocytes results to internalization of oxLDL and clearance from plasma, converting adipocytes to an oxLDL-buffering pool [58]. Reduction of oxLDL in patients with CHD with atorvastatin 10mg parallel with an increase of adiponectin, which has anti-atherogenic [55], anti-inflammatory and anti-diabetic [55] properties through reduction of insulin resistance [55]. The CARDS study reported a significant degree of preventive activity of atorvastatin against myocardial infarction in eucholesterolemic diabetic patients, conceivably attributed to such improvement of insulin sensitivity [55]. Statins also diminish the expression of CD40 and CD40 ligand in vascular cells, smooth muscle cells and macrophages, which are promoted by oxLDL and are considered proatherogenic [59]. Other anti-inflammatory pathways include reduction of C-reactive protein [60], chemokines, major histocompatibility complex II molecules, matrix-degrading enzymes, and procoagulant tissue factor [59]. Atorvastatin reverses the oxLDL-mediated inhibition of vascular endothelial growth factor-induced endothelial progenitor cell differentiation via the phosphatidylinositol 3 kinase/Akt pathway [61], which restores the oxLDL-related inhibition of mature endothelial cells migration [61]. This could improve neovascularization and collateral vessel formation in response to tissue ischemia. Atorvastatin also suppresses platelet activity [62] by reducing the expression of CD36 and LOX-1, which are present in platelets [43,62], thus inhibiting the oxLDL-mediated platelet hyperactivity [62]. Statins reduce the oxLDL-derived expression of adhesion molecules (E- and P-selectins, vascular cell adhesion molecule 1 [VCAM-1] and intercellular adhesion molecule 1 [ICAM-1]) in human coronary artery endothelial cells [15], through up-regulation of eNOS expression [15], which regulates the expression of adhesion molecules in endothelial cells [15]. Statins also diminish the oxLDL-mediated activation of nuclear factor-κB (NF-κB) [15], which regulates the transcription of adhesion molecule genes [33]. In diabetic patients with dyslipidemia atorvastatin reduced CVD and markers of inflammation, adhesion and oxidation, such as CRP, soluble ICAM-1, soluble VCAM-1, E-selectin, matrix metalloproteinase 9, secretory phospholipase A2 (sPLA2), and oxLDL, the latter by 38,4% [60]. Moreover, the change of oxLDL levels correlated with the change of sICAM-1 and E-selectin levels, suggesting that statins could possibly counteract the oxLDL-associated increase of NF-κB, and therefore, the production of such cell adhesion molecules [60]. Statins also enhance scavenger receptor expression in macrophages [60], and increase plaque stability via reduction of metalloproteinases [60].

The reduction of oxidised LDL and of carotid stenosis in our study was relevant for both, smokers and non-smokers. However, during subgroup analysis showed that the beneficial effect of statin use concerns mostly the subgroup of mild smokers, while no such effect was noticed for moderate and heavy smokers. How smoking may diminish the beneficial effect of statins on oxidized LDL and carotid stenosis is not yet clarified in the literature. A reasonable assumption might be that, since smoking increases the oxidative stress, it contributes to enhanced LDL oxidation [63]. Moreover, studies in animal models, have demonstrated that smoking alters the immunologic response to oxidized LDL by reducing the production of antibodies against these molecules, i.e. causing a kind of immune suppression regarding the response to oxidized LDL. Thus, it has been shown to increase carotid IMT [64].

The Mercodia oxLDL detects the MDA-modified apoB [28]. It has been proposed that oxLDL looses its predictive value for CVD when adjustment for apoB level is performed [54]. In several studies though, a significant reduction of Mercodia oxLDL with atorvastatin 10mg was still detected even after adjustment for apoB, [10,31,54], while in other studies no adjustment for LDL or apoB levels was made [54,65]. In our study the oxLDL:apoB ratio remained unchanged, but in the multivariate analysis the reduction of oxLDL was still significant after adjustment for apoB and LDL levels.

In patients with familial hypercholesterolemia a lack of association between oxLDL and IMT was reported at baseline, however two years therapy with atorvastatin 80mg was associated with regression of carotid IMT [66]. The LDL subfraction profile and autoantibodies against oxLDL remained unchanged. Nevertheless, the rate of oxidation and the amount of dienes formed decreased and this was linked to lessening of atherosclerosis. In our study the reduction of carotid stenosis was associated with decreased oxLDL levels. Besides, the unchanged oxLDL autoantibodies levels do not preclude the reduction of oxLDL, as was indicated in another study involving dialysis patients, where atorvastatin therapy reduced plasma oxLDL, whereas oxLDL autoantibodies did not changed significantly [67].

Disadvantages of the study were the relatively small size, the lack of a control group comprising of patients with carotid stenosis not on statin therapy, which would be unethical, the fact that researchers were not blinded to the patients' status, the lack of randomization of the dose-schedules and the use of only one method to detect oxLDL.

5. Conclusion

This prospective, cross-sectional study with such a long observation period provided enough evidence to postulate a favourable effect of low-dose atorvastatin therapy on oxLDL, which was additionally associated with improvement of stenosis in patients with carotid atheromatosis. We thus, assume that oxidised LDL may represent a far more sensitive risk factor for carotid stenosis, than LDL itself or apoB. Further studying is required to confirm such findings and to establish a clear clinical and pathophsiologic link between oxLDL and carotid stenosis.

Acknowledgements

The authors wish to acknowledge Dr. Antonios Polydorou for performing the catheterizations and stenting of the cartotid arteries in the group of patients that underwent intervention prior entering the study. We also thank him for allowing us access to the records of the angioplasty lab. Finally we are grateful for valuable advice and reviewing this manuscript before publishing.

We also wish to acknowledge Dr. Ioannis Dermitzakis for the critical contribution in evaluating the degree of stenosis of our patient population, as director of the ultrasonography laboratory in our institution. Without his help and valuable assistance this whole project would not have been completed.

The authors finally acknowledge Mrs. Anna Zervou for carrying out the biochemical laboratory measurements with diligence and accuracy, overlooking tiredness, physical and emotional strain. We thank her for her personal commitment in the success of this research.

Author details

Elias Skopelitis, Dimitrios Levisianou, Helen Lydataki and Sofoklis Kougialis

General Hospital of Nikaia and Piraeus, Athens, Greece

References

[1] Assmann G, Schulte H. Relation of high density lipoprotein cholesterol and triglycerides to incidence of atherosclerotic coronary artery disease (the PROCAM experience). Am J Cardiol 1992;70:733–737.

[2] Hokanson JE, Autsin MA. Plasma triglyceride level is a risk factor for cardiovascular disease independent of high–density lipoprotein cholesterol level: a meta–analysis of population–based prospective studies. J Cardiovasc Risk 1996;3:213–219.

[3] Katsouras CS, Karabina SA, Tambaki AP, et al. Serum lipoprotein (a) concentrations and apoprotein (a) isoforms: association with the severity of clinical presentation in patients with coronary heart disease. J Cardiovasc Risk 2001;8(5):311-317

[4] Anderson TJ, Meredith IT, Charbonneau F, et al. Endothelium – dependant coronary vasomotion relates to the susceptibility of LDL to oxidation in humans. Circulation 1996;93:1647-1650

[5] Durrington P, Sniderman A. (2002) Epidemiology and pathophysiology. In: Hyperlipidemia. Durrington P, Sniderman A (Eds). p. 29–31 Health Press, Oxford, UK

[6] Corti Ro, Fuster Va, Fayad Za, et al. Lipid lowering by simvastatin induces regression of human atherosclerotic lesions: two years' follow–up by high–resolution non-invasive magnetic resonance imaging. Circulation. 2002;106:2884–2887

[7] Nissen SE, Tuzcu ME, Schoenhagen P, Brown GB, Ganz P, Vogel RA, Crowe T, Howard G, Cooper CJ, Brodie B, Grines CL, DeMaria AN. For the REVERSAL investigators. Effect of intensive compared with moderate lipid lowering therapy on progression of coronary atherosclerosis. A randomized controlled trial. JAMA March 3, 2004;291(9).

[8] Toshima S, Hasegawa A, Kurabayashi M, Itabe H, Takano T, Sugano J, et al. Circulating oxidized low density lipoprotein levels. A biochemical risk marker for coronary heart disease. Arterioscler Thromb Vasc Biol 2000;20(10):2243-7.Holvoet P, Harris TB, Tracy RP, Verhamme P, Newman AB, Rubin SM, et al. Association of high coronary heart disease risk status with circulating oxidized LDL in the well-functioning elderly: findings from the Health, Aging, and Body Composition study. Arterioscler Thromb Vasc Biol 2003;23(8):1444-8.

[9] Ehara S, Ueda M, Naruko T, Haze K, Itoh A, Otsuka M, et al. Elevated levels of oxidized low density lipoprotein show a positive relationship with the severity of acute coronary syndromes. Circulation 2001;103(15):1955-60.

[10] Holvoet P, Collen D, & Van de Werf F. Malondialdehyde-modified LDL as a marker of acute coronary syndromes. JAMA 1999;281(18):1718-21.

[11] Penny WF, Ben-Yehuda O, Kuroe K, Long J, Bond A, Bhargava V, et al. Improvement of coronary artery endothelial dysfunction with lipid-lowering therapy: heterogeneity of segmental response and correlation with plasma-oxidized low density lipoprotein. J Am Coll Cardiol 2001;37(3):766-74.

[12] Nishi K, Itabe H, Uno M, Kitazato KT, Horiguchi H, Shinno K, et al. Oxidized LDL in carotid plaques and plasma associates with plaque instability. Arterioscler Thromb Vasc Biol 2002;22(10):1649-54.

[13] Witztum JL, & Steinberg D. Role of oxidized low density lipoprotein in atherogenesis. J Clin Invest 1991;88(6):1785-92.

[14] Steinbrecher UP, Parthasarathy S, Leake DS, Witztum JL, & Steinberg D. Modification of low density lipoprotein by endothelial cells involves lipid peroxidation and degradation of low density lipoprotein phospholipids. Proc Natl Acad Sci USA 1984;81(12):3883-7.

[15] Li D, Chen H, Romeo F, Sawamura T, Saldeen T, & Mehta JL. Statins modulate oxidized low-density lipoprotein-mediated adhesion molecule expression in human coronary artery endothelial cells: role of LOX-1. J Pharmacol Exp Ther 2002;302(2):601-5.

[16] Steinberg D. Low density lipoprotein oxidation and its pathobiological significance. J Biol Chem 1997;272(34):20963-6.

[17] Steinberg D, Parthasarathy S, Carew TE, Khoo JC, & Witztum JL. Beyond cholesterol. Modifications of low-density lipoprotein that increase its atherogenicity. N Engl J Med 1989;320(14):915-24.

[18] Ross R. Atherosclerosis--an inflammatory disease. N Engl J Med 1999;340(2):115-26.

[19] Bellosta S, Ferri N, Bernini F, Paoletti R, & Corsini A. Non-lipid-related effects of statins. Ann Med 2000;32(3):164-76.

[20] Weber C, Erl W, Weber KS, & Weber PC. HMG-CoA reductase inhibitors decrease CD11b expression and CD11b-dependent adhesion of monocytes to endothelium and reduce increased adhesiveness of monocytes isolated from patients with hypercholesterolemia. J Am Coll Cardiol 1997;30(5):1212-7.

[21] Jarvisalo MJ, Toikka JO, Vasankari T, Mikkola J, Viikari JS, Hartiala JJ, et al. HMG CoA reductase inhibitors are related to improved systemic endothelial function in coronary artery disease. Atherosclerosis 1999;147(2):237-42.

[22] Giroux LM, Davignon J, & Naruszewicz M. Simvastatin inhibits the oxidation of low-density lipoproteins by activated human monocyte-derived macrophages. Biochim Biophys Acta 1993;1165(3):335-8.

[23] Aviram M, Rosenblat M, Bisgaier CL, & Newton RS. Atorvastatin and gemfibrozil metabolites, but not the parent drugs, are potent antioxidants against lipoprotein oxidation. Atherosclerosis 1998;138(2):271-80.

[24] Li DY, Chen HJ, & Mehta JL. Statins inhibit oxidized-LDL-mediated LOX-1 expression, uptake of oxidized-LDL and reduction in PKB phosphorylation. Cardiovasc Res 2001;52(1):130-5.

[25] Kwak BR, & Mach F. Statins inhibit leukocyte recruitment: new evidence for their anti-inflammatory properties. Arterioscler Thromb Vasc Biol 2001;21(8):1256-8.

[26] Robinson JG, Smith B, Maheshwari N, & Schrott H. Pleiotropic effects of statins: benefit beyond cholesterol reduction? A meta-regression analysis. J Am Coll Cardiol 2005;46(10):1855-62.

[27] Puccetti L, Pasqui AL, Pastorelli M, Bova G, Cercignani M, Palazzuoli A, et al. Time-dependent effect of statins on platelet function in hypercholesterolaemia. Eur J Clin Invest 2002;32(12):901-8.

[28] Holvoet P, Donck J, Landeloos M, Brouwers E, Luijtens K, Arnout J, et al. Correlation between oxidized low density lipoproteins and von Willebrand factor in chronic renal failure. Thromb Haemost 1996;76(5):663-9.

[29] Executive Summary of The Third Report of The National Cholesterol Education Program (NCEP) Expert Panel on Detection, Evaluation, And Treatment of High Blood Cholesterol In Adults (Adult Treatment Panel III). JAMA 2001;285(19):2486-97.

[30] Vasankari T, Ahotupa M, Toikka J, Mikkola J, Irjala K, Pasanen P, et al. Oxidized LDL and thickness of carotid intima-media are associated with coronary atherosclerosis in middle-aged men: lower levels of oxidized LDL with statin therapy. Atherosclerosis 2001;155(2):403-12.

[31] van Tits LJ, van Himbergen TM, Lemmers HL, de Graaf J, & Stalenhoef AF. Proportion of oxidized LDL relative to plasma apolipoprotein B does not change during statin therapy in patients with heterozygous familial hypercholesterolemia. Atherosclerosis 2006;185(2):307-12.

[32] Liu ML, Ylitalo K, Salonen R, Salonen JT, & Taskinen MR. Circulating oxidized low-density lipoprotein and its association with carotid intima-media thickness in asymptomatic members of familial combined hyperlipidemia families. Arterioscler Thromb Vasc Biol 2004;24(8):1492-7.

[33] Robbesyn F, Salvayre R, & Negre-Salvayre A. Dual role of oxidized LDL on the NF-kappaB signaling pathway. Free Radic Res 2004;38(6):541-51.

[34] Papathanasiou AI, Lourida ES, Tsironis LD, Goudevenos JA, & Tselepis AD. Short- and long-term elevation of autoantibody titers against oxidized LDL in patients with acute coronary syndromes. Role of the lipoprotein-associated phospholipase A2 and the effect of atorvastatin treatment. Atherosclerosis 2008;196(1):289-97.

[35] Hulthe J, & Fagerberg B. Circulating oxidized LDL is associated with subclinical atherosclerosis development and inflammatory cytokines (AIR Study). Arterioscler Thromb Vasc Biol 2002;22(7):1162-7.

[36] Harrison DG, Freiman PC, Armstrong ML, Marcus ML, & Heistad DD. Alterations of vascular reactivity in atherosclerosis. Circ Res 1987;61(5 Pt 2):II74-80.

[37] Keaney JF, Jr., Guo Y, Cunningham D, Shwaery GT, Xu A, & Vita JA. Vascular incorporation of alpha-tocopherol prevents endothelial dysfunction due to oxidized LDL by inhibiting protein kinase C stimulation. J Clin Invest 1996;98(2):386-94.

[38] Simon BC, Cunningham LD, & Cohen RA. Oxidized low density lipoproteins cause contraction and inhibit endothelium-dependent relaxation in the pig coronary artery. J Clin Invest 1990;86(1):75-9.

[39] Frostegard J, Nilsson J, Haegerstrand A, Hamsten A, Wigzell H, & Gidlund M. Oxidized low density lipoprotein induces differentiation and adhesion of human monocytes and the monocytic cell line U937. Proc Natl Acad Sci USA 1990;87(3):904-8.

[40] Cushing SD, Berliner JA, Valente AJ, Territo MC, Navab M, Parhami F, et al. Minimally modified low density lipoprotein induces monocyte chemotactic protein 1 in human endothelial cells and smooth muscle cells. Proc Natl Acad Sci USA 1990;87(13):5134-8.

[41] Mehta A, Yang B, Khan S, Hendricks JB, Stephen C, & Mehta JL. Oxidized low-density lipoproteins facilitate leukocyte adhesion to aortic intima without affecting endothelium-dependent relaxation. Role of P-selectin. Arterioscler Thromb Vasc Biol 1995;15(11):2076-83.

[42] Li H, Freeman MW, & Libby P. Regulation of smooth muscle cell scavenger receptor expression in vivo by atherogenic diets and in vitro by cytokines. J Clin Invest 1995;95(1):122-33.

[43] Sawamura T, Kume N, Aoyama T, Moriwaki H, Hoshikawa H, Aiba Y, et al. An endothelial receptor for oxidized low-density lipoprotein. Nature 1997;386(6620):73-7.

[44] Archbold RA, & Timmis AD. Modification of coronary artery disease progression by cholesterol-lowering therapy: the angiographic studies. Curr Opin Lipidol 1999;10(6): 527-34.

[45] Bellosta S, Bernini F, Ferri N, Quarato P, Canavesi M, Arnaboldi L, et al. Direct vascular effects of HMG-CoA reductase inhibitors. Atherosclerosis 1998;137 Suppl:S101-9.

[46] Rothe G, Herr AS, Stohr J, Abletshauser C, Weidinger G, & Schmitz G. A more mature phenotype of blood mononuclear phagocytes is induced by fluvastatin treatment in hypercholesterolemic patients with coronary heart disease. Atherosclerosis 1999;144(1):251-61.

[47] Fuhrman B, Koren L, Volkova N, Keidar S, Hayek T, & Aviram M. Atorvastatin therapy in hypercholesterolemic patients suppresses cellular uptake of oxidized-LDL by differentiating monocytes. Atherosclerosis 2002;164(1):179-85.

[48] Vasankari T, Ahotupa M, Viikari J, Nuotio I, Vuorenmaa T, Strandberg T, et al. Effects of statin therapy on circulating conjugated dienes, a measure of LDL oxidation. Atherosclerosis 2005;179(1):207-9.

[49] Mason RP, Walter MF, & Jacob RF. Effects of HMG-CoA reductase inhibitors on endothelial function: role of microdomains and oxidative stress. Circulation 2004;109(21 Suppl 1):II34-41.

[50] Tsimikas S, Witztum JL, Miller ER, Sasiela WJ, Szarek M, Olsson AG, et al. High-dose atorvastatin reduces total plasma levels of oxidized phospholipids and immune complexes present on apolipoprotein B-100 in patients with acute coronary syndromes in the MIRACL trial. Circulation 2004;110(11):1406-12.

[51] Balk EM, Lau J, Goudas LC, Jordan HS, Kupelnick B, Kim LU, et al. Effects of statins on nonlipid serum markers associated with cardiovascular disease: a systematic review. Ann Intern Med 2003;139(8):670-82.

[52] Mulder DJ, van Haelst PL, Wobbes MH, Gans RO, Zijlstra F, May JF, et al. The effect of aggressive versus conventional lipid-lowering therapy on markers of inflammatory and oxidative stress. Cardiovasc Drugs Ther 2007;21(2):91-7.

[53] Orem C, Orem A, Uydu HA, Celik S, Erdol C, & Kural BV. The effects of lipid-lowering therapy on low-density lipoprotein auto-antibodies: relationship with low-density lipoprotein oxidation and plasma total antioxidant status. Coron Artery Dis 2002;13(1):65-71.

[54] Ky B, Burke A, Tsimikas S, Wolfe ML, Tadesse MG, Szapary PO, et al. The influence of pravastatin and atorvastatin on markers of oxidative stress in hypercholesterolemic humans. J Am Coll Cardiol 2008;51(17):1653-62.

[55] Miyagishima K, Hiramitsu S, Kato S, Kato Y, Kitagawa F, Teradaira R, et al. Efficacy of atorvastatin therapy in ischaemic heart disease - effects on oxidized low-density lipoprotein and adiponectin. J Int Med Res 2007;35(4):534-9.

[56] Sakabe K, Fukuda N, Wakayama K, Nada T, Shinohara H, & Tamura Y. Effects of atorvastatin therapy on the low-density lipoprotein subfraction, remnant-like particles cholesterol, and oxidized low-density lipoprotein within 2 weeks in hypercholesterolemic patients. Circ J 2003;67(10):866-70.

[57] Zhu Q, McMaster J, Mymin D, Dembinski T, Hatch G, Choy PC, et al. Effects of atorvastatin treatment on the oxidatively modified low density lipoprotein in hyperlipidemic patients. Mol Cell Biochem 2000;207(1-2):9-17.

[58] Zhao SP, & Zhang DQ. Atorvastatin enhances cellular uptake of oxidized LDL in adipocytes from hypercholesterolemic rabbits. Clin Chim Acta 2004;339(1-2):189-94.

[59] Schonbeck U, Gerdes N, Varo N, Reynolds RS, Horton DB, Bavendiek U, et al. Oxidized low-density lipoprotein augments and 3-hydroxy-3-methylglutaryl coenzyme A reductase inhibitors limit CD40 and CD40L expression in human vascular cells. Circulation 2002;106(23):2888-93.

[60] Hogue JC, Lamarche B, Tremblay AJ, Bergeron J, Gagne C, & Couture P. Differential effect of atorvastatin and fenofibrate on plasma oxidized low-density lipoprotein, inflammation markers, and cell adhesion molecules in patients with type 2 diabetes mellitus. Metabolism 2008;57(3):380-6.

[61] Imanishi T, Hano T, Matsuo Y, & Nishio I. Oxidized low-density lipoprotein inhibits vascular endothelial growth factor-induced endothelial progenitor cell differentiation. Clin Exp Pharmacol Physiol 2003;30(9):665-70.

[62] Puccetti L, Sawamura T, Pasqui AL, Pastorelli M, Auteri A, & Bruni F. Atorvastatin reduces platelet-oxidized-LDL receptor expression in hypercholesterolaemic patients. Eur J Clin Invest 2005;35(1):47-51.

[63] Van Himbergen T, Roest M, De Waart F, De Graaf J, Voorbij H, Van Tits L, et al. Paraoxonase genotype, LDL-oxidation and carotid atherosclerosis in male life-long smokers. Free Radic Res 2004;38(6):553-60

[64] Tani S, Dimayuga PC, Anazawa T, Chyu KY, Li H, Shah PK, et al. Aberrant antibody responses to oxidized LDL and increased intimal thickening in apoE-/- mice exposed to cigarette smoke. Atherosclerosis 2004;175(1):7-14

[65] Sasaki S, Kuwahara N, Kunitomo K, Harada S, Yamada T, Azuma A, et al. Effects of atorvastatin on oxidized low-density lipoprotein, low-density lipoprotein subfraction distribution, and remnant lipoprotein in patients with mixed hyperlipoproteinemia. Am J Cardiol 2002;89(4):386-9.

[66] van Tits LJ, Smilde TJ, van Wissen S, de Graaf J, Kastelein JJ, & Stalenhoef AF. Effects of atorvastatin and simvastatin on low-density lipoprotein subfraction profile, low-density lipoprotein oxidizability, and antibodies to oxidized low-density lipoprotein in relation to carotid intima media thickness in familial hypercholesterolemia. J Investig Med 2004;52(3):177-84.

[67] van den Akker JM, Bredie SJ, Diepenveen SH, van Tits LJ, Stalenhoef AF, & van Leusen R. Atorvastatin and simvastatin in patients on hemodialysis: effects on lipoproteins, C-reactive protein and in vivo oxidized LDL. J Nephrol 2003;16(2):238-44.

Chapter 7

Cerebral Protection in Carotid Angioplasty – Is There a Need? Advantages and Disadvantages of Each Type of Protection Device

Antenor Tavares and José Guilherme Caldas

Additional information is available at the end of the chapter

http://dx.doi.org/10.5772/57154

1. Introduction

Currently, ischemic cerebral vascular accident (ICVA; stroke) is an illness with a high incidence and a high mortality rate [1,2]. In Brazil, depending on the state of the Brazilian Federation and the period analyzed, cerebrovascular disease is the leading cause of mortality [3]. Moreover, survivors present a continuous risk of developing serious complications [4]. Carotid atherosclerotic disease is the cause of approximately 15 to 20% of cerebrovascular accidents [5].

Carotid stenosis is present in 7% of men and 5% of women aged 65 years or older [6]. In serious cases (>70% stenosis), stenosis is an important cause of ICVA and transient ischemic attack (TIA). The estimated risk of ipsilateral ICVA in 5 years is 4% in the population without carotid stenosis; the risk increases to 18% in patients with asymptomatic stenosis above 75% and reaches 27% in symptomatic patients with stenosis >75% [7]. Several authors have described risk factors associated with carotid atherosclerosis, such as age, smoking, systemic arterial hypertension (SAH), hypercholesterolemia, coronary artery disease, peripheral vascular disease, and male gender [4,8,9].

2. Treatment of carotid stenosis

Treatment options for carotid stenosis include medication or surgery [10-12]. Clinical treatment includes antiplatelet agents and statins associated with the control of risk factors such as arterial hypertension, dyslipidemia, hyperglycemia, diabetes, and smoking [13]. Relevant studies comparing the outcomes of clinical treatment and surgery showed an important reduction in the risk of CVA among the patients selected for surgical treatment. In the NASCET study, the risk of CVA was significantly reduced by surgery (9% in the surgical group versus 26% in the medication treatment) [10]. In another classical trial with asymptomatic patients, surgical treatment was also associated with a better prognosis (4.8% versus 10.6% for medication treatment) [14].

The two main effective treatment options for patients with serious carotid stenosis are carotid endarterectomy (CEA) and carotid angioplasty with stent (CAS). CEA was the first surgical option developed. It is indicated for symptomatic patients with carotid stenosis >60% and in centers with surgical risk below 6%. In asymptomatic patients, a degree of stenosis >70% is considered an indication for surgical treatment, but surgeons must notice morbi-mortality lower than 3% [10,14-17].

The most recent surgical option is CAS, which consists of an approach to stenosis through a natural route within the vessels. A flexible guide wire and catheter are inserted into the arterial system through a peripheral venipuncture and are maneuvered to the stenosis site, where the narrow portion is opened using the stent and balloon dilation.

CAS is considered less invasive than traditional surgery (CEA) and does not require an incision on the lateral side of the cervical region [18]. CAS also has the advantages of being able to maintain a steady flow of blood to the brain during CAS with a filter, generally using local anesthesia, and allowing early hospital discharge [18]. Thus, the indications for CAS are the same as those for CEA and also encompass other situations, such as comorbidities, occlusion of the contralateral carotid artery, high carotid bifurcation, concomitant distally associated stenosis, postradiotherapy stenosis, and restenosis after carotid endarterectomy [9,19,20].

The CREST trial compared CAS and CEA, examining complications, such as CVA, myocardial infarction, or death during CAS and CEA, and CVA four years after these techniques were applied. The authors observed similar rates of complications between CAS and CEA and concluded that the techniques are equivalent in terms of short- and long-term clinical results, but CAS carries a higher risk of ICVA and CEA carries a higher risk of heart attack during the periprocedural period. This study also found that good results might be influenced by good treatment and the expertise of the interventionists and surgeons [12].

Currently, CAS is considered a safe and effective technique for treating stenosis in the carotid artery >70% in symptomatic patients, when assessed by noninvasive methods, and >50% when assessed by catheter angiography, as indicated by the guidelines of the American Stroke Association (ASA; Class I recommendation with evidence level B) [21].

The first angioplasty for carotid stenosis was performed by Mathis in 1979 in a patient with fibromuscular dysplasia that caused symptomatic carotid stenosis [22]. The first angioplasty for atherosclerotic lesions was reported in 1980 by Kerber et al. [23]. The first series of carotid angioplasties was published in 1987 by Theron et al. and included 11 patients [24]. At the beginning of the 1980s, publications regarding the use of balloon occlusion in the carotid artery to reduce embolic complications began to appear [24-26].

The first balloon-expandable stent was used in a carotid artery in 1989; however, these early stent models were prone to extrinsic compression and deformation. In this group of stents, adverse effects occurred in more than 10% of patients within the short 30-day follow-up [27,28]. Subsequently, deformation was avoided using the self-expandable Wallstent® stent [29] and later by self-expandable nitinol alloy stents. However, the risk of cerebral embolism remained, although it was reduced compared with the risk associated with the first stents. Restenosis, which occurred frequently after angioplasties without a stent, was reduced drastically. Currently, all manufacturers of endovascular intervention materials produce stents with rapid self-expanding technology compatible with the thin 0.014-inch guides common to most cerebral protection systems [13]. Nonetheless, carotid stenosis treatment with either CAS with cerebral protection or with CEA continues to carry an inherent risk of embolism.

3. Is there a difference between materials used in carotid angioplasty?

As the CREST Trial showed, the risk of ICVA in CAS is a technical problem that remains unsolved [12]. A heavily debated topic in the literature is the design of the metallic alloy used to outline the empty spaces, which are called cells. Different types of frames for the metal skeleton can promote plaque stabilization, depending on the size of the free area between the metal brackets. Stents with a braided metallic mesh, which are dense throughout, can be more effective at covering the plaque and reducing the risk of embolism [30]. These closed-cell stents are characterized by small cells (areas enclosed by metal) joined together (Figure 1). Segmental rings connected to each other by points that are welded together and large areas that are not covered by metal are called open-cell stents [30]. Hybrid stents, which have a closed-cell design in their central part and an open-cell design in their proximal and distal parts, can also be found. These stents are rarely used in practice.

There are several examples of closed-cell stents, such as Wallstent® (Boston Scientific), Xact® (Abbott), and NexStent® (Endotex). The Carotid Wallstent® is considered the prototype for closed-cell design stents. Examples of stents with an open-cell design include Protégé® (Ev3), Precise® (Cordis), Acculink® (Abbott), and Exponent® (Medtronic). The Carotid Wallstent® model is manufactured with a stainless steel alloy and a closed-cell mesh, which may help to prevent embolic complications. Because of its design, the Carotid Wallstent® (Boston Scientific) undergoes a shortening by approximately 30% [31], and caution must be used when estimating its length. The Precise® (Cordis) stent is a nickel and titanium alloy (nitinol®) mounted on rings, which promotes an open-cell aspect and offers great flexibility. The Protégé® (Ev3) stent also uses nitinol and an open-cell design, and both conical and straight versions are available. These last two stents cannot be collected after they begin to release; therefore, they should only be opened when the implant site is certain. However, these stents do not undergo shortening.

A study by Tadros et al. used photomicroscopy to analyze debris found in the filters after CAS and showed that open-cell stents are associated with a larger mean particle size compared with closed-cell stents [32].

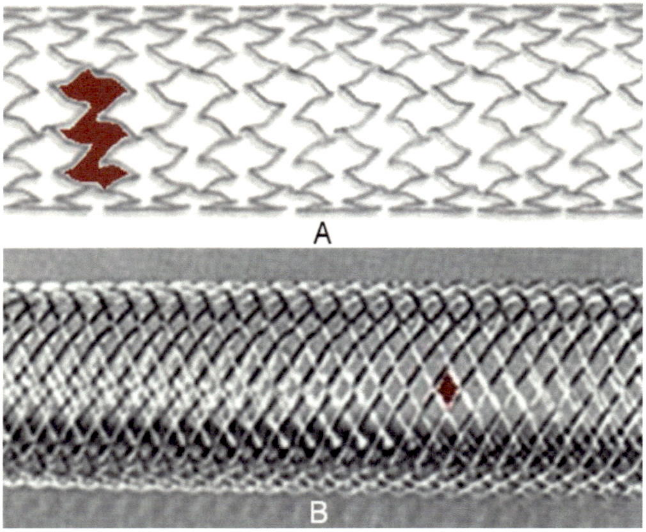

Figure 1. Typical arrangement of the metal mesh of an open-cell stent (A) and a closed-cell stent (B). The area of a cell in each type of stent is highlighted in red

The results for angioplasty should be analyzed considering that there are ongoing major evolutions in methods and materials. The results of angioplasties after the introduction of stents and cerebral protection systems cannot be compared with the results of studies conducted before the development of these materials [13,32-37].

Although the initial purpose of carotid stenosis treatment is the prevention of cerebral infarction, both CEA and CAS carry risks of causing infarcts [13]. The materials and techniques have been modified to reduce the risk of embolic complications during CAS. Several authors [32-38] have shown the rare relative incidence of cerebral embolism and death after carotid angioplasty with or without cerebral protection.

Our experience with carotid angioplasty began in 1998 and 2000. At that time, cerebral protection systems were not available in Brazil. During this period, 72 CAS were performed, and the combination of neurological complications and death reached 5.5%. In the subsequent period (2001 to 2007), 1215 CASs were performed with filters for cerebral protection, and our occurrence of neurological complications and death fell to 1.8% [38].

Although some authors defend the use of CAS without cerebral protection, we emphasize that symptomatic embolism is rare and that the use of safety devices, such as cerebral protection systems, functions as a reserve parachute: Although they are rarely needed, no one wants to jump without one (recommendation class IIa, level of evidence: C, [39]).

Currently, several devices are capable of providing cerebral protection during carotid stenosis treatment, but the morbimortality results differ for each device. The forms of protection for each device are also different. Nonetheless, other authors using various methods (most notably

Doppler and MRI) have shown that an enormous load of emboli to the brain may not determine symptoms. This phenomenon is called an asymptomatic embolism associated with CAS.

There are two types of cerebral protection systems: proximal and distal. The protection systems with filters are distal, and the protection devices with balloons can be proximal or distal. Proximal devices have the theoretical advantage of exerting protection during all phases of intervention, except during the positioning of the guide catheter or the long sheath. The proximal devices use temporary occlusion of the common carotid artery with a balloon, and a second balloon occludes the external carotid artery, resulting in the stagnation or reversal of the flow of the internal carotid artery (example: the PAES® Parodi antiembolism system). With this type of device, protection is initiated before the stenosis is crossed with the guide wire, which can reduce the risk of distal embolization. After the stent is implanted, the blood is aspirated from the carotid bifurcation to remove any fragments, and later, the proximal protection device is removed [40-42].

In contrast, with the distal devices, it is necessary to cross the stenosis with the microguide and then to use the distal device on the lesion. Therefore, the distal systems consist of a device (filter or balloon) with an integrated guide wire. This set-up allows the CAS to be performed along the guide wire. With the distal protection, embolization can occur when the guide catheter or sheath is positioned and during the passage of the guide wire through the stenosis before the distal device enters the action.

Distal protection systems allow two different forms of approach. One form is the occlusion of the distal cervical internal carotid artery by a balloon (example: PercuSurge®). With this type of system, there is a complete interruption of the antegrade flow, which provides protection for the particles that do not reach the brain. After the CAS, manual aspiration is performed, the balloon is deflated, and the system is removed [43,44].

The other form of distal protection is through the use of a filter (examples: EPI®, Angioguard®, Spider®). In this device, the filter (Figure 2) crosses the stenosis and is implanted in the distal cervical portion of the internal carotid artery. The stent and balloon are introduced over the guide to perform the CAS. There are different types of filters, but the aim of all of them is to retain particles, thereby preventing embolisms from reaching the brain and maintaining continuous blood flow. At the end of CAS, the filter is closed and removed from the patient with the embolic material inside [13]. In terms of design, the filters can be concentric (examples: Emboshield® and Angioguard® Cordis) or eccentric (examples: Filterwire EPI/EZ® Boston Scientific/Target and Spider®eV3). In concentric filters, the metallic guide occupies the center of the structure. In eccentric systems, the guide is outside the center of the protection device [45,46].

Thus, the two main types of cerebral protection devices used in CAS are filters that allow distal flow during the CAS and systems for the temporary occlusion of the carotid artery (balloons) that promote the inversion or paralysis of flow to the brain. Some authors defend filtering devices, but others defend the balloons because they are believed to offer more complete protection of the brain. Furthermore, the use of these cerebral protection systems is not supported in some patients.

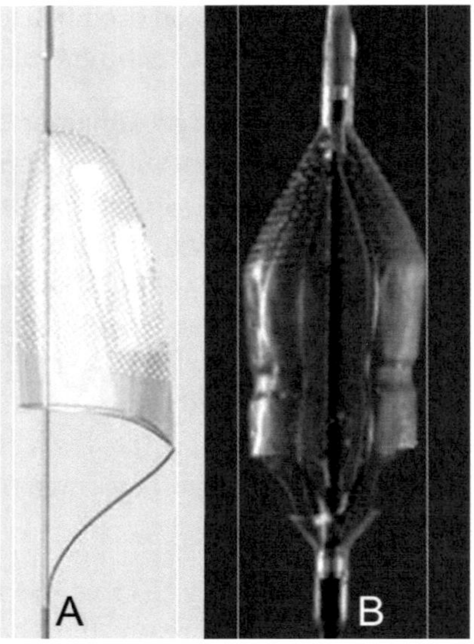

Figure 2. Examples of cerebral protection devices: eccentric design (A) in the EPI® filter and concentric design (B) in the Emboshield® system

Although all devices have a common goal of preventing the entry of particles into distal circulation, the perfect protection system does not exist [42]. Among proximal protection systems with balloons, arterial occlusion is the weakest point because patients might not tolerate it. Moreover, the contrast of vessels during the CAS is difficult because of flow stagnation, which makes positioning the stent difficult. Moreover, this system is more laborious and complex to use than filters. Additionally, proximal protection systems are very high profile and tend to lead to hemorrhaging complications at the puncture site. The device's advantages include its ability to initiate cerebral protection at an early stage and to avoid embolization during the initial passage of the wire through the stenosis [13,42].

The distal embolic protection devices with a balloon have the disadvantage of preventing antegrade flow, which renders some patients intolerant of this type of device. The balloon may also cause vascular lesions (example: pseudoaneurysm), and the affixture of the balloon may be lost during the CAS. Moreover, images cannot be easily obtained while the balloon is in use and, technically, the balloon is not very maneuverable. An advantage of distal protection devices is their ease of use compared with proximal occlusion balloons [13].

Among the disadvantages of distal embolic protection devices with filters is that they may not capture all particles and their delivery and recovery systems may cause embolisms. Some filters may attach to the stent because of bad handling. The advantages of filters include the preservation of antegrade flow to the brain during all stages of the CAS and the ability to obtain graphic images easily. Some systems allow the operator to select which guide wire to use to cross the lesion, which allows the filter to remain in contact with the arterial wall and the guide wire to be moved during the CAS without mobilizing the filter [13].

An advantage of using filters is their ability to maintain constant flow to the brain during all stages of the angioplasty, unlike protection balloons, which promote the temporary halt of flow to the brain. Carotid filters are also easier to use than occlusive or reverse flow protection balloons.

4. Cerebral embolism in the surgical treatment of carotid stenosis

Despite the advantages of cerebral protection systems, Mu®ller-Hu®lsbeck et al., in their 2005 study of ex vivo pig carotid arteries with four types of filters and one type of cerebral protection balloon, found that particles were passed with all of the protection systems tested [47]. Piñero et al. [48], using the transcranial Doppler technique, observed signs of embolism during several phases of CAS, including the initial unprotected phase. Similarly, Schimidt et al. [49] divided the carotid angioplasty into five phases from start to finish. This comparative study used one type of filter (EPI®) and one type of occlusive system with balloons (MO.MA®) and found that particles were passed in all phases of both systems.

The transcranial Doppler tool can help identify signs of embolism during an unprotected phase (before using the filter) or during the passage of the filter, and it can identify embolisms when the stent or balloon is applied or the filter is removed [50,51]. The transcranial Doppler can provide information about the flow in the polygon vessels [52] and show changes in the cervical segment after angioplasty [53]. However, the Doppler assessment has the disadvantage of evaluating only one vessel, usually the middle cerebral artery or the distal cervical internal carotid artery on the carotid stenosis side, leaving a vast territory of the brain uncovered during the evaluation of embolic phenomena. No correlation can be observed between the quantity of microemboli identified during ultrasound and new embolism outbreaks found during MRI [54]. In contrast, MRI can evaluate the entire encephalon, which is particularly important because embolic events may occur during the CAS or during the angiography preceding CAS in other areas of the brain supplied by the carotid undergoing CAS [46,48].

According to several authors, the use of cerebral protection systems is an important factor in reducing the risk of cerebral infarction during CAS [9,13,34,55]. However, although most patients are asymptomatic after CAS, signs of embolism can be detected using the transcranial Doppler technique and MRI [56] because of different factors, such as the existence of pores in the protection systems that allow particles up to 100 microns pass, the manipulation of the artery before the filter is opened, the filter not adapting to the artery wall, and crucially, a lack of proper training in handling the systems [46,48,49,54,57-63].

5. Imaging evaluation of cerebral embolism

We consider MRI an excellent method for evaluating cerebral ischemia in its various presentations. An MRI study of various acute neurological presentations of an ischemic nature includes several forms of ischemia presentation on the images [64].

Diffusion (DWI) is the best MRI technique to differentiate ischemia from chronic infarction. While the latter shows an increase in diffusion, the former classically restricts diffusion [65]. The identification of acute lesions in patients with multiple chronic lesions makes DWI a tool of unquestionable value in current imaging practice.

Water in tissues has a randomized translational movement ("Brownian motion") in its molecules caused by thermodynamic energy and the viscosity of the medium. This type of movement is related to CDA, and MRI uses DWI to evaluate it [66,67].

Diffusion imaging is sensitive to the microscopic movement of water protons. Water protons undergo a change during the transverse magnetization phase in the presence of a magnetic field gradient. Thus, areas with greater diffusion (faster movement) are subject to a high degree of signal attenuation compared with areas with lower diffusion (slow/restricted movement), which show lower signal attenuation. Animals subjected to occlusion of the middle cerebral artery (MCA) showed signs of ischemia in diffusion within 45 minutes. These findings are believed to reflect the restriction of water movement by the cellular membrane. MRI's greater sensitivity for detecting acute ischemia in diffusion is believed to be a result of the movement of water within the cell, which restricts the movement of water protons (cytotoxic edema), while the T2-weighted images show a signal change that results mainly from vasogenic edema. It is estimated that cytotoxic edema begins very soon after ischemic abuse, while the vasogenic edema begins to develop 6 hours after the ischemic incident.

Moseley et al. [65] argued that significant diffusion decrease (restriction or reduction) in ischemia reflects the deviation of an environment with extracellular water protons with a faster diffusion to a more restricted intracellular environment, in addition to the depletion of the sodium-potassium pump in the cellular membrane because of infarction. The cytotoxic edema is thus responsible for reducing diffusion during ischemia.

Nonetheless, the diffusion of ischemia areas can be reversed after early reperfusion and are potentially reversible if they occur after CAS. It has also been shown that ischemic lesions in diffusion might not leave changes that appear in later MRI scans after TIA frames.

The embolic complications identified in DWI occur more frequently than the apparent low rate of clinical complications would suggest. An MRI may quantify the ischemic foci, making it an important method for validating the advantages and complications of CAS.

To examine this issue more deeply, we conducted a prospective randomized study (patients chosen randomly from the outpatient neuroradiology service of INCOR) in a case-control setting [68]. We used angiographic exams and MRI studies that showed cerebral embolism represented by the diffusion sequence (DWI) before and after surgical endovascular treatment to quantify, locate, and measure new restriction foci in diffusion MRI and to correlate the new DWI restriction foci with demographic aspects (gender, age, side of the carotid treated, and symptoms), risk factors for cerebrovascular disease, aspects of the angioplasty technique used, and the presence of previous infarcts in MRI.

6. Methods

Our sample consisted of 40 patients presenting carotid stenosis of atherosclerotic origin. The patients were referred for MRI exams with diffusion techniques before and after CAS. All of the patients in this prospective study signed an informed consent form. The inclusion criteria were as follows: patients with serious carotid stenosis (shown by Doppler, ATC, or digital subtraction angiography [DSA]) who were referred for endovascular treatment for carotid atheromatous disease according to the local institutional guidelines, who agreed to participate in the research protocol, and who had MRI studies conducted with diffusion techniques at most 24 hours before and up to 72 hours after the CAS with a protection filter.

Exclusion criteria were the following: intra-arterial thrombi observed in the angiography before CAS; patients with disabling complications from previous cerebral infarcts; contraindications for the MRI scan, such as a cardiac pacemaker or claustrophobia, patients with macroemboli in the DSA after CAS, clinical conditions compatible with ischemia after CAS, angiographic exam showing stenosis <60%, MRI exams with movement artifacts, and imaging studies with serious stenosis in the contralateral cervical carotid, vertebral arteries, or intracranial arteries.

Three patients out of 40 were excluded because they showed stenosis <60%, and one patient was excluded for having exceeded the maximum time established for MRI after CAS because of coronary angina and hemodynamic instability.

The MRI studies were performed using commercially available single high-field equipment (1.5 T, LX Horizon®, General Electric Healthcare) with a skull coil ("birdcage transmit/receive quadrature").

The MRI scans before and after CAS followed the same sequencing protocol:

- Locator: 256x128 matrix, FOV 27 cm, 10 mm thickness, 5 mm spacing, number of acquisitions ("nex"): 1
- DWI: 128X128 matrix, FOV 22 cm, 5 mm thickness, 0 mm spacing, TE minimum 72.8 ms, TR 9000 ms, "b-value" 0 and 1000, diffusion direction: "all", number of acquisitions: 2
- Coefficient of apparent diffusion: map of "ADC"
- T2W, axial, 288x224 matrix, FOV 22 cm, 6 mm thickness, 0.6 mm spacing, TE 102 ms, TR 4750 ms, echo train length 23, bandwidth 31.25 and number of acquisitions: 2
- T1W, axial, 256x192 matrix, FOV 22 cm, 6 mm thickness, 0.6 mm spacing, TE 14 ms, TR 475 ms, bandwidth 15.63 and number of acquisitions: 2
- Fluid-attenuated inversion recovery (FLAIR): axial, 256x192 matrix, FOV 22 cm, 6 mm thickness, 0.6 mm spacing, TE 96 ms, TR 10000 ms, TI 2.100 ms and number of acquisitions: 1
- T2W, coronal, 288x224 matrix, FOV 22 cm, 6 mm thickness, 0.6 mm spacing, TE 102 ms, TR 4750 ms, bandwidth 31.25 and number of acquisitions: 2

New foci (NF) of ischemia were defined as the presence of a hypersignal (restriction) in diffusion after CAS that was not present in the same sequence before CAS. These foci were considered recent, additional infarcts compared with the first MRI.

The opposite of a recent infarction caused by DWI after CAS is an old infarction that is present in the T2W sequencing of the MRI before CAS. Chronic cerebral infarction is the end result of prolonged ischemia. Areas of hypersignal in the cerebral parenchyma in the T2 sequence with areas corresponding to the variable signal in T1 (with the tendency to be isointense compared with the fluid in T1 and T2) without restriction in DWI and with no enhancement after paramagnetic contrast were considered old infarctions ("T2W infarction"). Other diseases that may have a signal aspect similar to that of old infarctions (for example: porencephalic cysts, arachnoid cysts, low-grade astrocytoma) were excluded from the count because of their topographic characteristics, their appearance on the edge of the lesion, or their appearance on the surrounding tissue or because they showed a signal that differed from that of the fluid in the other sequences in the MRI study.

The MRI images were analyzed by the consensus of two experienced neuroradiologists using the eFilm® software without access to the clinical data or angiography and CAS data. If there were discrepancies between the two neuroradiologists' findings, the studies were analyzed by a third observer to reach a consensus.

The NF were correlated with age, gender, side of carotid artery treated, presence of previous symptoms related to carotid stenosis, risk factors for atherosclerosis and ICVA (diabetes mellitus, systemic arterial hypertension, hypercholesterolemia, ischemic coronary artery disease, arrhythmia, ischemic peripheral vascular disease, transient ischemic attack [TIA], and ischemic cerebrovascular accident [ICVA]), percentage of carotid stenosis, presence of ulcers in the atheromatous plaque, previous infarction noted on the MRI, number of catheters used, number of arteries on which angiographies were performed, contralateral carotid occlusion, endovascular access technique used to reach the common carotid artery on the side of the angioplasty, type of filter, type of stent, volume of contrast used in the CAS and angiography, fluoroscopy time spent during the procedure, and the localization, number, and diameter of these NF. These parameters were also correlated between patients with only one NF and those with multiple NFs.

The localization (laterality) of the encephalic NF was defined as ipsilateral if it coincided with the area supplied by the carotid artery undergoing angioplasty. The localization of the NF was defined as contralateral if the cerebral area did not coincide with the side of the CAS, meaning the area was nourished by the carotid artery contralateral to the angioplasty or the area located on the posterior fossa. In cases when it was impossible to determine laterality, the patient was excluded from the analysis, which occurred with two patients. Patients 16 and 27 showed stenosis in the carotid artery (left) and contralateral occlusion (right), with NF identified in the area supplied by the right carotid artery. Under this condition, the flow to the carotid area can use the anastomotic Willis polygon or openings in other collateral pathways can be determined (for example: flow through the vasa vasorum or retrograde flow through the ophthalmic artery). Thus, with NF in the area of the occluded artery, it is not possible to say with certainty whether the embolism originated directly in the CAS or migrated through the anastomosis of areas that revascularized the cerebral territory of the occluded carotid artery. Because of the difficulty of relating the localization of the embolism precisely with the artery that underwent angioplasty, we decided not to include these two cases in the analysis of laterality.

The diameter of each NF was noted using the maximum diameter of the lesion in the DWI sequence through a metric analysis determined manually in the software (eFilm®). For comparison, the NFs were divided into three groups of diameters (<5 mm, between 5 and 10 mm and >10 mm) according to the stratification method published by other authors [69,70].

The patients with carotid occlusion contralateral to the CAS were noted. To mark the occlusion of the internal carotid artery, we used DSA or MRI. In the absence of DSA in the carotid artery, we defined occlusion using MRI when there was no "flow-void" phenomenon and a high intravascular signal in the FLAIR sequence, compatible with thrombus in sections focusing on the internal intracranial carotid artery. Both imaging methods were accepted as sufficient for proving that a vessel was occluded.

Areas with DWI restriction after CAS (ischemia indicators) were correlated with demographic aspects, aspects of the angioplasty technique, stenosis characteristics, and the presence of previous infarctions on MRI. The quantification of stenosis in the carotid bulb studied was using the NASCET method [10] with DSA in all cases.

7. Angioplasty technique used

The patients were divided into two groups: "brief" angiography and "complete" angiography. An angiographic exam before CAS is conventionally called a brief angiography when the exam only includes an angiography of the carotid artery that is a candidate for treatment. A complete angiography includes the study of other cervical arteries or the aortic arch.

Antiplatelet therapy was standardized, and all patients received 75 mg clopidogrel and 100 mg acetylsalicylic acid orally on a daily basis, beginning at least five days before the procedure.

In the preparation of the materials, all of the introducers, catheters, and sheaths were pre-washed with physiologic saline flow and subsequently packed in a sterile container with physiologic serum and heparin before arterial puncture.

Under local anesthesia and light sedation from the anesthesiologist, arterial puncture was performed and the valved introducer was deployed in the common femoral artery, which was fixed to the skin with a wire suture for safety. If there was significant tortuosity of the iliac and femoral vessels, long introducers were sufficient to help stabilize the catheter and the catheter guide in the common carotid arteries.

A bolus injection of 10,000 units of heparin was administered intravenously after the valved introducer was installed. An atropine solution was prepared before the angioplasty and stored until the stent's release. Intermittent verbal communication was maintained with the patient during the procedure by the doctors performing the CAS, as in the eventual clinical tests.

In all cases, the angiography of the carotid artery undergoing CAS was initially performed with a 5 Fr angiographic catheter to confirm the stenosis shown with other methods. At this point in the procedure, angiographies of the cerebral vessels nourished by the carotid artery were performed, and they were repeated at the end of the CAS to observe any possible arterial occlusion. In all cases, a noniconic contrast with low osmolarity was used.

In all cases (n=36), an 8 Fr-caliber guide catheter was introduced into the common femoral artery inside the valved introducer, and the distal extremity was positioned in the common carotid artery undergoing CAS a few centimeters below the atherosclerotic plaque.

The possible methods for positioning the catheter guide safely in the common carotid artery, close to the bulb, were defined as access techniques. The endovascular techniques for accessing the carotid artery to be treated included direct access (DA), an exchange with the guide wire in the external carotid artery (ECA), exchange with the guide wire in the common carotid artery (ECC), and triaxial access (TRI). For the direct access technique (DA), the catheter guide was introduced into the common carotid artery by sliding it over a guide wire (0.035 inches) that had previously been placed in the artery.

The technique involving exchange with the guide in the external carotid artery (EEC) was as follows: the tip of the guide wire (0.035 inches) was positioned in the external carotid artery using a diagnostic catheter with a 5-Fr caliber (figure 3). It remained safely in this position without colliding with the atheromatous plaque, providing a means for the catheter guide to advance over the guide until it reached the common carotid artery. The ECC technique was defined as when the guide was positioned in the common carotid artery, rather than the external carotid artery, with the help of a catheter guide contained within a diagnostic catheter. At this point, the catheter was removed, and the catheter guide reached the common carotid artery by going over the guide. The TRI technique involved using a guide catheter with a diagnostic catheter inside (the designs and materials varied for each case) and a guide (0.035 inches) placed inside the diagnostic catheter. The catheter was free to attempt several maneuvers before the catheter guide penetrated the carotid artery for the angioplasty.

After positioning the catheter guide in the common carotid artery, one of the closed filter cerebral protection systems can be extended beyond the stenosis by positioning it a few centimeters above the stenosis close to the base of the skull, preferably in a rectilinear segment open in this topography. We also observed whether the filter was adjusted to the size of the artery to avoid dislocating the filter system during the subsequent maneuvers.

"Rapid exchange" filter systems were used, which consisted of a 0.014-inch microguide with a polyurethane membrane filter with 100 to 140 μm pores (100 μm in AngioGuard® filters [Cordis], 110 μm in EPI FilterWire EPI/EZ® filters [Boston Scientific/Target], and 140 μm in EmboShield® filters [Abbott]).

All of the patients were scheduled for the primary technique (without prior dilation of the stenosis via a balloon) using a stent with an appropriate diameter (7 to 8 mm) for each case and sufficient length to cover the bulb and the entire atherosclerotic plaque distally and inferiorly (at least 1 cm).

Self-expandable stents (Carotid Wallstent®, Boston Scientific/Target; Precise®, Cordis; and Protégé®, ev3) designed for carotid use in a 0.014-inch guide system were used. Only the straight version of the Protégé® stent was used in our study.

After the stent was released, 0.5 mg of atropine was administered intravenously. After tachycardia was observed, a catheter balloon was inserted and inflated inside the stent. The angioplasty balloon had the function of shaping the stent smoothly. The same balloon size was used for all of the procedures: 6 mm in diameter and 20 mm in length (Gazele®, Boston Scietific/Target and Amiia®, Cordis). In this study, after the balloon was deflated, an immediate-control cervical angioplasty was conducted with a smooth manual injection of the contrast medium to avoid disturbing the filter and possibly mobilizing any waste that it retained.

Once control via cervical DSA at the end of the CAS was considered satisfactory (residual stenosis at a maximum of 30%), the filter was collected. Later, after the removal of the filter and the last stage of CAS, carotid angiographies for intracranial vascularization were performed in anteroposterior (AP) and profile to show that the artery subjected to CAS remained patent. Additionally, the intracranial vessels were thoroughly studied and compared with the preangioplasty angiograms to detect any macroemboli. The catheter guide was removed at the end of the CAS, leaving only the arterial introducer in the inguinal region. Heparin was not antagonized. After the CAS, the cases were monitored in the intermediate intensive care unit for 12 to 24 hours with attention to the patient's neurological state and especially his/her blood pressure.

All of the procedures were performed by an experienced neuroradiologist (with over 20 years of specialty experience) with the help of one or two residents. No patient showed any neurological or other symptoms after the CAS. The follow-up for clinical observations was the in-hospital period of four days.

The data were analyzed using several methods and logistic regression analysis. All cases were evaluated using SPSS (Version 15.0). A p-value <0.005 was considered statistically significant.

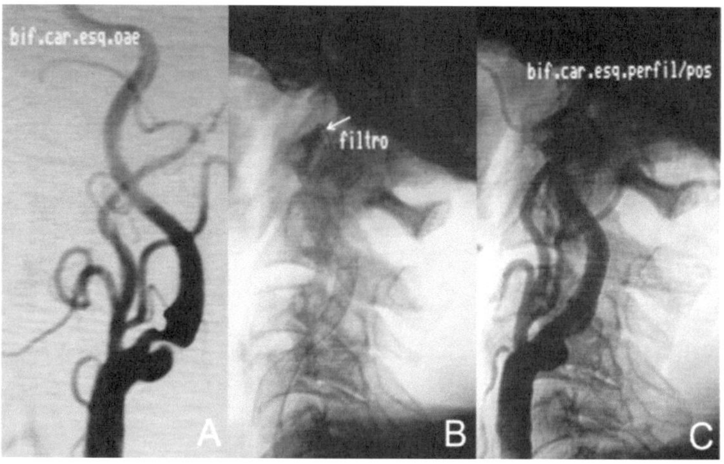

Figure 3. Patient number 2, 70 years old, male with diabetes, hypertension and coronary ischemia, displayed transient ischemic attack. . DWI exam after CAS (not shown) did not reveal micrusemboli. Angiography showed stenosis of 70% (A) in the left carotid artery with additional imaging (ulcer). EPI® open carotid filter (arrow) and Wallstent (7 x 40 mm) self-expandable stent (B). Control angiography after CAS (C)

8. Clinical and demographic data for patients before CAS

Of the 40 patients who began the study, 36 completed the protocol. Their ages varied from 54 to 87 years (average: 72.08 years).

	n (%)
n of patients	36 (100.00)
Male	25 (69.44)
Female	11 (30.56)
Right carotid artery	15 (41.67)
Left carotid artery	21 (58.33)
Symptomatic patients	27 (75.00)
Asymptomatic patients	09 (25.00)
Average age/standard deviation (years)	72.08 (±8.30)

Table 1. Distribution of demographic data for the 36 patients

Risk factors	**n (%)**
TIA	17 (47.22)
ICVA	11 (30.56)
TIA or ICVA	26 (72.22)
Arrhythmia	04 (11.11)
Ischemic coronary artery disease	09 (25.00)
Diabetes	12 (33.33)
Peripheral vascular disease	19 (52.70)
Hypercholesterolemia	12 (33.33)
Hypertension	32 (88.88)
TOTAL	116

Table 2. Distribution of risk factors (n=36 patients)

http://dx.doi.org/10.5772/57154

9. Data from the procedures and technical considerations of digital subtraction angiography and carotid angioplasty with a stent

Degree of stenosis[1] – average (variation)	76.31% (60-99%)
Ulcerated plaques – n (%)	14 (38.89%)
Contralateral carotid occlusion – n (%)	7 (17.95%)
"Broad" examn (%)	24 (66.67%)
"Brief" examn (%)	12 (33.33%)
Filter – n (%): Angioguard®	4 (11.11%)
Emboshield®	7 (19.44%)
EPI®	25 (69.44%)
Stent – n (%): Precise®	9 (25.00%)
Protégé®	5 (13.89%)
Wallstent®	22 (61.11%)
Catheterization technique – n Direct access	12
Exchange in the external carotid artery	10
Exchange in the common carotid artery	11
Triaxial	08
Fluoroscopy time (minutes; average)	665; 22.93 min/CAS[2]
N of catheters used (n; average)	83; 2.31 cat/patient
Contrast volume (milliliters; average)	5480 ml; 182.67 ml/CAS[3]
Vessels submitted to DSA (n; average)	106; average 2.94

[1] Percentage of stenosis evaluated by angiography

[2] Regarding fluoroscopy time, only 29 procedures were recorded (n=29). In seven patients, there were technical problems that prevented precise measurement.

[3] For contrast volume, only 30 procedures were recorded (n=30). In six patients, there were technical problems that prevented precise measurement.

Table 3. Technical aspects and characteristics of the angiographic exams (n=36)

10. Imaging results

10.1. Aspects of MRI before the CAS

The preliminary MRI study before CAS showed six restriction foci in diffusion in four (11.11%) patients (Table 4 and Figure 4). These foci were not recorded as NF after CAS.

	n (%) patients
Infarctions in T2	23 (63.9)
Foci of restriction in DWI (1ª MR)	4 (11.1)

Table 4. MRI data before CAS (n = 36)

Among the restriction foci in DWI before CAS, five out of six (83.33%) were ipsilateral to the carotid artery for CAS, and only one focus was not ipsilateral to the carotid that was treated (cerebellum). All hypersignal foci in DWI before CAS occurred in patients with symptomatic stenosis.

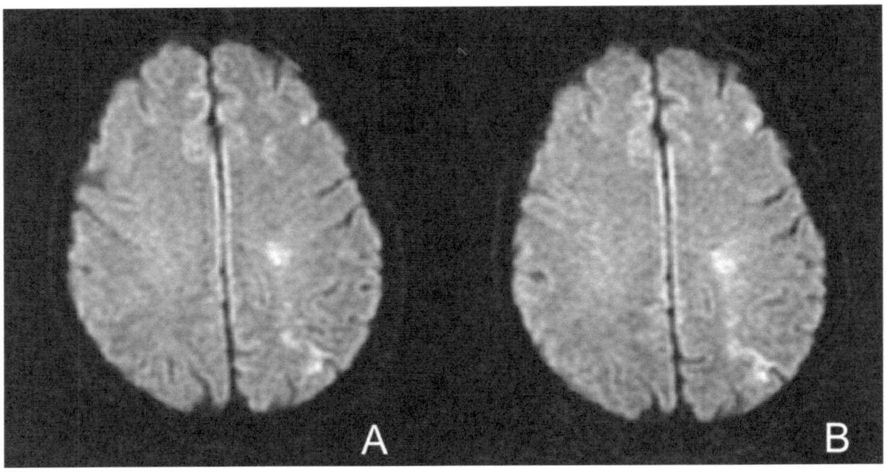

Figure 4. Patient number 7, male, 60 years old, underwent angioplasty of the left carotid artery. Restriction foci in DWI in the MRI scan before CAS (A). Manifestation found in 11.11% of patients. No NF were observed after CAS (B)

11. Aspects of MRI after CAS

There were no new areas of cerebral infarction after CAS in the analysis of conventional MRI sequences.

A comparison between the MRI diffusion sequences acquired before and after angioplasty showed 59 NF of restriction compatible with cerebral ischemia, which were distributed in 18/36 (50%) patients (Figures 5 and 6). The average NF in the 36 patients was 1.6 NF/patient (Table 5), and the diameter varied between 1 and 25 mm.

NF number	59 (18 patients)
NF size - n (%)	
<5 mm	35 (59.33)
5 – 10 mm	19 (32.21)
>10 mm	05 (8.46)
Vascular distribution (NF[1]) - n (%)	
Ipsilateral	44 (77.19)
Contralateral	13 (22.81)

pt – patient

[1] Two patients were excluded from the analysis of laterality

Table 5. Characteristics of new foci (NF) of hypersignal in DWI after angioplasty of the carotid artery

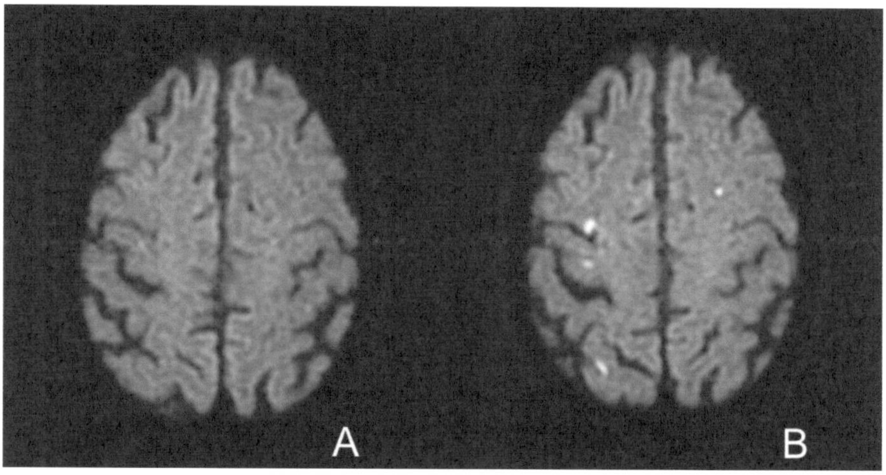

Figure 5. Patient number 9, 59 years old, underwent right CAS. DWI before CAS (A) without images of restriction. After CAS (B): ipsilateral NF (including primary motor rotation) and contralateral NF. Asymptomatic patient.

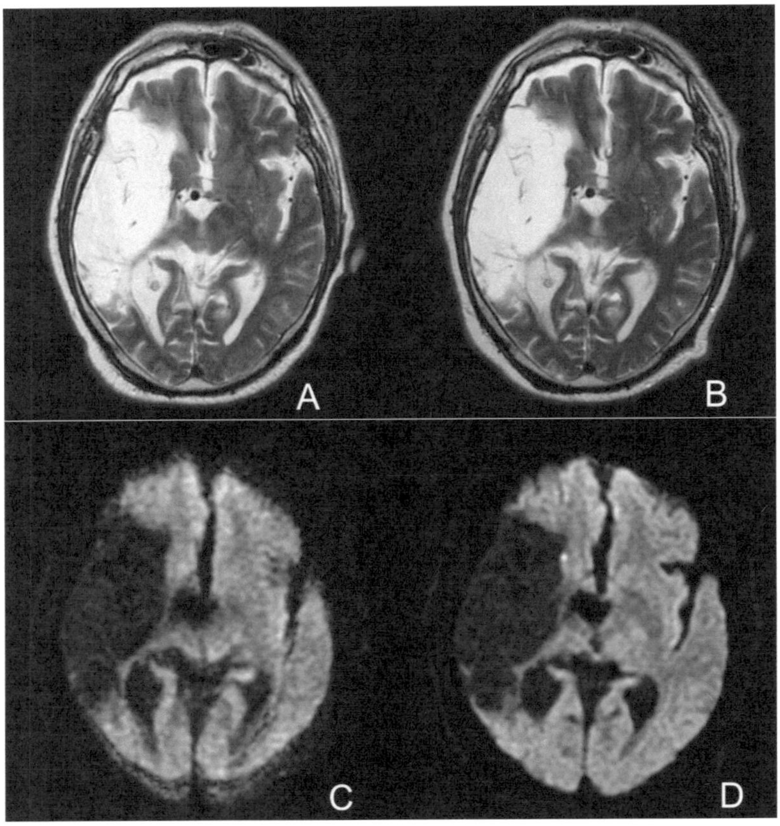

Figure 6. Patient 27, male, 73 years old with right carotid artery occlusion and stenosis of the left carotid artery estimated at 70% by DSA (not shown). Before CAS: T2 sequence (A) shows old infarction in the territory of the right MCA and diffusion sequence (C) without recent ischemia foci. The patient underwent DSA of both common carotid arteries and CAS of the left. In the MRI study, the T2 sequence was unchanged after CAS (B) and the DWI sequence showed NF in the head of the caudate nucleus to the right (D)

Laterality of NF	% of NF	n of NF	Average[2]	P
IP	77.19	44	2.75	
CL	22.81	13	0.81	0.063
Total	100.00	57	3.56	

CL – NF contralateral to the area for CAS; IP – NF ipsilateral to the area for CAS

[1] Two patients were excluded from the analysis of laterality.

[2] NF/patients

Wilcoxon test

Table 6. Number and average of NF by laterality (n=16 patients[1])

Presentation of NF per patient	n of NF	n of pt	Average (NF/pt)	SD	p
Single NF (1 nf/ pt)	9	9	1.00	0.00	
Multiple NF (≥2 nf/pt)	50	9	5.56	3.43	<0,001
TOTAL	59	18			

pt – patient

Mann-Whitney U test

Table 7. Distribution of NF (single or multiple)

Laterality	Number of patients	% of patients
IP pure	5	14.71
CL pure	5	14.71
Intersection (IP+CL in the same patient)	6	17.65

IP pure + intersection (IP+CL in the same patient)=11 patients=32.35%

IP pure: patients with only ipsilateral NF; CL pure: patients with only contralateral NF

[1] Two patients were excluded from the analysis of laterality.

No statistical test

Table 8. Distribution of NF based on laterality per patient (n=34 patients[1])

Laterality by patient	n of NF	Average[2]	p
IP pure	14 NF	2.80	
CL pure	5 NF	1.00	0.053
Bilateral	38 NF	6.33	

IP pure: patients with only ipsilateral NF; CL pure: patients with only contralateral NF; Bilateral: patients with both ipsilateral and contralateral NF

[1] Two patients were excluded from the analysis of laterality.

[2] NF per case

Kruskal-Wallis test

Table 9. Number and average of NF according to laterality per patient (n=34 patients[1])

NF after CAS	Average age (years)	SD	p
Without NF	71.83	9.03	
With NF	72.33	7.75	0.855

Mann-Whitney U test

Table 10. Average and standard deviation of age in the groups with and without NF in the DWI after CAS.

Factor	NF				p
	No		Yes		
	n	%	n	%	
AGE (years)					
<75	8	44.4	7	38.9	
≥75	10	55.6	11	61.1	0.855
TOTAL	18	100.0	18	100.0	
GENDER					
Male	15	83.3	10	55.6	
Female	3	16.7	8	44.4	0.080
TOTAL	18	100.0	18	100.0	
CAROTID ARTERY					
Right	8	44.4	7	38.9	
Left	10	55.6	11	61.1	0.735
TOTAL	18	100.0	18	100.0	

Logistic regression analysis

Table 11. Distribution of age, gender, and side of the carotid artery treated based on the appearance of NF in the DWI after CAS.

	NF				p
	Yes		No		
	n factors	SD[2]	n factors	SD[2]	
Risk factors[1](n=116)	60	1.75	56	1.18	
	n of patients	Average (NF/pt[3])	n patients	Average (NF/pt[3])	
Patients (n=36)	18	3.33	18	3.11	0.743

[1] Risk factors for atherosclerosis/ICVA

[2] Standard deviation for risk factors

[3] Patient

Mann-Whitney U test

Table 12. Correlation of all risk factors with NF after CAS

http://dx.doi.org/10.5772/57154

Risk factors	NF				p
	No		Yes		
	N	%	n	%	
TIA	8	44.44	9	50.00	0.800
ICVA	4	22.22	7	38.89	0.612
ICVA or TIA	12	66.67	14	77.78	0.845
ARR	2	11.11	2	11.11	1.000
COL	8	44.44	4	22.22	0.164
COR	4	22.22	5	27.78	0.701
DM	5	27.78	7	38.89	0.481
PVD	10	55.56	9	50.00	0.738
HBP	15	83.33	17	94.44	0.311

TIA: transient ischemic attack; ICVA: ischemic cerebral vascular accident; TIA or ICVA: cases with at least one ischemic condition; ARR: arrhythmia; COL: hypercholesterolemia; COR: ischemic coronary artery disease; DM: diabetes; PVD: peripheral vascular disease; HBP: high blood pressure

Logistic regression analysis

Table 13. Distribution of risk factors in relation to the appearance of NF after CAS

	NF				p
	No		Yes		
Patients	**n of pt[1]**	**% pt**	**n of pt**	**% pt**	
Asymptomatic (n=9)	7	77.8%	2	22.2%	
Symptomatic (n=27)	11	40.7%	16	59.26%	0.121

[1] Patient

Chi-squared test

Table 14. Occurrence of NF based on the presence of symptoms before CAS

Clinical status of the patient before CAS	n of NF	% of NF	p
Asymptomatic	11	18.6	
Symptomatic	48	81.4	0.263
TOTAL	59	100.0	

Mann-Whitney U test

Table 15. Correlation between the presence of carotid disease symptoms before the procedure and the number of NF after CAS

Infarct in T2	NF				p
	No		Yes		
	n pt[1]	%[2]	n pt	%	
Without	10	55.6	3	16.7	
With	8	44.4	15	83.3	0.037
TOTAL	18	100.0	18	100.0	

[1] Patient

[2] Percentage of patients in the group with NF (n=18)

Logistic regression analysis

Table 16. Distribution of NF according to the presence of previous cerebral infarct (in T2) in the first MRI

Infarct in T2	n of NF	%[1]	n of pt[2]	Average[3]	SD[4]	p
Without	3	5.08	13	0.23	0.44	
With	56	94.92	23	2.43	3.31	0.011
TOTAL	59	100.0				

[1] Percentage related to the complete NF group (n=59)

[2] Number of patients with cerebral infarct images on the initial MRI

[3] NF/patient

[4] Standard deviation

Mann-Whitney U test

Table 17. Distribution of the number of NF (after CAS) based on the presence of previous cerebral infarcts in T2 in the first MRI

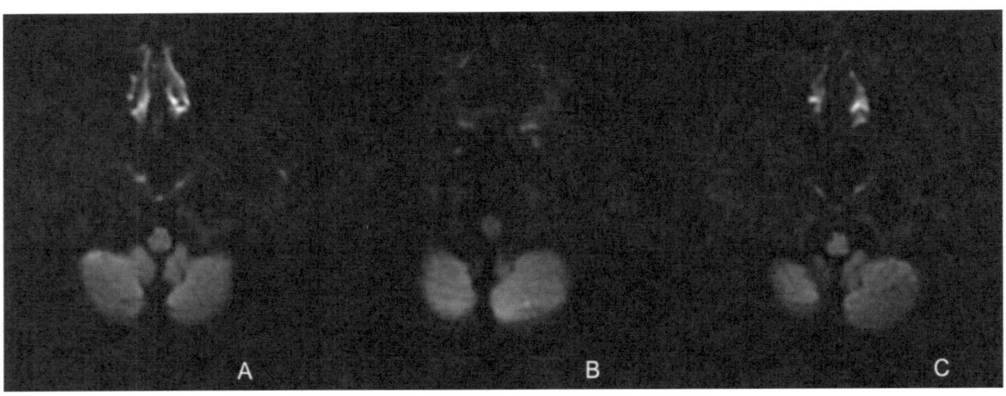

Figure 7. Patient number 19, 81 years old with bilateral stenosis in the carotid arteries. A DSA was performed in the aortic arch, common carotid arteries, left subclavian artery, and brachiocephalic trunk before the CAS of the left carotid artery. Diffusion study before the DSA and angioplasty (A). After DSA and CAS, an NF was identified in the DWI in the left hemisphere of the cerebellum (B). A new MRI performed 40 days after the CAS (not as part of the study protocol) showed the absence of lesions in the DWI (C) and in T2 (not shown).

One patient (Number 19) showed one NF in the cerebellum after angioplasty of the left carotid artery (Figure 7). Forty days later, the same patient was admitted for an angioplasty of the right carotid artery. Another MRI was performed at this opportunity (not as part of the research protocol), and it did not show diffusion lesions in the infarct area in T2 or in the enhancement, which is common for subacute cerebral infarctions.

12. Aspects of angiography and angioplasty

NF	N	Average	P
Yes	18	73.83	
No	18	78.78	0.239

Mann-Whitney U test

Table 18. Average degree of stenosis in the groups with and without NF after CAS

	NF				p
	No		Yes		
	N	%	N	%	
Ulcers	7	38.89	7	38.89	1.000

Logistic regression analysis

Table 19. Presence of ulcers and appearance of NF after CAS

	Occlusion of contralateral carotid artery				
NF	Yes		No		p
	N	%	n	%	
Yes	3	16.66	15	83.33	
No	4	22.22	14	77.77	0.674

Chi-squared test

Table 20. Distribution of NF according to the presence of contralateral carotid occlusion.

NF	Total time (min)	Average (min)	SD (min)	p
Without (n=14)	323	23.07	10.48	
With (n=15)	342	22.80	8.59	0.880

min: minute

Mann-Whitney U test

Table 21. Correlation of fluoroscopy time with NF after CAS

NF	Volume (ml)	Average (ml)	SD (ml)	p
Without (n=16)	2910	181.88	73.50	
With (n=14)	2570	183.57	54.01	0.918

ml: milliliter

Mann-Whitney U test

Table 22. Correlation of contrast volume used in the CAS and the appearance of NF after CAS

Patients	n of catheters[1]	Average[2]	p
Without NF	43	2.39	
With NF	40	2.22	0.462

[1] Total number of catheters used in each group

[2] Average catheter/patient

Mann-Whitney U test

Table 23. Number and average of catheters used in the CAS according to the presence of NF in the final MRI

Patients	n of vessels undergoing DSA	Average[1]	p
With NF	56	3.11	
Without NF	50	2.78	0.628

[1] Vessels subjected to angiography per patient

Mann-Whitney U test

Table 24. Number and average of vessels subjected to DSA according to the presence of NF after CAS

Arteries submitted to angiography	NF				p
	No (n=18)		Yes (n=18)		
	n	%	n	%	
RCCA	13	72.22	16	88.89	0.220
RSUB[1]	4	22.22	2	11.11	0.379
BAT	6	33.33	9	50.00	0.313
ARCH	4	22.22	5	27.78	0.701
LSUB[2]	8	44.44	10	55.56	0.506
LCCA	15	83.33	14	77.78	0.675

RCCA: right common carotid artery; LCCA: left common carotid artery; ARCH: aortic arch; RSUB: right subclavian artery; LSUB: left subclavian artery; BAT: brachiocephalic arterial trunk

[1] RSUB includes angiography of the ipsilateral vertebral artery

[2] LSUB includes angiography of the ipsilateral vertebral artery

Logistic regression analysis

Table 25. Number and percentage of each vessel subjected to DSA and the appearance of NF after CAS

Type of exam (n=36)	NF				p
	No		Yes		
	n of pt	% of exams	n of pt	% of exams	
"Brief" (n=12)	7	58.33	5	41.67	
"Broad" (n=24)	11	45.83	13	54.17	0.480

pt: patients

Logistic regression analysis

Table 26. Type of angiographic exam used and the appearance of NF after CAS

Technique used to access carotid	Catheterization techniques				p
	Without NF		With NF		
	n[1]	%[2]	n[1]	%[2]	
DA	6	50.00	6	50.00	1.000
ECC	5	50.00	5	50.00	1.000
EEC	4	36.37	7	63.64	0.283
TRI	6	75.00	2	25.00	0.124

DA: direct access; ECC: exchange in the common carotid artery; EEC: exchange in the external carotid artery; TRI: triaxial

[1] Number of times that each technique is used in the group with and without NF

[2] Percentage of access technique

Logistic regression analysis

Table 27. Correlation of catheterization techniques with NF after CAS

Brand of stent	NF				p
	No		Yes		
	n	%[1]	n	%[1]	
Precise®	4	44.45	5	55.56	
Protégé®	2	40.00	3	60.00	
Wallstent®	12	54.55	10	45.45	0.493

[1] Stent/brand

Chi-squared

Table 28. Correlation of types of stent with NF after CAS

Stent brand	n of stents with NF IP	NF IP	Average[1]	p
Precise®	9	18	2.00	
Protégé®	5	5	1.00	0.245
Wallstent®	20	21	1.05	

IP: ipsilateral

[1] NF IP/stent

NOTE: In this data analysis, CASs with NF outside the area where the stent was implanted were excluded.

Kruskal-Wallis test

Table 29. Correlation of stent brands with NF after CAS considering only the side where the stent was implanted

Stent design	n of stent with NF IP	NF IP	Average[2]	p
Closed cell	20	21	1.05	
Open cell	14	23	1.77	0.128

IP: ipsilateral

In this aggregation of the elements, CASs with NF outside the area where the stent was implanted were excluded

[1] Two patients were excluded from the analysis of laterality.

[2] NF IP/stent

Mann-Whitney U test

NOTE: Open-cell stent: Wallstent®; closed-cell stents: Precise® and Protégé®

Table 30. Correlation of stent designs with NF after CAS considering only the side where the stent was implanted (n=34 patients[1])

Filter brand	NF				p
	No		Yes		
	n	%	n	%	
Angioguard®	2	50.00	2	50.00	
Emboshield®	2	28.57	5	71.43	0.367
EPI®	14	56.00	11	44.00	

Chi-squared test

NOTE: 100 μm pores in AngioGuard®, 110 μm in EPI FilterWire EZ®, and 140 μm in EmboShield®

In this series, there was not a case in which excess thrombus or atheroma plaque materials determined acute occlusion of the filter during the CAS.

Table 31. Occurrence of NF based on filter brand (n=36)

Filter brand	n of uses	NF IP[2]	Average[3]	p
Angioguard®	4	9	2.250	
Emboshield®	6	12	2.000	
EPI®	24	23	0.958	0.582

[1] Two patients were excluded from the analysis of laterality.

[2] NF ipsilateral

[3] NFIP/filter brand

Kruskal-Wallis test

NOTE: 100 μm pores in AngioGuard®, 110 μm in EPI FilterWire EZ®, and 140 μm in EmboShield®

Table 32. Distribution of NF ipsilateral to the use of the filter, considering the different models (n=34 filters[1])

Filter design	n of uses	NF IP[2]	Average[3]	p
Eccentric	24	23	0.958	
Concentric	10	21	2.100	0.515

[1] Two patients were excluded from the analysis of laterality.

[2] NF ipsilateral

[3] NF IP/filter system protection design

NOTE: Eccentric, EPI®; Concentric, Angioguard® and Emboshield®

Mann-Whitney U test

Table 33. Distribution of NF ipsilateral to the use of the filters, considering filter design (n=34 filters[1])

In summary, our DWI MRI study after CAS found that 50.00% of patients showed NF of restriction/ischemia in DWI after CAS. All of the NF were clinically silent (100%). These NF were located in a cerebral area fed by the cerebral artery subjected to CAS in 77.19% of patients and an area smaller than 10 mm in 91.53% of patients. The NF in cerebral areas not fed by the cerebral artery undergoing angioplasty corresponded to 22.81% of NFs. The presence of previous cerebral infarcts on the MRI influenced the appearance of NF (p=0.037).

13. Discussion

13.1. Aspects of MRI imaging before CAS

The MRI scan before CAS showed great variety in the changes in the 36 patients, with special attention to ischemic aspects. We found four (11.1%) patients with hypersignal foci (a total of six foci) in the DWI MRI before CAS. These foci are considered recent ischemia foci, and they are not reported as NF involved with CAS, although most remained after treatment. This rate is similar to that reported by Jaeger et al. [56] In a study involving 70 CAS, the authors discovered hypersignal lesions in diffusion before CAS in 10 (14%) of the patients, with a total of 24 foci [56]. Images of ischemia in DWI were detected in 10 (19%) patients before CAS by Hammer et al. [61]. Hammer et al. [61] suggested that recent ischemia foci presented by some patients on the initial MRI indicate the relevance of performing an MRI scan before CAS to guarantee that any foci in the MRI after CAS are related to the procedure.

Piñero et al. [48] found lesions in the DWI ipsilateral to the carotid artery undergoing CAS in 11% of the patients. In our data, 88.33% of the lesions found in the DWI before the CAS were ipsilateral to the carotid artery treated. This result supports the idea that these plaques are constantly forming emboli that can be sent to the brain.

Our data showed that carotid atherosclerotic plaques are probable causes of hypersignal lesions in DWI before CAS and can be considered causes of ischemia symptoms. This finding is corroborated by the fact that most patients were symptomatic (75.0%). Most of the patients (63.9%) showed old cerebral infarcts in the T2 sequence of the MRI before CAS. In our series, a strong correlation between the rates of old infarcts and positive symptoms was found (75.0%).

13.2. Diffusion MRI study after CAS

According to Bates et al. [13], while the primary purpose of revascularizing the carotid artery is preventing cerebral infarction, current treatments, both CAS and endarterectomy, carry a risk of triggering brain infarction.

All interventional procedures performed in craniofacial vascular regions carry an inherent risk of causing embolisms to the brain with different levels of severity. In these cases, the diffusion MRI technique is the most efficient tool for detecting acute focal cerebral ischemia [46,71,72].

Angioplasty is certainly the interventional procedure in the craniofacial region that carries the greatest risk of embolism. This risk is well documented in various studies and varies greatly among the different groups that it effects [35,37,73].

The institution wherein the present study was conducted published data pertaining to 1,037 carotid angioplasties with stent implantation and cerebral protection in 2006. The incidence of disabling neurological complications and death was 2.2% [38]. Despite the low morbi-mortality of the method, the real incidence of embolism is not known because the patients remained asymptomatic.

We found restriction foci in the diffusion MRIs of 18 of the 36 (50%) patients in our series. These NF in the DWI after CAS are additional to those in the first MRI, which implies that the procedure or some aspect of it is related to the appearance of NF. The fact that all of the patients in this series were asymptomatic after CAS and remained so during the intrahospital observation period should also be taken into account.

The percentage of patients with NF in DWI in similar studies is quite variable: 9 to 78% (9% [74]; 15.8% [71]; 17.3% [48]; 20.4% [75]; 29% [56]; 30% [36]; 40% [61]; 41.5% [73]; 42% [46]; 42.6% [69]; 43% [59]; 49% [34]; 52% [35], 54% [58], 59.2% [76]; 9 and 78% [77]; 70% [70]).

The comparison of different studies is very difficult because even a small variation in the period after the CAS during which DWI was conducted might affect the result. In the study by Rapp et al. [77], a total of 23 patients underwent two MRI exams after the CAS. The first MRI scan was performed immediately after the procedure (1 to 2 h) and the second exam was performed 48 h later. The results indicated only two (9%) cases with NF in the DWI immediately after the procedure and 18 (78%) cases with NF 48 h later [77]. In a recent meta-analysis that included studies that followed the evolution of CAS by DWI (1,363 CAS), NF were found in 37% of patients [37].

The study that is most similar to ours is Kastrup et al. (2006); this study found microembolia in 49% of patients with cerebral protection. Two years later, the authors updated their series and published that NF occurred after CAS with a cerebral protection filter in 52% of patients [35].

du Mesnil de Rochemont et al. [46] found NF in 42% of CAS and, similar to our study, found no neurological deficit. In addition to this study, several others [35,37,48,61,69,73] have found that most patients remained asymptomatic after CAS, despite the presence of NF. These findings encouraged us to look for factors that lead to ischemic changes.

Jaeger et al. [56] demonstrated that smaller NF are less likely to become definitive lesions. His study showed that of the 59 restriction foci in the diffusion after CAS, only 17 (29%) were observed in the T2 sequence. They found that 17% of the lesions smaller than 5 mm in the DWI were visible in T2; 36% of the lesions in DWI between 5 and 10 mm were observed in T2, and 100% of the larger lesions (larger than 10 mm) were apparent in T2 [56]. As in Tedesco et al. [70], we considered the hypersignal images in T2 as already defined and permanent ischemia foci, unlike the lesions in DWI, which may be reversible.

In a series of 59 CASs, Jaeger et al. [56] found that 75% of NF were smaller than 5 mm; in the series by Piñero [48], the lesions were smaller than 5 mm in 57% of patients. However, in a series of 22 CASs in Roh et al. [78], all of the NF were smaller than 10 mm. In our study, small NF (<10 mm) corresponded to a large majority (91.53%) of the NF, while large NF (>10 mm) composed only 8.46% of the NF; this result shows that the eventual emboli caused by the procedure are small in size.

According to several authors, some lesions in DWI after CAS also occur in vascular regions independent from the CAS and are most likely related to the catheterization procedure [35,37,61,73]. Our data showed that most (77.19%) of the NF occurred in the region of the carotid artery that underwent angioplasty. However, a significant difference was not observed between the side of the CAS and the contralateral side in relation to NF.

In the publication by Piñero et al. [48], 67.9% of the NF were in the vascular area compatible with the CAS. However, Hammer et al. [61] found a similar number by studying 53 carotid angioplasties: 60% of the NF were in an ipsilateral situation to CAS and 40% occurred in contralateral topography.

By studying carotid angioplasty, Poppert et al. [58found NF in DWI in area of contralateral carotid or vertebral artery in 9.7% of patients. Poppert et al. [58] stated that during catheterization, to reach the right internal carotid artery, the materials must pass the aortic arch at the origin of other cerebral arterial trunks, such as the common carotid artery and left subclavian artery, in addition to the brachiocephalic trunk next to the right vertebral artery. Thus, material from plaques along this route can cause emboli in various brain regions beyond the area nourished by the carotid artery undergoing CAS [58].

Maleux et al. [73] described their surprise at finding that 35.3% of the NF (26.3% in contralateral anterior circulation and 9% in the cerebellum) occurred in regions not nourished by the carotid artery ipsilateral to the CAS. They considered the manipulation of the guide wire, catheter, or guide catheter in the aortic arch as a possible cause of the lesions [73].

A meta-analysis with data collected from CAS studies between 2000 and 2007 found lesions in diffusion in 14.5% of CAS outside the region treated, and NF were observed in 35% of the procedures in the region of the carotid artery treated by CAS [37]. Thus, catheterization was one of the main causes of the microemboli.

In our study, half of the patients with NF had a single lesion (single NF), and the other half showed multiple foci (varying from 2 to 11 NF), which totaled 50 NF. Thus, patients with multiple NF accounted for 84.75% of the NFs found in diffusion. Our study reproduced the finding of Piñero et al. [48]. These studies found a single focus in DWI in 53.6% of patients, and multiple foci were found in 46.4% of the patients in diffusion after CAS [48].

In our study, we found five patients who showed ipsilateral NF, five patients who showed contralateral NF, and another six who showed ipsilateral and contralateral NF simultaneously. Thus, the ipsilateral situation was the main localization of the NF occurrence in absolute terms, but the most common presentation was associated to the contralateral NF than isolated. A similar distribution of laterality was found in a retrospective study by Tedesco et al. [70] of 27 CAS. Similar numbers were also observed by Hammer et al. [61], who, in a series of CAS under cerebral protection, found eight cases with only ipsilateral NF, seven cases with exclusively contralateral NF, and six cases with a combination of ipsilateral and contralateral NF. According to these authors, these events can be related to the doctor's skill in catheterizing the aortic arch and the supra-aortic trunks and to the prevention of emboli formation beyond the collateral circulation by the Willis polygon or other routes [61].

When patients with NF in an area other than the carotid artery for angioplasty are excluded (i.e., emboli resulting from catheterization), our risk of cerebral embolism from angioplasty alone is reduced from 50.00% (18 patients) to 32.35% (11 patients).

du Mesnil de Rochemont et al. [46] found an average of one NF per patient in the ipsilateral area, while Jaeger et al. found that the average number of NF ipsilateral to the CAS was 2.6 per patient and that the average number of NF contralateral to the CAS was 1.2 per patient [56]. In our study, the average number of ipsilateral NF was 2.8 per patient, and the average number of contralateral NF was 1.0 per patient.

The highest mean (6.33) NF per patient was for the presentation of ipsilateral and contralateral NF simultaneously. This finding justifies the idea that the initial angiography or the catheterization technique and the CAS are involved in the high average number of bilateral NF.

Our average number of NF per patient, which was higher than that reported by most authors, may reflect the fact that most (66.7%) of our cases underwent a broad diagnostic exam before the angioplasty. Thus, the hypothesis can be applied that, because most of the cases had bilateral NF, these NF were more likely related to the catheterization than to the angioplasty itself.

Because of the risk of embolism during angiographic exams (diagnostic) and in interventional procedures such as CAS, we believe that the exams should be performed by certified and experienced neuroradiologists only. This statement is supported by other authors [71,79].

Moreover, modern noninvasive methods can be used with good reproducibility in some centers, allowing a definition of the anatomy, degree of stenosis, and intracranial circulation, which enables decisions about the CAS to be made without the use of a broad angiography before the CAS.

Several other authors [8,48,56,58,71,80-82] studied risk factors for the occurrence of atherosclerotic disease and ICVA, including diabetes, hypertension, coronary artery disease, ischemic peripheral vascular disease, hypercholesterolemia, arrhythmia, previous ischemic stroke, previous TIA, vasculitis, and hemorrhagic cerebrovascular accident. Most authors did not find significant differences related to the appearance of hypersignal foci in DWI. Some authors found some relevant factors, but those were not confirmed by other authors.

Clinical risk factors were not significant determinants of the formation of NF after CAS in our study. The only risk factor statistically proven to be involved in the creation of lesions in DWI after CAS was a radiological factor: old cerebral infarcts shown on MRI images, especially in T2W.

Our study found a tendency toward a greater number of NF in older patients (≥75 years) and those who underwent angioplasty of the left carotid artery. Hammer et al. [61] identified a tendency for NF to be found in patients with advanced age (>75 years); however, as in our study, they failed to prove it statistically ($p=0.1$).

du Mesnil de Rochemont et al. [46] confirmed this trend by finding that age above 70 years old was a predictor for the occurrence of foci in diffusion, and they wondered whether this finding could be related to the fact that more elderly patients have more diffuse atherosclerosis compared with younger patients. These authors did not find a significant correlation for factors such as gender, degree of stenosis, type of stent, type of filter, and risk factors, such as hypertension, diabetes, smoking, hypercholesterolemia, coronary heart disease, and peripheral arterial occlusive disease [46].

Generally, our group without NF showed fewer risk factors (56 factors) than the group with NF after CAS did (60 factors). While not significant, the difference shows a tendency that the more comorbidities the patient has, the greater his or her risk of developing NF in a CAS. The difference was also not significant for the clinical conditions of previous ischemic cerebrovascular accident and transient ischemia attack. Similarly, for the risk factor of cerebral ischemia, which was associated with both TIA and ICVA, the difference was also not significant.

In our group (n=36), which was characterized by advanced age (average of 72 years), serious stenosis (average narrowing of 76.31%) and symptoms of previous ischemic conditions in most patients (72.22%), the subgroup of previously asymptomatic patients showed a lower risk of NF: only 18.6% of the observed NF. Moreover, a large majority, 48/59 (81.4%) of the NF occurred in symptomatic patients. Despite this tendency, there was not a significant difference. Hammer et al. [61], in a series of 53 CAS, identified a tendency to find NF in symptomatic patients, although no statistical proof was found.

According to Kastrup et al. [35], it is conceivable that the high prevalence of active plaques with thrombotic activity in recently symptomatic patients may determine the high rate of NF in this group. When our patients are regrouped into asymptomatic (9 patients) and symptomatic (27 patients) groups to evaluate the interference of previous symptoms with the occurrence of NF, the hypothesis is confirmed. The asymptomatic patients did not develop NF in most (77.8%) of the CAS cases, while the symptomatic patients showed NF in most cases (59.3%). Again, the analysis did not prove a significant difference ($p=0.121$), but it confirms the tendency for symptomatic patients to be at greater risk in the procedure. Piñero et al. [48] also showed an increased risk of embolism in angioplasty for symptomatic patients in their series (19.8%) compared to asymptomatic patients (10%; $p = 0.155$). This ratio is approximately 2:1, while ours was approximately 2.7:1.

We found a significant difference in the NF lesions in DWI after CAS in patients with previous infarcts (based on the T2 sequence) compared with those without. Cerebral infarct was present in 63.9% of patients in our entire series. It was observed that most (83.3%) of the patients with NF after CAS showed cerebral infarcts on the MRI before the CAS. Nonetheless, the patients who did not show cerebral infarcts on the MRI before the CAS mostly evolved (55.6%) without NF in the DWI after CAS ($p=0.037$). Again, the average number of NF varies enormously in relation to whether the patient had or not a previous infarct on T2 (initial MRI). The average NF in the group with a previous cerebral infarct was 2.43 NF/patient, while the average in the group without a previous infarct was only 0.23 NF/patient ($p=0.011$).

This association makes it clear that a definitive ischemic lesion in imaging (in T2W) is a great risk factor for developing microembolic complications during carotid angioplasty. Thus, the patients who have infarcts caused by embolism or other factors are the same patients who present NF after CAS. Additionally, the tendency for symptomatic patients (who do not necessarily always present infarcts on MRI) to exhibit more NF after CAS indicates that the main cause of microemboli during CAS may be the patients' condition, including the plaque composition, risk factors, and how the atherosclerosis presents in their bodies. It is possible that the NF are signs of the underlying disease, and they may be exacerbated during CAS. Our idea about the vulnerability of plaque is shared by Piñero at al. [71], who evaluated the composition of the material found in the filters after CAS and stated that the atheromatous plaque and the vessel wall are the main sources of microemboli during CAS.

Despite several publications on signs compatible with microemboli after CAS and CEA, no consensus can be found among authors regarding the real clinical representation of NF. According to some authors [62,69], the clinical value of NF after CAS is not adequately clear. In our study, although 50% of patients showed foci compatible with ischemia in the diffusion after angioplasty, none showed ischemic neurological syndrome. Some published series have obtained a similar result, meaning most patients with NF after CAS were asymptomatic [46,54].

While the brain shows some tolerance for microemboli [83,84], the fact that subclinical deficits promoted in the NF areas after CAS may cause long-term neurological deterioration cannot be neglected. Long-term studies on cognitive function are needed.

The clinical impact of these clinically "silent" lesions in the brain that do not cause motor, sensory, or linguistic deficits (i.e., in non-eloquent brain areas) was debated by Bendszus [63, 80]. According to these authors, there is evidence that the cumulative load of ischemic brain injury can cause neuropsychological deficits or aggravate vascular dementia.

However, the discrepancy between the clinical safety of CAS and the number of NF of ischemia is intriguing. It is known that there can be TIA abnormalities in DWI that undergo regression and do not cause lesions that remain as ischemic scares in T2. Despite the normalization of DWI after TIA, structural damage caused by late neuronal apoptosis may be present, even in the absence of tissue necrosis [63]. For these authors, DWI shows the entire picture of emboli during different procedures, and the ischemic conditions are only the visible tip of the iceberg [63].

Studying the DWI sequence in patients with clinical conditions of TIA, Kidwell et al. showed that in five of nine patients with ischemia foci in DWI after TIA, no evidence of infarcts was found in follow-up imaging scans, indicating that almost half of the lesions from DWI in TIA may be completely reversible on imaging [85]. Thus, we most likely overestimate the true incidence of cerebral ischemic lesion after CAS when we base it only on DWI of MRI.

Although not part of research protocol, an MRI scan was conducted 40 days after CAS in a patient who showed NF in the MRI after CAS. The third MRI scan did not show ischemic lesions in the DWI or in T2. Thus, the NF indicated in the MRI after CAS proved evanescent (like short-lived). This suggests that small lesions in the DWI that occur after CAS and are clinically silent may not be definitive ischemic lesions.

Similarly, a small study (seven patients) from Schlüter et al. [86] identified reversal on imaging in 76% (5/21) of the NF after CAS at an average MRI follow-up four months later. A recent study showed that 92.1% of the signs of microemboli disappeared and that 5.2% remained in an MRI study three months after the CAS [72]. Thus, the NF after CAS are potentially reversible on imaging and without neurological developments [60,75,86].

Some authors [69,87] correlated the neurological deficits after CAS with the diameter of the foci of ischemia in the DWI. Small lesions were associated with good clinical evaluation. Small NF (>5 mm) were reported as having the highest chance of not becoming definitive ischemic lesions in later MRI scans compared with NF larger than 5 mm [75]. In addition to the size of the foci in DWI, the topography may also determine whether the lesion will be clinically silent or not [56,71].

For Piñero et al. [48], the position of the lesions in the diffusion was predominantly cortical and subcortical in 67.9%.The study by Jaeger et al. showed that 95% of the NF had a cortical/subcortical localization, mainly in the area of the ACA and MCA. Jaeger et al. considered this distribution to be more compatible with standard cerebral embolism than with types of cerebral ischemia [56].

Similar to Piñero et al. [48] and Jaeger et al. [56], the predominant pattern of the NF in our study were lesions with small diameters and apparently random distribution. This finding is compatible with the topography of the distal arteries, including the cortical and subcortical vessels and perforating branches. There was also no predominance in border ("watershed") areas of vascularization.

Although we found NF in various areas, such as the motor cortex and basal ganglia, the patients presented no clinical deficit during the hospitalization period. It may be that because the NF had a small volume, they were less relevant for clinical lesions due to collateral circulation, despite being in eloquent area. Nonetheless, improvement in cerebral perfusion was shown after CAS in publications by Tavares and Caldas and may counterbalance clinical damage resulting from microemboli that occur after CAS [68,88,89].

13.3. Aspects of angiography, angioplasty, and cerebral protection

In addition to maintaining a constant flow to the brain in all phases of CAS, cerebral protection with a filter is likely to be used in all cases (unlike the occlusive balloon technique, which is reserved for patients who are candidates for temporary carotid occlusion) [42]. Other limitations of techniques that use balloon for cerebral protection include severe tortuosity of the cervical and thoracic arteries and increased diameter of the external carotid >6 mm [72]. These were our reasons for choosing filters as a means of protection in our cases.

Angiographic factors and factors in the angioplasty, such as percentage of stenosis, presence of ulceration in the plaque, and number of catheters used, did not show a statistically significant difference in our study with respect to the appearance of NF after CAS. In contrast to our findings, Ohki et al., studying ex vivo angioplasty with stent, found that the greatest number of particles during the procedure was associated with serious stenosis >90% [90]. Gauvrit et al. [74], similar to our findings, did not find a significant difference between the degree of stenosis in groups of patients with and without NF after CAS. Schnaudigel et al. [37], in a meta-analysis, considered that the degree of stenosis influenced the incidence of NF after CAS; however, it was difficult to compare the articles because of great variation in the diagnostic methods (DSA, CTA, MRA, and Doppler) and methodologies (NASCET, ECST or not mentioned) used to grade the stenosis [37]. Roh et al. [78] found NF after CAS in eight of 22 (36%) cases. Thus, similar to us, they did not find a significant difference in the presence of NF in relation to the presence or absence of ulcers in the plaque. Among our patients, the percentages with ulcers were identical in the groups with and without embolism in CAS.

We note that ulcers did not influence the result of embolism, although one of the steps, overcoming the ulcerated stenosis by the still-closed closed filter, occurred without cerebral protection. This fact may suggest the safety of filters in crossing stenotic lesions, even anatomically complex ones, such as ulcerated plaques. More studies are needed to prove this hypothesis. Lacroix et al. [69], in a series of 61 CASs, analyzed technical conditions such as the procedure duration and presence of ulcers in atheromatous plaque. They did not find a correlation between these elements and the frequency of NF in DWI.

We did not find a significant difference between contralateral occlusion and the occurrence of NF after CAS. This finding confirms the clinical reasoning that patients with carotid stenosis and contralateral carotid occlusion have an embolism risk similar to that of other patients during CAS treatment. This fact contrasts with endarterectomy, for which the clinical results are materially negatively influenced by the presence of contralateral carotid occlusion [10,91-93].

The fluoroscopy time used in CAS may reflect the technical difficulty of the procedure as this time is equivalent to the set of short intervals in which X-ray was applied during the maneuvers necessary for the catheters, guides, balloons, stents, and other materials [82]. Pinheiro et al. [48] used fluoroscopy for 21 min (average) per CAS, a result similar to our series (22.93 min per CAS). As in our study, Tedesco et al. [70] did not find a correlation between long fluoroscopy times or greater amounts of contrast and the appearance of NF after CAS. Conversely, Rapp et al. [77] found an increase in NF after CAS depending on the fluoroscopy time used. However, the fact that we did not find a significant difference in the fluoroscopy time between the groups with and without embolism suggests that cases in which the angioplasty is technically difficult may require longer times for the interventionist, but theoretically, the increased time does not increase in the risks of embolism. The CASs in this study were always conducted by an individual with a considerable amount of experience. The only way to exclude this bias would be to evaluate the learning curve of a technician in training, which may explain the results of [77].

Although each contrast injection has an unknown theoretical risk of carrying emboligenic particles, this was not proven in our series, but there was not a significant difference in volume between the groups with and without NF. Nonetheless, we remember that, in medical services such as ours with a neuroradiology practice, the cases of embolism are possibly not due to the technique used because the contrast volume and the fluoroscopy time are similar for both groups. Moreover, it is possible that the risk of embolism may be endogenous to patients at a neuroradiology institution where the iatrogenic embolism factor is studied and controlled. The study by Kato et al. [94], as well as ours, did not find a significant difference in the groups with and without NF regarding contrast volume, duration of the procedure, and the use of additional catheters.

In our series, greater number of angiographies was found in the group that showed NF, and the occurrence of NF varied based on the type of exam applied. Most of the exams defined as broad were associated with emboli, and most of the brief exams did not show any NF after CAS. However, there was no statistical confirmation.

Following the same trend, the average DSA per patient was greater in the patients with NF (average 3.11) than among patients (average 2.78) without NF. Despite the theoretical risk of increasing embolism with the diagnostic exam, the statistical analysis was not sufficient to prove this hypothesis. Thus, the greater the number of vessels on which angiographies were performed, the higher the occurrence of NF. The logical deduction is that conventional angiography has the same responsibility for causing NF as angioplasty alone.

The catheter itself is a potential source of embolism, although complication rates are low [95], and most complications are asymptomatic ischemic complications [61]. Bendszus et al. were the first to publish diffusion MRI as a detection method for clinically silent emboli after cerebral angiographies. They found 42 hypersignal foci in the DWI in 23 out of 100 (23%) patients after DSA with manual injection of the contrast, all without neurological deficits [80].

Britt et al., in a short series, estimated an incidence of less than 9% of asymptomatic cerebral infarcts in diffusion in patients undergoing cerebral angiography for diagnostic purposes [96]. Kato et al. [94], in a study of 50 patients, observed NF in the diffusion after DSA in 8 of the 41 (19.51%) patients. Chuah et al. [97] found NF after angiographies in 3 of 20 (15%) patients, all of which were smaller than 10 mm and occurred at a rate of only one per patient.

Angiography of the aortic arch before CAS was associated with a high risk of microemboli, according to a publication of 27 CASs by Tedesco et al. [70]. This study reports that the aortography by catheter was avoided in cases where ulcers or stenosis were identified in the aortic arch during the revision of exams conducted immediately before CAS. Some authors have reduced the use of aortography by catheter. After the inclusion of MRI angiography in the protocol by Rapp et al. [77], digital angiography by catheter was abolished in 81% of CASs.

In the detailed statistical analysis using logistic regression of our data, we did not find a significant difference between DSA of the aortic arch ($p = 0.701$) and the appearance of NF in diffusion after CAS. In addition to CAS and DSA, several other catheter techniques show risks of cerebral embolism during the procedure. Rordorf et al. [98] found lesions in diffusion in 8 of 14 (57%) patients after embolization of unruptured cerebral aneurysms. In this series, the majority, with the exception of one new focus, was ipsilateral to the treated aneurysm [98]. Cronqvist et al. [99] published a series of 21 patients suffering from cerebral arteriovenous malformation who underwent 50 embolization procedures. In their study, NF were less frequent (22% of procedures). Of the 35 NF found in DWI, 23 (66%) were of ischemic origin, 8 (23%) represented perinidal venous clots, and 4 (11%) were of uncertain origin [99].

Brain catheterization is not the only cause of brain embolism. In prospective studies, there was an incidence of up to 15% for cerebral NF after cardiac catheterization [100]. Ischemia foci in

DWI are found in a substantial number of carotid surgeries (endarterectomy), heart and coronary surgeries, and interventions with cerebral angiographies [63,101,102]. Cardiac bypass surgery may induce NF for cerebral ischemia in up to 45% of patients [103].

Willinsky et al. [82] point to mechanisms related to brain catheterization, such as thromboembolism resulting from the withdrawal of the guide within the catheter. The withdrawal causes the empty space of the catheter to fill with blood. This space is subjected to stagnation, unnoticed by the inexperienced practitioner, and causes the formation of emboli [79]. Other mechanisms cited are the dissection and fracture of plaques; the fragmentation of plaques with catheters, guide catheters and guide wires; platelet activation; changes in clotting factors; and the introduction of air bubbles [36,46].

Willinsky et al. [82] published a five-year retrospective study of 2,899 cerebral angiographies and found neurological complications in 39 (1.3%), 20 of which were transitory (0.7%), five (0.2%) were reversed, and 14 (0.5%) were permanent. Neurological events in angiography were significantly more frequent in older patients (>55 years) and patients with concomitant cardiovascular disease and when the fluoroscopy was longer [82]. Kaufmann et al. [95] published the widest series of cerebral angiographies that resulted in clinical complications by evaluating 19,827 consecutive patients in a 22-year retrospective study at the Mayo Clinic. They found neurological complications in 2.63% of patients, permanent infarcts in 0.14%, and deaths in 0.06% [95]. Hematoma at the puncture site was the most common occurrence (4.2%). The independent factors identified as associated with neurological complications included atherosclerotic cerebrovascular disease, transient ischemic attacks, and subarachnoid hemorrhage [95].

Therefore, we assume that there is a theoretical risk of brain embolism, including possible severe ischemic events, with all of the interventional procedures.

According to some authors, the diffusion MRI technique is the most efficient tool for detecting acute focal brain ischemia [68,71,76].

Among the interventional procedures, carotid angioplasty achieved a significant reduction in embolism with the introduction of protection systems, but emboli were not avoided completely [35,37,46,68,73]. Good practice in neuroradiology procedures appears to be a mitigating factor for embolic damage during carotid angioplasty procedures. Consistent with our idea, Verzini et al. and Piñero et al. said that the interventionist's experience is a factor for reducing periprocedural complications [68,71,104]. For du Mesnil de Rochemont et al. [46], unintentional movement of the filter during the intervention is a potential cause of microemboli and mainly occurs during the initial learning curve. This movement can largely be avoided with improved interventional technique and new materials [46,68]. We believe that the learning curve for CAS might be long and could exceed 200 cases.

Tedesco et al. [70] stated that their CAS program was modified to include the omission of the aortic arch. This change began when MRI images provided sufficient anatomic detail and initiated anticoagulation before the passage of guides and catheters in the ascending and transverse aorta [70]. Thus, these authors state that aortography should be reserved for patients for whom the MRI before CAS does not provide anatomic details to guide the catheter. In contrast, these same authors affirm that more complex and challenging aortic arches (described as Type II and Type III) were not identified as high risk for embolization [70]. Most authors describe rates of non-symptomatic NF in DWI in the area contralateral to CAS that are similar to brain angiography rates.

The initial catheterization of CAS cannot be excluded because the procedures cannot be separated. Although the catheterization occurs alone for diagnostic purposes [80], angiography is a mandatory initial stage for all angioplasties [36]. Bendszus et al. [105] subsequently published that the use of heparin and air filters materially reduced ischemic events in brain catheterization.

Most studies on the relationship between NF in DWI and CAS only mention the material used; few describe a single access technique for the common carotid artery, usually direct access. In all cases, we used a standardized form for the highest-caliber (8 Fr) guide catheter, believing that the good stabilization of the system achieved by this material facilitates the manipulation of materials (filter, stent, balloons).

In our experience, direct access without exchanges is preferable only in technically simple cases with favorable anatomy. According to our review, our study is the only one that comparatively analyzes the catheterization access technique with the guide catheter in the carotid artery undergoing angioplasty. The risk for each technique to be involved with embolism was 50.00%, 50.00%, 63.64%, and 25.00%, respectively, for direct access, exchange in the external carotid artery, exchange in the common carotid artery, and triaxial. Thus, the triaxial technique showed a tendency for greater safety, possibly by having a more gradual progression of size (from the guide wire to the guide catheter) and causing less aggravation of the aortic arch and supra-aortic trunks. We can add that the triaxial technique should be used as a first attempt when technically possible.

Because the triaxial form of access showed a small number of NF, although without statistical significance, it is possible to predict that replacing the set (a short-valved introducer and guide catheter) with a long sheath (110 cm), which is currently available, in a single product that is also used triaxially (introducer, sheath, and guide) may reduce the index of embolic complications. More comparative studies of compatible techniques (guide, catheter, sheath) and other techniques are needed to prove this trend.

Although the filter is the central focus of discussion in most articles cited here for preventing embolization during CAS, the stent is the material used to effectively treat plaque to prevent embolic ischemic conditions in the long run. Our data do not show important significant differences between the brands of stent tested and the brands of protection filters used, as in Kastrup et al. [35] and Palombo et al. [75]. However, it is possible to identify a tendency for a smaller number of NF with a closed-cell stent (Wallstent®) compared with the open-cell stents. The Protégé® stent showed a reasonable resolve for the appearance of NF ipsilateral to CAS, but the small number of times this material was used precludes reliable statements about this relationship.

Schillinger et al. [30], studying the impact of open-cell versus closed-cell stents, reviewed data from 10 European centers totaling 1,684 patients and did not identify a significant difference regarding neurological complications and death up to 30 days after CAS. Additionally, du Mesnil de Rochemont et al. [46] found a tendency for a greater number of ischemic lesions with the use of segmented nitinol stents (open cells) compared to Wallstent®. They suggested that open-cell stents are used in more technically complex cases with marked vascular tortuosity. In our study, we obtained the same result, but the types of stents were used without differentiation regarding tortuosity. A prospective study by Sahin at al. analyzing patients with closed-cell and open-cell stents showed that open-cell stents were less associated with clinical events of brain ischemia [106]. Moreover, Hart et al. [45], studying 701 CASs, stated that closed-cell stents and eccentric filters had lower rates of TIA/ICVA/death combination 30 days after the procedure in symptomatic patients and patients with echolucent plaques in ultrasound. Our results and from other authors led to the theory that these stent and filter designs may be intrinsically more effective at preventing brain embolism from fractured plaque or other thrombogenic material.

The retrospective analysis of 3,179 consecutive CASs by Bosiers et al. [107] showed a significant difference with a greater rate of neurological complications (symptomatic or not) with open-cell stents. Using DWI specifically to study NF after CAS, the recent meta-analysis from Schnaudigel et al. [37] shows that the incidence of NF after CAS was significantly greater in open-cell stents than in closed-cell stents. Thus, our study is in agreement with those of other authors [32,37] and supports the idea that closed-cell stents are sufficient to cover plaque and prevent the embolization of large plaque particles post-CAS through the struts of the stent.

Several studies with separated groups with and without cerebral protection support the effectiveness of protection systems [34,35,37]. Kastrup et al. [33] found a combined frequency of CVA and death after 30 days of 1.8% for the group with protection and 5.5% for the group without protection ($p<0.001$). Additionally, a lower incidence of serious neurological complications was found when a filter was used (2.2%) than without a filter (5.5%) [38]. By studying groups with and without protection and the relationship with NF formation, Kastrup et al. found emboli in 49% of patients with cerebral protection and 67% of patients without protection [34]. Two years later, this group updated their data and published the occurrence of NF after CAS without a filter in 68% of patients and 52% of patients with a filter [35].

As expected, the meta-analysis by Schnaudigel et al. [37] found a lower index of foci ipsilateral to the CAS in DWI in patients with the use of cerebral protection systems (33%) than in patients without the use of protection (45%). The same authors cited no change in the risk of NF occurrence in the contralateral area with or without cerebral protection (respectively, 14% and 13%; $p=0.6$) [37]. In our study, all cases were performed with a protection filter. The use of a control group without a filter would be considered unethical according to our research group. However, different types of filters were compared, and the technique used to place the guide catheter was analyzed.

In addition to innovation of materials, proper training is needed for each type of filter. Attention to the correct apposition of the filter device should be a mandatory stage in the CAS [108], as it requires experience in executing the procedure because of the natural tortuosity of carotids. Positioning can be hampered by vascular tortuosity, which is sometimes excessive.

The choice of filter is also important because, if it has a smaller diameter than the vessel, blood and particles pass between the filter and the artery wall [46,104,109].

Two articles from Müller-Hulsbeck et al. [47,57] using an animal model of the carotid artery showed that miniscule particles of debris smaller than 100 μm can pass the pores of the filters [57]. Additionally, the filters can damage the vessel walls [47], which may subsequently result in the displacement of fragments and thrombi due to accidental movement of the filtering device. Other authors claim that we cannot exclude the possibility that when the filters are closed and removed, the collection system may swing the tool and loosen some of the captured particles, freeing them in the vessel lumen [46,68].

It is possible that because the stent and balloon use a microguide for the devices, in the case of the EPI/EZ® and Angioguard® filters used in this study, they may mobilize the filter and release free particles. The Emboshield® device does not carry this theoretical risk because it stays no fixed to the guide while it is in action. However, in our study, the Emboshield® device has an average appearance of NF similar to the other concentric device, Angioguard®, and both have a higher average than the eccentric device EPI®. This result reflects the need for training with each device because the only way of preventing the displacement of materials is the correct use of the devices.

In 2000, Coggia et al. [110] published the passage of particles in all stages of CAS in an ex vivo study. Most of the particles were smaller than 60 μm, and the pores of the commercially available filters were approximately 100 μm. The passage of these particles through the protection devices and entrapment in capillaries or cerebral arteries is possible [110]. Angelini et al. [50] showed through electronic microscopy that 83.7% of filters have particles adhered to them and, on average, the filters contained 33.7 particles (24 to 46). In that study, the average diameter of the fragments captured in the filters was 289.5 μm (1.08 to 5043.5 μm). The main particles found by this group were soft acellular material, lipid-laden macrophages, and cholesterol clefts. Less frequently, they found calcium particles and platelet aggregates. All of these materials are typically identified in atherosclerotic plaques, whether they are complicated or not. When a protective balloon was used, similar materials were found [50].

In 2009, Piñero et al. [111] published a structural analysis of the material contained in filters after angioplasties and stated that atherosclerotic plaques and vessel walls are the main sources of microemboli during CAS [71,111]. However, a study on the action of cerebral protection devices found that 88% of particles were retained in the filters in an ex vivo simulation of CAS [112]. Piñero et al. [48,71,111] considered filter diameter to be very important but not the only factor in the formation of NF. They claimed that bad positioning of the filter on the carotid wall due to tortuosity, displacement of the filter while handling the materials, and high profile crossover are technical difficulties that await future studies and improvements in materials. Rough handling can promote the formation of emboli during the positioning and removal of the filter.

Some authors explain that the size of debris removed from the filters differs from the real size at the moment of embolization and that most of the small emboli may be the result of the fragmentation of particles trying to pass through the grid of the filter [113]. Thus, continuous flow predisposes the fragmentation of content retained in the filter. Physician experience and speed are necessary to reduce the time of the procedure and avoid this fragmentation and potential emboli between the pores [68].

The filters that were used in the protocol of this study had mesh with pores from 100 to 140 μm, reducing the migration of cholesterol crystals and clots, platelet aggregations, and macrofragments of atheromatous plaques through filtering. The diameter of the filter pores used was smaller than the particles described by Theron et al. [114] and Ohki et al. [90] and than most of the particles described by Angelini et al. [50].

Our series showed an average of 1.6 NF per patient, a number well below the average of 33 particles found adhered to filters in the study by Angelini et al. [50]. It is possible that filters provide real protection, given the disparity between these numbers. Nonetheless, the action of each individual's thrombolysis system cannot be excluded as also drastically, or at least partially, reducing the permanence of emboli at its distal point.

The disparity between the low number of ischemic events after CAS [33,38] and the relatively high frequency of multiple small restriction foci in diffusion after CAS [35,69,70,73] that are compatible with embolism suggests that filters mainly act by retaining large particles that could evolve into clinical conditions of ischemia, rather than by grasping small particles. In our series, the eccentric filter EPI® had embolism in diffusion in 44% of cases, suggesting apparently superior protection compared to other models. The Angioguard® filter contained emboli in 50% of cases, while the Emboshield® device showed the highest rate of emboli (71.43%) in the group. Our data establish a strong tendency for superior protection measured in the eccentric filter (0.958 NF ipsilateral) compared to the concentric designs (2.100 NF ipsilateral). A study from Tedesco et al. [70] found a high rate of NF (70% of patients). These authors used a combination of the concentric filter and the open-cell stent, which may have contributed to the high rate of emboli. While there may be unequal protection between these filters, the difference shown in this series is not statistically significant. Our data cannot completely indicate greater protection of the eccentric model compared to the concentric model. Furthermore, poor distribution among types of filters with very small groups (Angioguard®, n=4) was observed. Thus, we avoid speculative comparison regarding the safety of each device.

A retrospective study of 3,160 CAS published Iyer et al. [115] found that the type of protection (nine different systems, including concentric and eccentric filters and proximal and distal occlusion balloons) had no influence on the clinical result. However, these authors did not study the brain using MRI after CAS.

For Piñero et al. [48,111], the difficulty of correctly positioning the filter on the wall of tortuous vessels, the displacement of material during the release, the creation of emboli by the relatively high-profile crossover and low flexibility, the loss of accumulated particles during the removal of the filter, and the diameter of the filter's pores appear to be very important to the appearance of ischemia related to embolization. This finding should lead to future studies that help to perfect protection systems [48,111].

In 2006, du Mesnil de Rochemont et al. [46] found three (6%) occlusions of filters by debris or clots in a series of 50 CASs. In a series of 162 CASs, Piñero et al. found filter occlusion in four (2.5%) patients during the procedure [48]. It is predicted that these cases will become significant infarcts due to the large size of the particles because it was sufficient to obstruct the filter pores up to total occlusion of the flow. Piñero et al. [48] assume that, without the use of a filter in these cases, the morbidity of their series would increase from 4 to 6.5%.

There was no case of filter occlusion by debris or thrombi in our series. Vasospasms related to the filtering devices were short-lived and without hemodynamic impairment. Other complications related to the filters were not found in this series. Filter occlusion leading to a stopped flow is a rare occurrence. It was more observed with the use of the first generation of EPI® filters, where the diameters of the pores were only 80 μm [46,116].

While the first step in CAS, which includes catheterization, the positioning of the guide catheter and the passage of the filter over the stenosis, occurs without protection, the phases with the greatest number of emboli released from plaque are the implantation of the stent and the angioplasty by balloon. An overload of the filter protection system is the angioplasty by balloon. Piñero at al. [111] showed that the more balloon dilations are applied to CAS, the greater the load of emboli found in the filters. Therefore, physician experience is necessary to use the balloon as delicately as possible.

Unfortunately, the other technique currently used in the treatment of carotid stenosis – CEA – also has ischemic complications [59] and more brain emboli than CAS [37,83]. Another common complication in CEA is lesions to the cranial nerves and cardiac infarction [117,118].

Comparative studies between CEA and CAS found a greater number of NF after CAS than after CEA. However, the lesions in the DWI after CAS are significantly smaller than after the endarterectomy. Analyzing the NF in the DWI after CAS and endarterectomy, Roh et al. [78] reasoned that the lesions in diffusion after CAS are generally asymptomatic and that the lesions in DWI associated with symptoms are more frequent in CEA [37,78]. In recent years, the materials used in CAS have been improved to reduce complications. DWI can be used as a tool in this evolving analysis of materials and also in the technical improvement of neurointervention.

Our study shows some limitations. Data collection of a control group without the use of cerebral protection to prove the device's effectiveness is incorrect based on our ethical views of the procedure, but it is a limitation of the study. However, other published studies that conducted CAS with and without protection systems clearly show a smaller number of NF [35,37] and lower risk of ischemic events [33,38] after CAS in the groups where the devices were used.

The formation of emboli can be impeded by antiplatelet and anticoagulant medications [76], but this is not the focus of our research shown here. In neuroradiology procedures, the prevalence of resistance to aspirin varied from 2 to 21%, and resistance to clopidogrel varied from 43 to 52% [119-121]. This result is extremely important because atheromatous plaques and superimposed thrombi are the main source of microemboli during CAS. A recent study from Song et al. [76] using the VerifyNow system showed that the frequency of resistance to clopidogrel was significantly higher in patients with foci of microemboli in DWI after CAS than in patients without foci of microemboli in MRI after CAS. In their series, all the patients who showed clinical ischemic events had resistance to antiplatelets [76].

A randomized prospective study evaluated platelet activation after coronary stents in pigs and showed that the closed-cell stent produced less intimal prolapse and thus a smoother stent-vessel wall interface than the stent with open-cells and that platelet activation was greater during the 30 days following implantation of an open-cell versus a closed-cell stent [122].

Our study concentrates on the designs of stents and filters, but other particularities of constructing the materials can interfere in the safety of CAS, such as the type of filtering element. A study considered that perforated membrane filters have greater resistance to cerebral blood flow [123], but it did not evaluate whether there was greater capture of emboli. Our study also had a relatively short follow-up time. We only used the period when the patients were hospitalized, generally three to four days. We consider that this peri-procedure period is sufficient to evaluate the late appearance of NF because the disappearance of NF is described in some cases [60,68,75].

14. Conclusions

The use of protection systems aims to avoid massive embolism, which occasionally happens. However, a perfect cerebral protection system is not commercially available. While cerebral protection with filters is effective, it is necessary to develop new protection devices that are more effective and can be occlusive systems with a lower profile and greater ease of use. Both techniques, angioplasty with stent (with filter or flow occlusion systems) and endarterectomy, are involved in cases of intracranial embolism per treatment.

New restriction foci (NF) in diffusion were present in half of the patients after CAS with cerebral protection and were most frequently located in the ipsilateral area (77.19%), suggesting that the filters did not prevent all microemboli. New restriction foci in DWI after CAS were located in regions (22.81%) different than in the angioplasty and were associated with diagnostic catheterization. Therefore, long neurointerventionist medical training should be required before CASs are performed.

The NF in DWI after CAS were mostly small in diameter (<10 mm in 91.53%) and were always clinically silent (100%) in our study.

The presence of cerebral infarcts in the T2 sequence in the initial MRI was the only factor that significantly predisposed the appearance of new restriction foci in DWI after CAS. Thus, the risk of microemboli was directly related to intrinsic factors of the patient. Other demographic factors and aspects related to the angioplasty technique were not statistically significant to the occurrence of NF in our study. There was a tendency for other factors, such as the triaxial access technique, asymptomatic patients, and an eccentric filter, to be involved in the appearance of a smaller number of NF after CAS.

The appearance of microemboli attributed to catheterization and not angioplasty with stent shows that proper training for medical specialists in cervical and cerebral circulation (neuro-interventionists) can be key to reducing risks for patients. General specialists in vessels (vascular surgeons) and coronary circulation (cardiologists) generally do not have specific training for cervicocerebral circulation; most of their training focuses on the aorta and coronary arteries, respectively. We therefore recommend that angiographies to diagnose cervical and cerebral circulation and carotid angioplasty be conducted by interventional neuroradiologists to reduce the risk of emboli.

To maintain cerebral flow during the endovascular carotid treatment, CAS with filter is the first choice in cases of serious stenosis. The use of occlusive systems is promising but requires more technical development to reduce the risks associated current systems.

Acknowledgements

We are grateful for the help of Cláudio Campi de Castro (who conducted the project and IRM evaluation), Paulo Puglia Jr, Francisco Ramos Jr (who designed the study protocol), Michel Eli Frudit, Hélio Leitão, Maurício Jory, Leandro Assis Barbosa, Guilherme Abrão, Carlos Pereira Silva, Mateus Miranda, Fausto Motta Ferraz, Carlos Hagioto, Salassiê Mansur, Rodrigo Peres Ignácio, Eduardo Figueiredo (for the application of RM evaluation), and professor Gercino Monteiro Filho (for statistical analysis). The present research was supported by the Fundação de Amparo à Pesquisa do Estado de São Paulo (FAPESP).

Author details

Antenor Tavares[1*] and José Guilherme Caldas[2]

*Address all correspondence to: antenorts@gmail.com

1 Universidade de São Paulo, UniEvangélica University, and Hospital Geral de Goiania, Brazil

2 Universidade de São Paulo, Hospital Síro-Libanes, Brazil

References

[1] American Heart Association. Heart disease and stroke statistics-2004 Update. Dallas: American Heart Association; 2003

[2] Roger VL, Go AS, Lloyd-Jones DM, Adams RJ, Berry JD, Brown TM, et al. Heart Disease and Stroke Statistics-2011 Update: A Report From the American Heart Association. Circulation 2011;123(4) e18-e209.

[3] Gagliardi RJ, André C, Fukujima MM, Melo-Souza SE, Zétola VF. Abordagem da doença carotídea na fase aguda do acidente vascular cerebral [Management of carotid disease in acute phase of stroke: national opinion]. Arquivos de Neuro-psiquiatria 2005;63(3a) 709-712.

[4] Goldstein LB, Adams R, Alberts MJ, Appel LJ, Brass LM, Bushnell CD, et al. Primary Prevention of Ischemic Stroke: A Guideline From the American Heart Association/ American Stroke Association Stroke Council: cosponsored by the atherosclerotic peripheral vascular disease interdisciplinary working group; Cardiovascular Nursing Council; Clinical Cardiology Council; Nutrition, Physical Activity, and Metabolism Council; and the Quality of Care and Outcomes Research Interdisciplinary Working Group: The American Academy of Neurology affirms the value of this guideline. Stroke 2006;37(6) 1583-1633.

[5] Petty GW, Brown Jr RD, Whisnant JP, Sicks JD, O'Fallon WM, Wiebers DO. Ischemic stroke subtypes: a population-based study of incidence and risk factors. Stroke 1999;30 2513-2516.

[6] O'Leary DH, Polak JF, Kronmal RA, Kittner SJ, Bond MG, Wolfson SK Jr, et al. Distribution and correlates of sonographically detected carotid artery disease in the Cardiovascular Health Study. The CHS Collaborative Research Group. Stroke 1992;23(12) 1752-1760.

[7] Inzitari D, Eliasziw M, Gates P, Sharpe BL, Chan RKT, Meldrum HE, et al. The causes and risk of stroke in patients with asymptomatic internal-carotid-artery stenosis. North American Symptomatic Carotid Endarterectomy Trial Collaborators. New England Journal of Medicine 2000;342(23) 1693-1700.

[8] Laris MR, Arteaga A, Cuevas A, Rigotti A. HDL cholesterol: a new target in the treatment of lipid disorders and atherosclerosis? Revista Médica de Chile 2005;133(7) 823-832.

[9] Caldas JGMP, Puglia Jr P, Barbosa LA. Tratamento da doença carotídea oclusiva. In: Carnevale FC. (ed.) Radiologia intervencionista e cirurgia endovascular. Rio de Janeiro: Revinter; 2006. p165-182.

[10] NASCET 1991. The North American Symptomatic Carotid Endarterectomy Trial Collaborators. Beneficial effect of carotid endarterectomy in symptomatic patients with high-grade carotid stenosis. N Engl J Med. 1991; 325: 445–53.

[11] Yadav JS, Wholey MH, Kuntz RE, Fayad P, Katzen BT, Mishkel GJ, Mishkel GJ, Bajwa TK, Whitlow P, Strickman NE, Jaff MR, Popma JJ, Snead DB, Cutlip DE, Firth BG, Ouriel K. For the Stenting and Angioplasty with Protection in Patients at High Risk

for Endarterectomy Investigators Protected carotid-artery stenting versus endarterectomy in high-risk patients. N Engl J Med. 2004;351:1493-501

[12] Mantese VA, Timaran CH, Chiu D, Begg RJ, Brott TG, CREST Investigators. The Carotid Revascularization Endarterectomy versus Stenting Trial (CREST): stenting versus carotid endarterectomy for carotid disease. Stroke 2010;41(10 Suppl) S31-S34. doi: 10.1161/STROKEAHA.110.595330.

[13] Bates ER, Babb JD, Casey DE Jr, Cates CU, Duckwiler GR, Feldman TE, et al. ACCF/SCAI/SVMB/SIR/ASITN 2007 clinical expert consensus document on carotid stenting: a report of the American College of Cardiology Foundation Task Force on Clinical Expert Consensus Documents (ACCF/SCAI/SVMB/SIR/ASITN Clinical Expert Consensus Document Committee on Carotid Stenting). Journal of the American College of Cardiology 2007;49(1) 126-170.

[14] ACAS 1995. Executive Committee for the Asymptomatic Carotid Atherosclerosis Study. Endarterectomy for asymptomatic carotid artery stenosis. Endarterectomy for asymptomatic carotid artery stenosis. Journal of the American Medical Association 1995;273(18) 1421-1428.

[15] Biller J, Feinberg WM, Castaldo JE, Whittemore AD, Harbaugh RE, Dempsey RJ, et al. Guidelines for carotid endarterectomy: a statement for healthcare professionals from a special writing group of the Stroke Council, American Heart Association. Stroke 1998;29(2) 554-562.

[16] Barr JD, Connors III JJ, Sacks D, Wojak JC, Becker GJ, Cardella JF, et al. Quality improvement guidelines for the performance of cervical carotid angioplasty and stent placement. Journal of Vascular and Interventional Radiology 2003;14(9 Pt 2) S321-S335.

[17] Chaturvedi S, Bruno A, Feasby T, Holloway R, Benavente O, Cohen SN, et al. Carotid endarterectomy — an evidence-based review. Report of the Therapeutics and Technology Assessment Subcommittee of the American Academy of Neurology. Neurology 2005;65(6) 794-801.

[18] Menon D, Stafinski T. Cerebral protection devices for use during carotid artery angioplasty with stenting: a health technology assessment. International Journal of Technology Assessment in Health Care 2006;22(1) 119-129.

[19] Bonamigo TP, Lucas ML. Análise crítica das indicações e resultados do tratamento cirúrgico da doença carotídea [Critical analysis of indications and outcomes of surgical treatment for carotid disease]. Jornal Vascular Brasileiro 2007;6(4) 366-377.

[20] Gurm HS, Nallamothu BK, Yadav J. Safety of carotid artery stenting for symptomatic carotid artery disease: a meta-analysis. European Heart Journal 2008;29(1) 113-119.

[21] Furie KL, Kassner SE, Adams RJ, Albers GW, Bush RL, Fagan SC, et al. Guidelines for the prevention of stroke in patients with stroke or transient ischemic attack: a

guideline for healthcare professionals from the American Heart Association/American Stroke Association. Stroke 2011;42(1) 227-276.

[22] Mathias K. Perkutane transluminale katheter-behandlung supraaortaler arterienobstruktionen. Angiology 1981;3 47-50.

[23] Kerber CW, Hornwell LD, Loehden OL. Catheter dilatation of proximal carotid stenosis during distal bifurcation endarterectomy. American Journal of Neuroradiology 1980;1(4) 348-349.

[24] Theron J, Raymond J, Casasco A, Courtheoux F. Percutaneous angioplasty of atherosclerotic and postsurgical stenosis of carotid arteries. American Journal of Neuroradiology 1987;8(3) 495-500.

[25] Bockenheimer SA, Mathias K. Percutaneous transluminal angioplasty in arteriosclerotic internal carotid artery stenosis. American Journal of Neuroradiology 1983;4(3) 791-792.

[26] Theron J, Courtheoux P, Alachkar F, Bouvard G, Maiza D. New triple coaxial catheter system for carotid angioplasty with cerebral protection. American Journal of Neuroradiology 1990;11(5) 869-874.

[27] Marks MP, Dake MD, Steinberg GK, Norbash AM, Lane B. Stent placement for arterial and venous cerebrovascular disease: preliminary experience. Radiology 1994;191(2) 441-446.

[28] Diethrich EB, Ndiaye M, Reid DB. Stenting in the carotid artery: initial experience in 110 patients. Journal of Endovascular Surgery 1996;3(1) 42-62.

[29] Roubin GS, New G, Iyer SS, Vitek JJ, Al-Mubarak N, Liu MW, et al. Immediate and late clinical outcomes of carotid artery stenting in patients with symptomatic and asymptomatic carotid artery stenosis: a 5-year prospective analysis. Circulation 2001;103(4) 532-537.

[30] Schillinger M, Gschwendtner M, Reimers B, Trenkler J, Stockx L, Mair J, et al. Does carotid stent cell design matter? Stroke 2008;39(3) 905-909.

[31] Connors III JJ, Wojak JC. Tools of the trade. In: Connors III JJ, Wojak JC. (eds.) Interventional Neuroradiology: Strategies and Practical Techniques. Philadelphia: W.B. Saunders; 1999. p1-37.

[32] Tadros RO, Spyris CT, Vouyouka AG, Chung C, Krishnan P, Arnold MW, et al. Comparing the embolic potential of open and closed cell stents during carotid angioplasty and stenting. Journal of Vascular Surgery 2012;56(1) 89-95.

[33] Kastrup A, Gröschel K, Krapf H, Brehm BR, Dichgans J, Schulz JB. Early outcome of carotid angioplasty and stenting with and without cerebral protection devices: a systematic review of the literature. Stroke 2003;34(3) 813-819.

[34] Kastrup A, Nägele T, Gröschel K, Schmidt F, Vogler E, Schulz J, et al. Incidence of new brain lesions after carotid stenting with and without cerebral protection. Stroke 2006;37(9) 2312-2316.

[35] Kastrup A, Gröschel K, Nägele T, Riecker A, Schmidt F, Schnaudigel S, et al. Effects of Age and Symptom Status on Silent Ischemic Lesions after Carotid Stenting with and without the Use of Distal Filter Devices. American Journal of Neuroradiology 2008;29(3) 608-612.

[36] Cosottini M, Michelassi MC, Puglioli M, Lazzarotti G, Orlandi G, Marconi F, et al. Silent cerebral ischemia detected with diffusion-weighted imaging in patients treated with protected and unprotected carotid artery stenting. Stroke 2005;36(11) 2389-2393.

[37] Schnaudigel S, Gröschel K, Pilgram SM, Kastrup A. New brain lesions after carotid stenting versus carotid endarterectomy: a systematic review of the literature. Stroke 2008;39(6) 1911-1919

[38] Caldas, JG. Carotid angioplasty with stent placement under filter protection: experience with 1037 cases. e-Mémoires de l'Académie Nationale de Chirurgie 2006;5(4) 1-4.

[39] Brott TG, Halperin JL, Abbara S, Bacharach JM, Barr JD, Bush RL, et al. 2011 ASA/ACCF/AHA/AANN/AANS/ACR/ASNR/CNS/SAIP/SCAI/SIR/SNIS/SVM/SVS guideline on the management of patients with extracranial carotid and vertebral artery disease: executive summary: a report of the American College of Cardiology Foundation/American Heart Association Task Force on Practice Guidelines, and the American Stroke Association, American Association of Neuroscience Nurses, American Association of Neurological Surgeons, American College of Radiology, American Society of Neuroradiology, Congress of Neurological Surgeons, Society of Atherosclerosis Imaging and Prevention, Society for Cardiovascular Angiography and Interventions, Society of Interventional Radiology, Society of NeuroInterventional Surgery, Society for Vascular Medicine, and Society for Vascular. Journal of the American College of Cardiology 2011;57(8) 1002-1044.

[40] Parodi JC, La Mura R, Ferreira LM, Mendez MV, Cersósimo H, Schönholz C, et al. Initial evaluation of carotid angioplasty and stenting with three different cerebral protection devices. Journal of Vascular Surgery 2000;32(6) 1127-1136.

[41] Reimers B, Sievert H, Schuler GC, Tubler T. Proximal endovascular flow blockage for cerebral protection during carotid artery stenting: results from a prospective multicenter registry. Journal of Endovascular Therapy 2005;12(2) 156-165.

[42] Grunwald IQ, Papanagiotou P, Struffert T, Politi M, Krick C, Romaike BFM, et al. Reversal of flow during carotid artery stenting: use of the Parodi antiembolism system. Neuroradiology 2007;49(3) 237-241.

[43] Schlüter M, Tübler T, Mathey DG, Schofer J. Feasibility and efficacy of balloon-based neuroprotection during carotid artery stenting in a single-center setting. Journal of the American College of Cardiology 2002;40(5) 890-895.

[44] Henry M, Henry I, Klonaris C, Masson I, Hugel M, Tzvetanov K, et al. Benefits of cerebral protection during carotid stenting with the PercuSurge GuardWire system: midterm results. Journal of Endovascular Therapy 2002;9(1) 1–13.

[45] Hart JP, Peeters P, Verbist J, Deloose K, Bosiers M. Do device characteristics impact outcome in carotid artery stenting? Journal of Vascular Surgery 2006;44(4) 725-730.

[46] du Mesnil de Rochemont R, Schneider S, Yan B, Lehr A, Sitzer M, Berkefeld J. Diffusion-weighted MR imaging lesions after filter-protected stenting of high-grade symptomatic carotid artery stenoses. American Journal of Neuroradiology 2006;27(6) 1321-1325.

[47] Müller-Hülsbeck S, Stolzmann P, Liess C, Hedderich J, Paulsen F, Jahnke T, et al. Vessel wall damage caused by cerebral protection devices: ex vivo evaluation in porcine carotid arteries. Radiology 2005;235(2) 454-460.

[48] Piñero P, Gonzalez A, Mayol A, Martinez E, González-Marcos JR, Boza F, et al. Silent ischemia after neuroprotected percutaneous carotid stenting: a diffusion-weighted MRI study. American Journal of Neuroradiology 2006;27(6) 1338-1345.

[49] Schmidt A, Diederich KW, Scheinert S, Bräunlich S, Olenburger T, Biamino G, et al. Effect of two different neuroprotection systems on microembolization during carotid artery stenting. Journal of the American College of Cardiology 2004;44(10) 1966-1969.

[50] Angelini A, Reimers B, Barbera MD, Saccà S, Pasquetto G, Cernetti C, et al. Cerebral protection during carotid artery stenting collection and histopathologic analysis of embolized debris. Stroke 2002;33(2) 456-461.

[51] Vos JA, van den Berg JC, Ernst SM, Suttorp MJ, Overtoom TT, Mauser HW, et al. Carotid angioplasty and stent placement: comparison of transcranial Doppler US-data and clinical outcome with and without filtering cerebral protection in 509 patients. Radiology 2005;234(2) 493-499.

[52] Barbosa MF, Abdala N, Carrete Jr H, Nogueira RG, Nalli DR, Fonseca JRF, et al. Doppler transcraniano convencional em voluntários assintomáticos: variabilidade e valores de referência para parâmetros de fluxo sangüíneo [Reference values for measures of blood flow velocities and impedance indexes in healthy individuals through conventional transcranial Doppler]. Arquivos de Neuro-psiquiatria 2006;64(3B) 829-838.

[53] Fregni F, Castelo-Branco LEC, Conforto AB, Yamamoto FI, Campos CR, Puglia Jr P, et al. Treatment of subclavian steal syndrome with percutaneous transluminal angioplasty and stenting. Arquivos de Neuro-psiquiatria 2003;61(1) 95-99.

[54] Rosenkranz M, Fiehler J, Niesen W, Waiblinger C, Eckert B, Wittkugel O, et al. The amount of solid cerebral microemboli during carotid stenting does not relate to the

frequency of silent ischemic lesions. American Journal of Neuroradiology 2006;27(1) 157-161.

[55] Tinoco ECA, Silva LF, Luquini BB, Campanha R, Nascimento M, Horta L. Estudo prospectivo comparativo entre a endarterectomia e a angioplastia com stent e proteção cerebral no tratamento das lesões ateroscleróticas carotídeas: resultados em 30 dias. Jornal Vascular Brasileiro 2006;5(4) 257-262.

[56] Jaeger HJ, Mathias KD, Hauth E, Drescher R, Gissler HM, Hennigs S, et al. Cerebral ischemia detected with diffusion-weighted MR imaging after stent implantation in the carotid artery. American Journal of Neuroradiology 2002;23(2) 200-207.

[57] Müller-Hülsbeck S, Jahnke T, Liess C, Glass C, Grimm J, Heller M. Comparison of various cerebral protection devices used for carotid artery stent placement: an in vitro experiment. Journal of Vascular and Interventional Radiology 2003;14(5) 613-620.

[58] Poppert H, Wolf O, Resch M, Theiss W, Schmidt-Thieme T, von Einsiedel HG, et al. Differences in number, size and location of intracranial microembolic lesions after surgical versus endovascular treatment without protection device of carotid artery stenosis. Journal of Neurology 2004;251(1) 1198-1203.

[59] Flach HZ, Ouhlous M, Hendriks JM, van Sambeek MRHM, Veenland JF, Koudstaal PJ, et al. Cerebral ischemia after carotid intervention. Journal of Endovascular Therapy 2004;11(3) 251-257.

[60] Hauth EAM, Jansen C, Drescher R, Schwartz M, Forsting M, Jaeger HJ, et al. MR and clinical follow-up of diffusion-weighted cerebral lesions after carotid artery stenting. American Journal of Neuroradiology 2005;26(9) 2336-2341.

[61] Hammer FD, Lacroix V, Duprez T, Grandin C, Verhelst R, Peeters A, et al. Cerebral microembolization after protected carotid artery stenting in surgical high-risk patients: results of a 2-year prospective study. Journal of Vascular Surgery 2005;42(5) 847-853.

[62] Oppenheim C, Lamy C, Touzé E, Calvet D, Hamon M, Mas JL, et al. Do transient ischemic attacks with diffusion-weighted imaging abnormalities correspond to brain Infarctions? American Journal of Neuroradiology 2006;27(8) 1782-1787.

[63] Bendszus M, Stoll G. Silent cerebral ischaemia: hidden fingerprints of invasive medical procedures. Lancet Neurology 2006;5(4) 364-372.

[64] Cooper JA. Extracranial atherosclerosis, subacute cerebral infarction, chronic cerebral infarction, lacunar infarction. In: Osborn AG, Blaser S, Salzman K. (eds.) Diagnostic Imaging: Brain. Salt Lake City: Amirsys; 2004. pI-4-28-I-4-35; pI-4-80-I-4-91.

[65] Moseley ME, Butts K. Diffusion and perfusion. In: Stark DD, Bradley Jr WG. (eds.) Ressonância magnética. 3a ed. Rio de Janeiro: Revinter; 2005. p1515-1538.

[66] Jensen MC, Brant-Zawadzki MN, Jacobs BC. Isquemia. In: Stark DD, Bradley Jr WG. (eds.) Ressonância magnética. 3a ed. Rio de Janeiro: Revinter, 2005. p1255-1276.

[67] Otaduy MCG, Toyama LMN, Amaro Jr E. Técnicas de obtenção de imagens em neurorradiologia. In: Leite CC. (ed.) Neurorradiologia Diagnóstico por imagem das alterações encefálicas. Rio de Janeiro: Guanabara Koogan; 2008. p1-48.

[68] Sá Júnior, AT de. Alterações de difusão e perfusão cerebral por RM em angioplastia carotídea com "stent" sob proteção cerebral por filtros [Changes in diffusion and perfusion weighted magnetic resonance imaging in carotid angioplasty with stenting under cerebral protection by filters]. PhD thesis. University of São Paulo; 2009.

[69] Lacroix V, Hammer F, Astarci P, Duprez T, Grandin C, Cosnard G, et al. Ischemic cerebral lesions after carotid surgery and carotid stenting. European Journal of Vascular and Endovascular Surgery 2007;33(4) 430-435.

[70] Tedesco MM, Lee JT, Dalman RL, Lane B, Loh C, Haukoos JS, et al. Postprocedural microembolic events following carotid surgery and carotid angioplasty and stenting. Journal Vascular Surgery 2007;46(2) 244-250.

[71] Piñero González de la Peña P, González García A, Moniche Álvarez F, Mayol Deyá A, González Marcos JR, Cayuela Domínguez A, et al. Contenido en filtros tras angioplastia y colocación de stent carotídeo: relación con lesiones isquémicas en la resonancia magnética de difusión. Radiología 2012;54(2) 155-164.

[72] de Castro-Afonso LH, de Oliveira L, Pontes-Neto OM, Fábio SR, Wajnberg E, Abud DG. Carotid artery stenting performed with a flow-reversal technique: improved technical performance. Journal of Neuroradiology 2013;40(1) 29-37.

[73] Maleux G, Demaerel P, Verbeken E, Daenens K, Heye S, Sonhoven F, et al. Cerebral ischemia after filter-protected carotid artery stenting is common and cannot be predicted by the presence of substantial amount of debris captured by the filter device. American Journal of Neuroradiology 2006;27(9) 1830-1833.

[74] Gauvrit JY, Delmaire C, Henon H, Debette S, al Koussa M, Leys D, et al. Diffusion/perfusion-weighted magnetic resonance imaging after carotid angioplasty and stenting. Journal of Neurology 2004;251(9) 1060-1067.

[75] Palombo G, Faraglia V, Stella N, Giugni E, Bozzao A, Taurino M. Late evaluation of silent cerebral ischemia detected by diffusion-weighted MR imaging after filter-protected carotid artery stenting. American Journal of Neuroradiology 2008;29(7) 1340-1343.

[76] Song TJ, Suh SH, Min PK, Kim DJ, Kim BM, Heo JH, et al. The influence of anti-platelet resistance on the development of cerebral ischemic lesion after carotid artery stenting. Yonsei Medical Journal 2013;54(2) 288-294. doi: 10.3349/ymj.2013.54.2.288.

[77] Rapp JH, Wakil L, Sawhney R, Pan XM, Yenari MA, Glastonbury C, et al. Subclinical embolization after carotid artery stenting: new lesions on diffusion-weighted mag-

netic resonance imaging occur postprocedure. Journal of Vascular Surgery 2007;45(5) 867-872.

[78] Roh HG, Byun HS, Ryoo JW, Na DG, Moon WJ, Lee BB, et al. Prospective analysis of cerebral infarction after carotid endarterectomy and carotid artery stent placement by using diffusion-weighted imaging. American Journal of Neuroradiology 2005;26(2) 376-384.

[79] CAVATAS Investigators. Endovascular versus surgical treatment in patients with carotid stenosis in the Carotid and Vertebral Artery Transluminal Angioplasty Study (CAVATAS): a randomised trial. Lancet 2001;357 1729-1737

[80] Bendszus M, Koltzenburg M, Burger R, Warmuth-Metz M, Hofmann E, Solymosi L. Silent embolism in diagnostic cerebral angiography and neurointerventional procedures: a prospective study. Lancet 1999;354(9190) 1594-1597.

[81] Rabelo LM, Viana RM, Schimith MA, Patin VG, Valverde MA, Denadai RC, et al. Risk factors for atherosclerosis in students of a private university in São Paulo-Brazil. Arquivos Brasileiros de Cardiologia 1999;72(5) 575-580.

[82] Willinsky RA, Taylor SM, TerBrugge K, Farb RI, Tomlinson G, Montanera W. Neurologic complications of cerebral angiography: prospective analysis of 2,899 procedures and review of the literature. Radiology 2003;227(2) 522-528.

[83] Crawley F, Stygall J, Lunn S, Harrison M, Brown MM, Newman S, et al. Comparison of microembolism detected by transcranial Doppler and neuropsychological sequelae of carotid surgery and percutaneous transluminal angioplasty. Stroke 2000;31(6) 1329-1334

[84] Smith JAM. Operator experience versus embolic protection in the carotid arteries. Endovascular Today 2006;8 75-78.

[85] Kidwell CS, Alger JR, Di Salle F, Starkman S, Villablanca P, Bentson J, et al. Diffusion MRI in patients with transient ischemic attacks. Stroke 1999;30(6) 1174-1180.

[86] Schlüter M, Tübler T, Steffens JC, Mathey DG, Schofer J. Focal ischemia of the brain after neuroprotected carotid artery stenting. Journal of the American College of Cardiology 2003;42(6) 1007-1013.

[87] van Everdingen KJ, van der Grond J, Kapelle LJ, Ramos LM, Mali WP. Diffusion-weighted magnetic resonance imaging in acute stroke. Stroke 1998;29(9) 1783-1790.

[88] Tavares A, Caldas JG, Castro CC, Puglia P Jr, Frudit ME, Barbosa LA. Changes in perfusion-weighted magnetic resonance imaging after carotid angioplasty with stent. Interventional Neuroradiology 2010;16(2) 161-169.

[89] Tavares A., Caldas JC. Decreased Cerebral Perfusion in Carotid Artery Stenosis, Carotid Angioplasty and Its Effects on Cerebral Circulation. In: Balestrino M. (ed.) Advances in the Treatment of Ischemic Stroke. Rijeka: InTech; 2012. p183-212. Available from http://www.intechopen.com/books/advances-in-the-treatment-of-ischemic-

stroke/cerebral-perfusion-and-interaction-with-carotid-angioplasty (accessed 20 August 2013).

[90] Ohki T, Marin ML, Lyon RT, Berdejo GL, Soundararajan K, Ohki M, et al. Ex vivo human carotid artery bifurcation stenting: correlation of lesion characteristics with embolic potential. Journal of Vascular Surgery 1998;27(3) 463-471.

[91] Sabeti S, Schillinger M, Mlekusch W, Nachtmann T, Lang W, Ahmadi R, et al. Contralateral high-grade carotid artery stenosis or occlusion is not associated with increased risk for poor neurologic outcome after elective carotid stent placement. Radiology 2004;230(1) 70-76.

[92] Lee JH, Choi CG, Kim DK, Kim GE, Lee HK, Suh DC. Relationship between circle of Willis morphology on 3D time-of-flight MR angiograms and transient ischemia during vascular clamping of the internal carotid artery during carotid endarterectomy. American Journal of Neuroradiology 2004;25(4) 558-564.

[93] Kastrup A, Gröschel K. Carotid endarterectomy versus carotid stenting: an updated review of randomized trials and subgroup analyses. Acta Chirurgica Belgica 2007;107(2) 119-128.

[94] Kato K, Tomura N, Takahashi S, Sakuma I, Watarai J. Ischemic lesions related to cerebral angiography: Evaluation by diffusion weighted MR imaging. Neuroradiology 2003;45(1) 39–43.

[95] Kaufmann TJ, Huston III J, Mandrekar JN, Schleck CD, Thielen KR, Kallmes DF. Complications of diagnostic cerebral angiography: evaluation of 19,826 consecutive patients. *Radiology* 2007;243(3) 812-819.

[96] Britt PM, Heiserman JE, Snider RM, Shill HA, Bird CR, Wallace RC. Incidence of Postangiographic Abnormalities Revealed by Diffusion-Weighted MR Imaging. American Journal of Neuroradiology 2000;21(1) 55-59.

[97] Chuah KC, Stuckey SL, Berman IG. Silent embolism in diagnostic cerebral angiography: detection with diffusion-weighted imaging. Australasian Radiology 2004;48(2) 133-138.

[98] Rordorf G, Bellon RJ, Budzik Jr. RF, Farkas J, Reinking GF, Pergolizzi RS, et al. Silent thromboembolic events associated with the treatment of unruptured cerebral aneurysms by use of guglielmi detachable coils: prospective study applying diffusion-weighted imaging. American Journal of Neuroradiology 2001;22(1) 5-10.

[99] Cronqvist M, Wirestam R, Ramgren B, Brandt L, Romner B, Nilsson O, et al. Endovascular treatment of intracerebral arteriovenous malformations: procedural safety, complications, and results evaluated by MR imaging, including diffusion and perfusion imaging. American Journal of Neuroradiology 2006;27(1) 162-176.

[100] Busing KA, Schulte-Sasse C, Fluchter S, Suselbeck T, Haase KK, Neff W, et al. Cerebral infarction: incidence and risk factors after diagnostic and interventional cardiac

catheterization--prospective evaluation at diffusion-weighted MR imaging. Radiology 2005;235(1) 177-183.

[101] Shannon P, Billbao JM, Marotta T, Terbrugge K. Inadvertent foreign body embolization in diagnostic and therapeutic cerebral angiography. American Journal of Neuroradiology 2006;27(2) 278-282.

[102] Grunwald IQ, Papanagiotou P, Politi M, Struffert T, Roth C, Reith W. Endovascular treatment of unruptured intracranial aneurysms: occurrence of thromboembolic events. Neurosurgery 2006;58(4) 612-618.

[103] Knipp SC, Matatko N, Wilhelm H, Schlamann M, Massoudy P, Forsting M, et al. Evaluation of brain injury after coronary artery bypass grafting. A prospective study using neuropsychological assessment and diffusion-weighted magnetic resonance imaging. European Journal of Cardio-Thoracic Surgery 2004;25(5) 791-800.

[104] Verzini F, Cao P, De Rango P, Parlani G, Maselli A, Romano L, et al. Appropriateness of learning curve for carotid artery stenting: an analysis of periprocedural complications. Journal of Vascular Surgery 2006;44(6) 1205-1211.

[105] Bendszus M, Koltzenburg M, Bartsch AJ, Goldbrunner R, Gunthner-Lengsfeld T, Weilbach FX, et al. Heparin and air filters reduce embolic events caused by intra-arterial cerebral angiography: a prospective, randomized trial. Circulation 2004;110(15) 2210-2215.

[106] Sahin M, Açar G, Özkan B, AlIcI G, YazIcIoglu MV, Bulut M, et al. Comparison of short-term outcomes after carotid artery stenting according to different stent designs. Postępy w Kardiologii Interwencyjnej 2013;9,2(32) 121-125. doi: 10.5114/pwki.2013.35445.

[107] Bosiers M, De Donato G, Deloose K, Verbist J, Peeters P, Castriota F, et al. Does free cell area influence the outcome in carotid artery stenting? European Journal of Vascular and Endovascular Surgery 2007;33(2) 135-141.

[108] Siewiorek GM, Wholey MH, Finol EA. A Comparative Analysis of Bench-Top Performance Assessment of Distal Protection Filters in Transient Flow Conditions. Journal of Endovascular Therapy 2012;19(2) 249-260.

[109] Lin PH, Zhou W, Kougias P, Sayed HE, Lumsden AB. Assessing the learning curve of CAS. Endovascular Today 2006;8 68-74.

[110] Coggia M, Goëau-Brissonnière O, Duval JL, Leschi JP, Letort M, Nagel MD. Embolic risk of the different stages of carotid bifurcation balloon angioplasty: An experimental study. Journal of Vascular Surgery 2000;31(3) 550-557.

[111] Piñero P, González A, Martínez E, Mayol A, Rafel E, González-Marcos JR, Moniche F, et al. Volume and composition of emboli in neuroprotected stenting of the carotid artery. American Journal of Neuroradiology 2009;30(3) 473-478. doi: 10.3174/ajnr.A1407.

[112] Ohki T, Roubin GS, Veith FJ, Iyer SS, Brady E. Efficacy of a filter device in the prevention of embolic events during carotid angioplasty and stenting: An ex vivo analysis. Journal of Vascular Surgery 1999;30(6) 1034-1044.

[113] Wittkugel O, Fiehler J, Koch C, Eckert B, Kilic E, Frahm M, et al. Endovascular treatment of internal carotid artery stenosis: effect of primary stent application on debris particle release in human cadaveric specimens. Radiology 2003;229(3) 855-860.

[114] Theron JG, Payelle GG, Coskun O, Huet HF, Guimaraens L. Carotid artery stenosis: treatment with protected balloon angioplasty and stent placement. Radiology 1996;201(3) 627-636.

[115] Iyer V, de Donato G, Deloose K, Peeters P, Castriota F, Cremonesi A, et al. The type of embolic protection does not influence the outcome in carotid artery stenting. Journal of Vascular Surgery 2007;46(2) 251-256.

[116] Berkefeld J, du Mesnil de Rochemont R, Sitzer M, Zanella FE. Distale Protektionsverfahren beim Karotisstent60 [Distal protection devices in carotid stent]. Der Radiologe 2004;44(10) 991-997.

[117] Astor FC, Santilli P, Tucker HM. Incidence of cranial nerve dysfunction following carotid endarterectomy. Head & Neck Surgery 1983;6(2) 660-663.

[118] Rodriguez-Lopez JA, Diethrich EB, Olsen DM. Postoperative morbidity of closely staged bilateral carotid endarterectomies: an intersurgical interval of 4 days or less. Annals of Vascular Surgery 2001;15(4) 457-464.

[119] Prabhakaran S, Wells KR, Lee VH, Flaherty CA, Lopes DK. Prevalence and risk factors for aspirin and clopidogrel resistance in cerebrovascular stenting. American Journal of Neuroradiology 2008;29(2) 281-285.

[120] Reavey-Cantwell JF, Fox WC, Reichwage BD, Fautheree GL, Velat GJ, Whiting JH, et al. Factors associated with aspirin resistance in patients premedicated with aspirin and clopidogrel for endovascular neurosurgery. Neurosurgery 2009;64(5) 890-895.

[121] Lee DH, Arat A, Morsi H, Shaltoni H, Harris JR, Mawad ME. Dual antiplatelet therapy monitoring for neurointerventional procedures using a point-of-care platelet function test: a single-center experience. American Journal of Neuroradiology 2008;29(7) 1389-1394

[122] Gurbel PA, Callahan KP, Malinin AI, Serebruany VL, Gillis J. Could stent design affect platelet activation? Results of the Platelet Activation in STenting (PAST) study. Journal of Invasive Cardiology 2002;14(10) 584-589.

[123] Hendriks JM, Zindler JD, van der Lugt A, Pattynama PM, van Sambeek MR, Bosch JL, et al. Embolic Protection Filters for Carotid Stenting: Differences in Flow Obstruction Depending on Filter Construction. Journal of Endovascular Therapy 2006;13(1) 47-50. doi: 10.1583/04-1325.1.

Chapter 8

Management of Atherosclerotic Carotid Artery Stenosis

David J. Padalino and Eric M. Deshaies

Additional information is available at the end of the chapter

http://dx.doi.org/10.5772/57156

1. Introduction

Ischemic stroke is a leading cause of morbidity and mortality worldwide. Common etiologies of ischemic stroke include cardioembolic events, intracranial arterial stenosis, extracranial large vessel dissection (spontaneous and traumatic), genetic or familial causes such as Moya-Moya Disease and fibromuscular dysplasia, and carotid artery stenosis. The latter is responsible for a significant percentage of ischemic strokes due to carotid atherosclerotic disease and will be the focus of this chapter. Diagnosis is often made based on physical exam by the primary care physician and routine ultrasonic or radiographic screening. Detection of carotid artery stenosis typically results in the eventual referral to a general vascular surgeon or a cerebrovascular neurosurgeon when revascularization is indicated for intervention. Selecting candidates for medical treatment or revascularization is guided by data obtained from excellently performed trials including the *North American Symptomatic Carotid Endarterectomy Trial (NASCET)* and the *Asymtomatic Carotid Artery Stenosis (ACAS) Trial*. Treatment depends upon the severity of carotid stenosis and the absence or presence of stroke symptoms. Medical management, carotid endarterectomy, and carotid artery stenting with angioplasty, each have important roles in the appropriate treatment of carotid stenosis. It is the surgeon's responsibility to assess the patient's history, physical exam findings, imaging studies, and risk factors, to make appropriate recommendations on the best treatment for the patient at hand. The purpose of this chapter is to review the management of atherosclerotic carotid artery disease based on available data in the literature and to provide information useful in daily practice.

2. Epidemiology

Approximately 750,000 persons in the United States alone experience an ischemic stroke each year [1]. Stroke care expense for the United States healthcare system was 74 billion dollars based on 2010 economic data and with the aging American population and higher incidence of obesity and diabetes in young adults, this cost to the American economy will increase [2]. An interesting analysis was published demonstrating that approximately 120 million neurons (equivalent to 714 kilometers or 444 miles of myelinated fibers) are lost each hour after a large arterial occlusion, thereby accelerating brain aging by 3.6 years per hour of ischemia time [3]. This neuronal loss often translates into permanent and devastating neurological sequelae.

It has been estimated that 20-30% of ischemic strokes result from extracranial carotid artery stenosis secondary to atherosclerotic disease [4,5]. Atherosclerosis is a chronic progressive process associated with modifiable risk factors that promote chronic inflammatory events within the arterial wall. Progression of atherosclerotic plaque formation causes ischemic stroke generally by one of two mechanisms: either a flow-limiting stenosis of the arterial lumen resulting in cerebral hypoperfusion typically in the watershed territories or more commonly, thromboembolic events from ruptured atherosclerotic plaque. Until one of these events causes a stroke, carotid stenosis remains asymptomatic and often goes undetected.

The prevalence of carotid stenosis can vary widely with geographic location due to cultural, genetic, and socioeconomic differences. The acquired nature of atherosclerotic disease implies that several of the risk factors that contribute to its development can be modified by individual changes in lifestyle, diet, and medical management.

3. Risk factors

Important modifiable risk factors for developing carotid atherosclerotic disease include smoking, hypertension, dyslipidemia and poor glycemic control in diabetic patients. Smoking is strongly associated with development of carotid atherosclerotic disease whereby comparing age-matched non-smokers, former smokers and current smokers, the prevalence of clinically significant carotid stenosis (>50%) was seen in 4.4%, 7.3% and 9.5% ($P<0.0001$), respectively. Treatment of hypertension has been associated with reduced risk of developing carotid stenosis and stroke. For every 20mmHg increase in systolic blood pressure the odds ratio of developing moderate carotid stenosis is 2.11. Additionally, every 10mg/dL increase in serum cholesterol level was associated with an odds ratio of 1.10 for developing hemodynamically significant carotid stenosis. Strict control of postprandial glucose levels in diabetic patients has been associated with a reduction of carotid intimal media thickness and may also help to reduce the incidence of stroke from carotid stenosis [6].

4. Histopathology of atherosclerotic disease

It has been well established that carotid stenosis tends to occur at the bifurcation, which corresponds to vascular shear stresses as determined by *in vivo* measurements and *in vitro* flow models. The healthy artery is composed of three distinct layers, the tunica intima, tunica media and tunica adventitia, as seen from the lumen to the outer vessel wall. The tunica intima is composed of a luminal endothelial layer consisting of an internal elastic lamina and a fibro-collagenous tissue layer, the latter two of which are thrombogenic. This tissue layer is covered externally by the tunica media consisting of smooth muscle cells followed by a fibrocollagenous layer composed of the external elastic lamina and an external fibrous serosa layer, which composes the tunica adventitia layer. Carotid stenosis is thought to form as a result of intimal endothelial injury by mechanical hemodynamic shear stresses and metabolic and inflammatory processes. The plaque material often contains macrophages, inflammatory cells, calcium, lipid and cholesterol deposits, thought to be formed as part of the healing process after endothelial injury [1].

After disruption of the arterial endothelial lining, expression of inflammatory cell adhesion markers such as VCAM-1, ICAM and other receptors are upregulated [1,7]. Additionally, platelets adhere to the disrupted endothelium after balloon angioplasty and they degranulate, thereby releasing various cytokines and growth factors including transforming growth factor beta (TGF-β), epidermal growth factor (EGF) and platelet derived growth factor (PDGF) [1,8]. These result in migration and proliferation of the vascular smooth muscle cells of the tunica media to form a neointimal layer in an attempt to heal the disrupted endothelium. This neointima becomes more permeable to inflammatory cells as degranulated platelets adhere and remodel the site of the injured intima [1,9,10]. T-cells, monocytes and lipid laden macrophages are seen in these plaques as they become more chronic, and calcium is often deposited during this process in an attempt to stabilize the plaque. Plaques with less calcification tend to be more vulnerable to rupture or thrombosis, indicating that the deposition of calcium appears to be protective and helps to stabilize the plaque by encasing the inflammatory materials, rather than leaving them exposed for further exacerbation of the inflammatory process [1,11].

The proliferation of smooth muscle cells is accompanied by an increase in matrix metalloproteinases (MMPs) such as MMP-2 and MMP-9, which help to remodel the vessel by dilating the stenotic segment, thereby initially compensating for the loss of intimal diameter by the early plaque. However, with progression of the plaque thickness, the vessel eventually can no longer dilate further to compensate once the plaque occupies about 40-50% of the luminal diameter, and the lumen becomes progressively more narrowed [1].

Vascular stenosis alone does not appear to correlate well with predicting which asymptomatic plaques will result in cerebrovascular symptoms, and therefore additional information about the plaque characteristics are important to assess the vulnerability of the plaque to progress and become symptomatic. Factors which appear to be important in identifying vulnerable plaques include echolucency of the plaque on high resolution B-mode ultrasound, absence of calcification, presence of intraplaque hemorrhage, surface irregularity, fibrous cap thickness, plaque volume and presence and location of a necrotic core [12].

5. Presentation and radiographic evaluation

The history alone can often give a great clue to the underlying cause of the carotid stenosis, once identified. Atherosclerotic disease is the most common cause of carotid stenosis, and is more prevalent in older patients. In patients with a history of head and neck cancer and exposure to radiation therapy, intimal hyperplasia and other radiation changes would be the most likely underlying cause of the stenosis, and are typically more difficult to treat compared with atherosclerotic lesions [13]. Patients involved in a recent trauma or neck manipulation may have an arterial dissection that can lead to significant arterial stenosis or occlusion [14]. All of these causes could present with or without symptoms, and although the likelihood of symptoms may be more prevalent in higher degrees of stenosis, it is important to correlate the clinical history and presentation with the radiographic findings when evaluating carotid stenosis, as this will help to drive the decisions for conservative or invasive treatment of lesions identified. Currently, the US Preventive Services Task Force recommends against screening for carotid stenosis in the general asymptomatic population [15].

Several clinical trials have been performed to evaluate the patient populations who will benefit from various treatment options, including medical management, surgical intervention with carotid endarterectomy (CEA) or carotid angioplasty with or without stent placement (CAS), and also with or without distal embolic protection devices for endovascular treatments.

One publication from the Netherlands reviewed four major population based studies for a meta-analysis to determine the prevalence of moderate (50-70%) and severe (>70%) carotid stenosis in men and women at various ages [16]. The investigators determined that the prevalence of asymptomatic moderate carotid stenosis ranged from 0.2% (95% CI, 0.0% to 0.4%) in men aged <50 years to 7.5% (5.2% to 10.5%) in men aged ≥80 years, and severe carotid stenosis ranged from 0.1% (0.0% to 0.3%) in men aged <50 years to 3.1% (1.7% to 5.3%) in men aged ≥80 years. For women, the prevalence of asymptomatic moderate carotid stenosis ranged from 0% (0% to 0.2%) in those aged<50 years to 5.0% (3.1% to 7.5%) in women aged ≥80 years, while severe asymptomatic carotid stenosis for women ranged from 0% (0.0% to 0.2%) to 0.9% (0.3% to 2.4%), between these age groups. Although this data helps to understand the prevalence of this condition, it can only be applied to this particular population that was studied.

Traditionally, patients who presented with stroke or TIA symptoms would undergo diagnostic catheter angiography for the diagnosis of carotid stenosis. With the advent of current non-invasive vascular imaging since the 1980's such as carotid duplex ultrasound, MRA and CTA, the most common presentation of carotid stenosis is an incidental finding of asymptomatic stenosis noted on one of these imaging studies which could be performed for a variety of reasons other than for stroke or TIA, including screening imaging studies performed to follow up clinical exam findings such as auscultation of a carotid bruit. The sensitivity and specificity of auscultation of a carotid bruit when used to evaluate for carotid stenosis are extremely poor. One study compared the sensitivity and specificity of detecting carotid or vertebral stenosis with duplex ultrasound evaluation compared with the gold standard catheter angiogram and also reviewed the presence or absence of a cervical bruit on examination. This study showed that the location and estimated degree of stenosis was accurately identified in 97% of carotid and 90% of vertebral stenosis cases with duplex ultrasound compared with catheter angiography, but the presence of a bruit on exam would only correctly diagnose 27.6% of patients with confirmed hemodynamically significant stenosis, and was falsely positive in 22.6% of patients with confirmed normal vasculature, making the positive and negative predictive correlation of a cervical bruit auscultated on physical exam extremely unreliable [17].

CTA and MRA imaging modalities can often have a greater than 95% sensitivity and specificity for detecting hemodynamically significant vascular stenosis when compared with diagnostic catheter angiography as the gold standard imaging modality [18]. These non-invasive imaging studies have shown to be of benefit in screening for and following stability or progression of vascular stenosis, but it should be noted that in evaluating the accuracy of each of these imaging modalities and comparing with that of digital subtraction angiography (DSA) using an *in vitro* stenosis model, Smith et al found that the CTA and MRA studies tended to underestimate the stenosis whereas the DSA tended to overestimate the stenosis when evaluating the >70% stenosis model, while there was no significant difference between these imaging studies in the estimated stenosis when evaluating the <70% stenosis model [19].

6. Treatment options

The medical management of carotid stenosis has revolved around anti-inflammatory and anti-platelet agents as the drugs of choice. Marquardt et al studied the UK population and documented the frequency of ipsilateral ischemic stroke in the setting of asymptomatic carotid stenosis ≥50% [20]. It was reported that with adequate medical management, the risk was 0.34% for any ipsilateral non-disabling stroke, 0.0% for severe disabling stroke, and 1.78% for ipsilateral TIA. These results would support best medical management for all asymptomatic carotid stenosis, irrespective of the degree of stenosis. Aspirin is known to have anti-inflammatory properties by irreversible blockade of the cyclooxygenase (COX)-1 and COX-2 pathways of arachidonic acid metabolism. Carotid fibrous plaque formation and remodeling are influenced by several factors including MMPs secreted by leukocytes in the intima which remodel the extracellular matrix, and this results in thrombosis with vulnerable plaques in which the fibrous cap has become significantly thinned and embolic events resulting in TIA and stroke may ensue [1]. The Clopidogrel and Aspirin for the Reduction of Emboli in Symptomatic Carotid Stenosis (CARESS) trial evaluated the use of aspirin alone vs aspirin with clopidogrel in symptomatic carotid stenosis >50% and found that combination therapy reduced the frequency of asymptomatic microembolization as detected by transcranial doppler ultrasound more effectively than aspirin alone [21].

Several major trials evaluating asymptomatic carotid stenosis include the Veterans Administration Trial (VA, 1993 [22]), the Asymptomatic Carotid Surgery Trial (ACST, 1994 [23]) and the Asymptomatic Carotid Artery Stenosis Trial (ACAS, 1995 [24]). The VA trial looked at medical management alone with aspirin 650mg po BID versus combined medical management with the same aspirin dose and with CEA for asymptomatic carotid stenosis of 50% or greater in 444 men in the VA medical system. This study failed to show any statistically significant differences in clinical outcome between these two groups [22]. The ACST group evaluated the timing of CEA for patients with asymptomatic carotid stenosis of 60% or greater. Patients were treated with best medical management and the treatment group received CEA as soon as possible. The second group only received CEA if symptoms developed while on medical therapy. A total of 3120 patients were enrolled and this study failed to show any statistically significant differences in long term clinical outcome between groups [23]. In 1995, the ACAS trial was published which reviewed the results of 1662 asymptomatic patients with >60% carotid stenosis. Patients were randomized into two groups, the first consisting of medical therapy alone with aspirin 325mg daily and the second group treated with medical therapy and CEA within 2 weeks of randomization [24]. This trial found a reduced 5-year stroke risk from 11.0% in the medical arm to 5.1% in the surgical arm with a 3% perioperative morbidity and mortality.

Catheter based diagnostic cerebral angiography remains the gold standard imaging modality for diagnosing and measuring carotid stenosis. The risk of stroke for asymptomatic patients is 2-3% annually and 12% in symptomatic stroke patients [20,25]. Clinical trials have demonstrated measurable differences in the treatment strategy for symptomatic versus asymptomatic carotid stenosis. A majority of data advocates best medical management for asymptomatic carotid stenosis because of the very low incidence of ipsilateral stroke, regardless of the degree of stenosis. According to the ACAS and NASCET trial results, revascularization is recommended for symptomatic male patients with ≥50% ipsilateral cervical internal carotid artery stenosis, while revascularization is not recommended for symptomatic female patients until the severity of ipsilateral cervical carotid stenosis reaches ≥70% [26], however, this difference between men and women has remained somewhat controversial and these results have not been consistently reproduced [27]. Currently, carotid endarterectomy continues to be the gold standard for revascularization. If the patient has significant risk factors placing them at a high risk for endarterectomy, then revascularization via carotid angioplasty and stenting is an alternative therapy. Such risk factors typically include: previous ipsilateral carotid endarterectomy, recent myocardial infarction within previous thirty days, contralateral carotid occlusion, radiation to the neck, chronic obstructive pulmonary disease, and previous carotid stent.

Carotid stent placement is offered to patients who have no contraindications to long-term antiplatelet agent use and who are at a high risk for surgery. Distal embolic protection devices are generally used to lower the risk of embolic events from stent placement and balloon angioplasty, but recent recommendations vary; cases where there is a reasonably high potential for distal embolic events during the angioplasty procedure may benefit from distal protection devices [28–32]. Carotid angioplasty alone without stent placement is associated with a very high rate of re-stenosis. The CAVATAS trial examined the treatment of carotid stenosis with angioplasty alone (N=145) versus carotid angioplasty and stent placement (N=50) vs carotid endarterectomy (N=213). This trial showed that carotid endarterectomy resulted in significantly lower rates of carotid re-stenosis >70% 5 years after treatment compared with endovascular therapy (30.7% vs 10.5%). Additionally, in the endovascular treatment group, the patients treated with angioplasty alone had a higher rate of re-stenosis >70% compared with those treated with stent placement (36.2% vs 16.6%) [33]. With the placement of a stent, the in-stent re-stenosis rate has been reported to be as low as 5% after four years [34]. Risk factors that may increase the likelihood of recurrent stenosis after carotid angioplasty, stent or endarterectomy have been examined and in a report from Skelly et al, these risk factors include prior stroke, transient ischemic attack, amaurosis fugax, and prior neck cancer [35].

Large trials designed to evaluate surgical versus medical treatment for symptomatic carotid stenosis include the Veterans Administration 309 Trial (VA309, 1991 [36]), the European Carotid Surgery Trial (ECST, 1998 [37]), and the North American Symptomatic Carotid Endarterectomy Trial (NASCET, 1998 [26]). VA309 evaluated the results of treating 189 symptomatic patients with >50% carotid stenosis ipsilateral to the symptoms with best medical management or a combined approach of best medical management with CEA. The study found a statistically significant reduction in the stroke risk over 11.9 months for the surgical arm compared to the medical arm (7.7% vs 19.4%, P=0.11) [36]. In 1998, both ECST and NASCET were published. ECST evaluated 3024 patients with some degree of symptomatic carotid stenosis that was determined by varying modality and varying quality vascular imaging studies. The trial randomized 1811 patients to the surgical arm and 1213 patients to the medical arm, and the overall risk of surgery was determined to be about 7%, which did not vary with the degree of stenosis. For symptomatic carotid stenosis (as measured by the ECST method) of greater than 80%, the three-year major stroke or death rate was 14.9% for the surgical arm and 26.5% in the medical arm, revealing a statistically significant benefit for surgery in that group [37]. NASCET evaluated 1108 patients with symptomatic carotid stenosis in the CEA arm and 1118 demographically similar patients in the best medical management arm. The results showed no benefit for surgery below 50% stenosis, some benefit particularly in men with moderate stenosis (50-69%) and clear benefit for surgery with severe stenosis (>70%). The rate of any ipsilateral stroke over five-year follow up for moderate carotid stenosis (50-69%) was 15.7% in the surgical arm and 22.2% in the medical arm (P=0.045), with the immediate perioperative stroke or death risk being reported as 2% [26].

The Carotid Revascularization Endarterectomy versus Stenting Trial (CREST) evaluated 2502 symptomatic and asymptomatic carotid stenosis patients who were randomly assigned to CEA or CAS [38]. The study found no significant differences in combined stroke, myocardial infarction and death risk over 4 year follow up between these groups, however, there was a trend toward more myocardial infarctions in the surgical arm (6.8% vs 7.2%, CAS vs CEA, P=0.51) and a statistically significant higher rate of periprocedural stroke in the endovascular arm (6.4% vs 4.7%, CAS vs CEA, P=0.03). A study published in February 2013 evaluated the effect of these perioperative complications on long term survival. According to this trial, having a stroke within the first year resulted in a two-fold lower survival rate (HR=6.6; CI=3.7-12) than those patients who suffered a perioperative myocardial infarction two years after intervention (HR=3.6;CI=2-6.8), but this difference becomes negligible at 5 years (HR=2.7; CI=1.7-4.3 vs HR=2.8; CI=1.8-4.3) [39].

The Carotid and Vertebral Transluminal Angioplasty Study (CAVATAS) examined the treatment of carotid stenosis with carotid endarterectomy (N=213) vs endovascular treatment with angioplasty alone (N=145) or angioplasty and stent placement (N=50). The rate of recurrent stenosis >70% after endovascular therapy for all patients treated with or without stent placement was about 3 times higher than the restenosis rate after endarterectomy after 5 years of follow up (30.7% vs 10.5%, p=<0.0001). However, of the endovascular treated patients, the occurrence of restenosis >70% in the angioplasty alone group compared to the stent group was more than twice as frequent (36.2% vs 16.6%, p=0.04). Of all patients with >70% restenosis in the first year after treatment with CEA or CAS compared to the patients with <70% restenosis in this same time period, there was a trend toward a higher ipsilateral stroke rate in the greater stenosis group, but this result did not reach clinical significance (9.7% vs 5.4%, p=0.4) [33]. These results suggest that CEA provides the greatest durability of treatment with fewer cases of hemodynamically significant recurrent stenosis compared with stent placement, although stent placement is significantly superior to angioplasty alone for long-term durability. Treated patients should be followed for recurrent stenosis, and although the greater stenosis group did not have a statistically significant increase in the number of ipsilateral stroke events, it would be wise to more closely monitor these patients, be more aggressive with medical management with anti-platelet agents, or even offer repeat treatment for those patients with progressively worsening stenosis during the follow up period.

7. Operative techniques for carotid endarterectomy

Patients with symptomatic carotid stenosis >50% or asymptomatic carotid stenosis >70%, or who had a stroke ipsilateral to the carotid stenosis while on best medical management should be offered a carotid revascularization procedure. CEA remains the gold standard of care for carotid stenosis. It should be considered for those patients who have a low medical risk for general anesthesia, have not had prior radical neck surgery or radiation to the neck and who have a surgically accessible carotid bifurcation.

Because the surgery involves clamping the carotid artery temporarily, some surgeons will decide to place a silicone tubing to shunt the blood and allow continuous carotid flow throughout the operation, however, this can be associated with a higher rate of thromboembolic events and some surgeons will choose to place a shunt in only select cases [40,41]. If the surgeon chooses to selectively shunt only those patients who do not tolerate carotid clamping for the surgery, he or she can decide to perform this surgery either awake under local anesthesia allowing for intra-operative neurological exams or under general anesthesia with neuromonitoring to evaluate for changes in somatosensory evoked potentials (SSEPs) and motor evoked potentials (MEPs) while the carotid artery is clamped. If the surgeon chooses to shunt all carotids, then the routine use of neuromonitoring would not typically be required or justified. Some surgeons will measure stump pressures from the external carotid artery (ECA) after clamping to help determine if the patient will require selective placement of a carotid shunt, however, this has not been shown to be a good predictor of whether a patient will go on to have a stroke from the surgery. The authors here routinely use neuromonitoring for all patients under general anesthesia in order to choose the patients who will require selective shunting.

Pre-operative medical preparation is important, and patients undergoing CEA should be taking an anti-platelet such as aspirin daily. The use of clopidogrel, although not required, would not necessarily prevent the surgeon from performing the CEA, although there is a slightly higher risk of local hematoma for patients taking combination anti-platelet agents. A drain is often recommended in selected cases, particularly if the patient is taking both aspirin and clopidogrel at the time of the surgery, and if it is difficult to maintain a dry surgical field at the time of the operation.

The approach to the carotid sheath for the CEA begins with positioning the patient in the supine position on the operating table with the head turned slightly toward the contralateral side and the neck slightly extended for optimum exposure. The planned incision line should be marked with a skin marker along the anterior border of the sternocleidomastoid muscle, which would be approximately parallel to the expected course of the carotid artery, for optimum exposure. The neck should be prepped behind and below the ear from just above the mastoid down to the upper chest, just below the clavicle, and from midline out laterally to the anterolateral border of the trapezius muscle above the shoulder. After proper sterile technique for preparation and draping of the operative field, the skin is incised along the previously marked incision site. The platysma muscle is encountered and split parallel to the muscle fibers, which is also parallel to the incision. The omohyoid muscle is separated as needed for adequate exposure of the common carotid artery (CCA) and at least 2-3cm of the ECA and internal carotid artery (ICA). If additional exposure is required superiorly, the superior aspect of the planned incision should be extended superiorly and posteriorly just below the mastoid, and care should be taken to not injure the hypoglossal nerve at this level during the deeper dissection. Care should be taken to avoid injury to the recurrent laryngeal nerve or the esophagus during the dissection to the carotid sheath. The carotid artery typically resides medially in the carotid sheath, the internal jugular vein typically lies lateral to the carotid artery, and the vagus nerve typically lies deep to both of these structures and between them.

The systolic blood pressure (SBP) is raised prior to placing the clamp, typically to 140-160 mmHg for patients who are normotensive at baseline, to help promote perfusion through collateral circulation. Generally, raising the SBP by about 20% of the baseline should allow for adequate collateral circulation. The carotid artery is then clamped in the following order when the surgeon is ready to perform the endarterectomy, with the ICA being clamped first followed by the CCA (typically with a Fogarty carotid clamp or other atraumatic clamp device), followed by the ECA. If neuromonitoring is used, these signals are also monitored continuously, and changes in the SSEP and or MEP signals that would be consistent with ischemia changes should prompt the surgeon to selectively place a shunt into that carotid artery.

The arteriotomy is performed with a #11 scalpel blade until a pair of Potts scissors can be inserted into the true lumen and the incision can be extended from the CCA to the ICA full thickness through the plaque. Care must be taken to identify the superior thyroid artery origin, especially if there is back-bleeding after performing the arteriotomy, as this may arise very near the carotid bifurcation, unless a temporary clip is applied to this arterial branch. The plaque is then carefully but quickly teased from the endothelial layer of the carotid artery and the plaque is transected as far as possible with the exposure and the carotid artery wall is inspected for loose debris which is carefully removed and irrigated with heparinized saline. The carotid artery is then sutured with 6-0 prolene in simple running fashion, using a minimal full thickness stitch to reapproximate the incised vessel edges without causing additional stenosis with the suturing. Multiple simple interrupted sutures can also be used, but this tends to be significantly more time consuming and is no more effective than the simple running suture. The use of heparinized saline throughout the procedure and back bleeding from the ECA to flush out any loose particles just prior to placing the last 6-0 prolene suture into the carotid artery is also recommended. The clamps are then removed in the reverse order that they were placed, with the ECA clamp removed first, followed by the CCA clamp, followed lastly by the ICA clamp. There are several standard techniques to close a cervical approach incision, which would typically include a subcutaneous layer of absorbable suture placed in inverted simple interrupted fashion followed by a cosmetic skin edge reapproximation with absorbable running subcuticular sutures, sterile adhesive strips or skin glue.

8. Interventional techniques for carotid angioplasty and stent

Patients who are not candidates for CEA due to high surgical risk factors are defined by Medicare guidelines, and include patients with recurrent stenosis after prior ipsilateral CEA, prior radiation therapy to the neck or previous ablative neck surgery such as radical neck dissection, surgically inaccessible cervical lesion above the C2 level, presence of a CCA lesion below the clavicle, contralateral vocal cord palsy, presence of a tracheostomy stoma, or patients with a contralateral ICA occlusion. Additionally, patients who are medically unstable and high risk for surgery, with COPD or other pulmonary condition which would make removal of the endotracheal tube at the end of the surgery difficult or dangerous for the patient, or recent acute myocardial infection within 30 days would also be considered high surgical risk, and a carotid artery stent procedure could be considered.

All patients receiving angioplasty of the carotid bulb should be prepared with cardiac defibrillator pads pre-procedurally, and atropine should be readily available for immediate injection in the event of severe bradycardia or asystole. Advanced cardiac life support (ACLS) materials should be readily available in the event of a potentially fatal cardiac arrhythmia that could occur as a result of the parasympathetic reflex from carotid bulb stretch during the angioplasty. The operator can choose whether to use distal embolic protection devices, however, there is no general recommendation available from the literature to support the use of distal embolic protection devices for all cases [28–32]. The authors here will routinely use a distal embolic protection filterwire device to allow continuous perfusion while providing a barrier to capture potentially large particulate matter during stent and angioplasty for carotid atherosclerotic disease when it is safe and feasible to place such a device. Additionally, Medicare requires that all carotid stent procedures be performed with distal embolic protection devices, whenever feasible.

The patient should be pre-medicated with anti-platelet agents such as aspirin and clopidogrel, and the authors here use 325mg aspirin and 75mg clopidogrel daily for 7 days prior to a scheduled elective stent placement, or a loading dose of 325mg aspirin and 300mg clopidogrel the day prior to a semi-urgent stent placement, or the day of an emergency stent placement with supplemental abciximab given as a bolus of 0.25mg/kg up to a maximum of 20mg bolus, followed by a continuous drip of 0.125mcg/kg/min to a maximum of 10mcg/min for 24h, and then followed by 325mg aspirin and 75mg clopidogrel daily for 3 months before the next follow up angiogram. At the time of the follow up angiogram, if there is no in-stent stenosis or other reason for additional procedures, then the clopidogrel can be stopped, and the patient is continued on low-dose aspirin 81mg daily indefinitely.

One potential complication with stent placement is thromboembolic events that have been found to occur in up to 10% of cases where the patient was found to not have adequate platelet inhibition with the standard anti-platelet therapy described above, and these individuals are described as "non-responders" [42]. It is now known that the incidence of non-responders to clopidogrel is potentially very high, ranging from 5-40% of treated patients, and appears to be more prevalent in the Asian population compared with the Caucasian or African populations. Clopidogrel is a pro-drug that is metabolized by the cytochrome P450 emzyme pathway in the liver into the active thiol metabolite. Factors such as platelet ADP receptor heterogeneity, poor drug absorption, drug-drug interactions, and differences in metabolism of the drug by the cytochrome P450 system, as well as patient non-compliance may all contribute to the variability of drug efficacy between individuals. Variant alleles of the CYP2C19 and CYP2C9 enzymes (CYP2C19 I331V, CYP2C9 R144C and CYP2C9 I359L) have been described to have a reduced conversion rate of the clopidogrel pro-drug into the active thiol metabolite [43]. Alternative anti-platelet agents such as prasugrel (Effient) may be used, as non-responders to clopidogrel typically will respond adequately to prasugrel. Other alternative anti-platelet agents should be evaluated with the most current pharmacological literature. A pharmacy consultation may be needed to find an effective alternative anti-platelet drug for patients who do not respond to a therapeutic level with these medications. It would be wise to test all patients who require elective pre-medication with aspirin and clopidogrel using a P2Y12 activity test before performing the procedure, whenever possible, in order to identify those patients who may be non-responders to the standard therapy.

The patient is placed in the supine position on the angiography table with the femoral artery access site prepared in the usual sterile fashion. Using the modified Seldinger technique, the femoral artery is accessed with a long access catheter typically with at least a 6F inner diameter (ID) to allow room for placement of a distal protection device and the stent device simultaneously, along with any additional 0.014 or 0.018 inch microwires, termed "buddy wires," which may be placed to improve the stability of the guide catheter in the CCA. The guide catheter is positioned in the CCA just proximal to the carotid bifurcation and appropriate digital subtraction angiography (DSA) is performed to optimally visualize the stenosis and the takeoff of the ICA. A 0.014 inch microwire is guided beyond the ICA stenosis using a road map. The distal protection device is deployed over the microwire into a straight segment of the ICA proximal to the petrous segment. Occasionally, the stenosis will be so severe that pre-dilation angioplasty of the stenosis with a balloon that has a low crossing profile, such as a 2.5mm x 30mm Maverick or Mini-Trek balloon, before the placement of the distal protection device or the stent may be required. Cardiovascular instability or arrhythmias are uncommon when inflating a small balloon such as this at the ICA origin. An appropriately sized stent is selected, which is typically about 30-40mm in length to cover the lesion completely and about 1-2mm greater diameter than the widest measured carotid diameter into which the stent will be deployed, typically at the bifurcation [44]. Because the carotid artery bulb is typically significantly larger than the cervical segment of the ICA, some carotid stents are designed with a tapered diameter, such as 6mm diameter distally and 8mm diameter proximally, to accommodate for this and to prevent the stent from being significantly oversized distally for an appropriately selected diameter for the proximal ICA. The appropriately selected stent is then positioned across the ICA stenosis, taking care to avoid placement of the distal end of the stent at a curved segment of the ICA, as some patients may have a relatively tortuous ICA course. This will help to avoid kinking of the stent or occlusion or dissection of the ICA. After the stent is deployed across the lesion, a DSA run is performed to confirm the location of the stent and to evaluate for residual stenosis. An appropriately selected balloon is then chosen and positioned along the center of the greatest stenosis. At the time of balloon inflation, care should be taken to watch the heart rate and blood pressure, as stretching of the carotid bulb could result in significant bradycardia or asystole. The balloon should be inflated only a few seconds, and should not remain inflated for more than 10-20 seconds during the initial post-stent angioplasty. The balloon may be left inflated longer as long as the patient remains asymptomatic with the occlusion of carotid blood flow, but this should not be done for longer than 1-2 minutes at a time. The distal protection device is then recovered, taking care to avoid inadvertently snagging on the stent tines and potentially dislodging the position of the stent. The femoral arteriotomy access site is then closed and the patient should remain flat with the accessed leg straight for at least 1 hour after placement of an arterial closure device, or for 4-6 hours with a sandbag or clamp to hold pressure on the femoral arteriotomy site if no closure device is used.

9. Conclusions

The NASCET evidence supports the treatment of symptomatic hemodynamically significant carotid artery stenosis of ≥50% by NASCET criteria for men, and ≥70% for women. The only trial that advocates surgical intervention for asymptomatic carotid stenosis is the ACAS trial, and surgical intervention for asymptomatic carotid artery stenosis ≥60% was supported, but other trials would support best medical management because of the very low incidence of ipsilateral stroke from asymptomatic carotid stenosis, regardless of the degree of stenosis. Carotid endarterectomy remains the gold standard treatment for patients who are medically stable enough to tolerate the surgery. Carotid angioplasty without stent placement has a high rate of recurrence of stenosis, and therefore with current devices available, patients in whom endovascular treatment has been chosen for carotid stenosis should be treated with stent placement and should be pre-medicated with anti-platelet agents such as aspirin and clopidogrel, or alternative drugs such as prasugrel in clopidogrel non-responder patients. These medications should be continued for at least 3 months post-procedurally and the low dose (81mg) aspirin should be continued indefinitely.

http://dx.doi.org/10.5772/57156

Author details

David J. Padalino and Eric M. Deshaies*

*Address all correspondence to: deshaiee@upstate.edu

Department of Neurosurgery, SUNY Upstate Medical University, Syracuse, New York, USA

References

[1] Hall HA, Bassiouny HS. Pathophysiology of Carotid Atherosclerosis. In: Nicolaides A, Beach KW, Kyriacou E, Pattichis CS, editors. Ultrasound Carotid Bifurc Atheroscler [Internet]. London: Springer London; 2011 [cited 2013 May 12]. p. 27–39. Available from: http://www.springerlink.com/index/10.1007/978-1-84882-688-5_2

[2] Lloyd-Jones D, Adams RJ, Brown TM, Carnethon M, Dai S, De Simone G, et al. Executive summary: heart disease and stroke statistics--2010 update: a report from the American Heart Association. Circulation. 2010 Feb 23;121(7):948–54.

[3] Saver JL, Fonarow GC, Smith EE, Reeves MJ, Grau-Sepulveda MV, Pan W, et al. Time to treatment with intravenous tissue plasminogen activator and outcome from acute ischemic stroke. Jama J Am Med Assoc. 2013 Jun 19;309(23):2480–8.

[4] Bluth E, Carroll B, Rumack CM. The Extracranial Cerebral Vessels. Diagn Ultrasound. 4th ed. Philadelphia, PA: Elsevier/Mosby; 2010.

[5] Miller JC PhD. Imaging for Carotid Stenosis. Radiol Rounds Mass Gen Hosp [Internet]. 2012 Sep [cited 2013 May 20];10(9). Available from: http://www.mghradrounds.org/index.php?src=gendocs&ref=2012_september

[6] Fazel P, Johnson K. Current Role of Medical Treatment and Invasive Management in Carotid Atherosclerotic Disease. Bayl Univ Med Cent Proc. 2008 Apr;21(2):133–8.

[7] Baumgartner HR, Studer A. [Effects of vascular catheterization in normo- and hypercholesteremic rabbits]. Pathol Microbiol (Basel). 1966;29(4):393–405.

[8] Bowen-Pope DF, Ross R, Seifert RA. Locally acting growth factors for vascular smooth muscle cells: endogenous synthesis and release from platelets. Circulation. 1985 Oct;72(4):735–40.

[9] Faggiotto A, Ross R, Harker L. Studies of hypercholesterolemia in the nonhuman primate. I. Changes that lead to fatty streak formation. Arter Dallas Tex. 1984 Aug;4(4): 323–40.

[10] Gerrity RG, Naito HK, Richardson M, Schwartz CJ. Dietary induced atherogenesis in swine. Morphology of the intima in prelesion stages. Am J Pathol. 1979 Jun;95(3): 775–92.

[11] Beckman JA, Ganz J, Creager MA, Ganz P, Kinlay S. Relationship of clinical presentation and calcification of culprit coronary artery stenoses. Arterioscler Thromb Vasc Biol. 2001 Oct;21(10):1618–22.

[12] Grønholdt ML, Nordestgaard BG, Schroeder TV, Vorstrup S, Sillesen H. Ultrasonic echolucent carotid plaques predict future strokes. Circulation. 2001 Jul 3;104(1):68–73.

[13] Houdart E, Mounayer C, Chapot R, Saint-Maurice JP, Merland JJ. Carotid stenting for radiation-induced stenoses: A report of 7 cases. Stroke J Cereb Circ. 2001 Jan; 32(1):118–21.

[14] Opeskin K. Traumatic carotid artery dissection. Am J Forensic Med Pathol. 1997 Sep; 18(3):251–7.

[15] U.S. Preventive Services Task Force. Screening for Carotid Artery Stenosis [Internet]. 2007. Available from: http://www.uspreventiveservicestaskforce.org/uspstf/uspsacas.htm

[16] De Weerd M, Greving JP, Hedblad B, Lorenz MW, Mathiesen EB, O'Leary DH, et al. Prevalence of asymptomatic carotid artery stenosis in the general population: an individual participant data meta-analysis. Stroke J Cereb Circ. 2010 Jun;41(6):1294–7.

[17] Hennerici M, Aulich A, Sandmann W, Freund HJ. Incidence of asymptomatic extracranial arterial disease. Stroke J Cereb Circ. 1981 Dec;12(6):750–8.

[18] Anzidei M, Napoli A, Zaccagna F, Di Paolo P, Saba L, Cavallo Marincola B, et al. Diagnostic accuracy of colour Doppler ultrasonography, CT angiography and blood-pool-enhanced MR angiography in assessing carotid stenosis: a comparative study with DSA in 170 patients. Radiol Med (Torino). 2012 Feb;117(1):54–71.

[19] Smith JC, Watkins GE, Smith DC, Palmer EW, Abou-Zamzam AM, Zhao CX, et al. Accuracy of digital subtraction angiography, computed tomography angiography, and magnetic resonance angiography in grading of carotid artery stenosis in comparison with actual measurement in an in vitro model. Ann Vasc Surg. 2012 Apr;26(3): 338–43.

[20] Marquardt L, Geraghty OC, Mehta Z, Rothwell PM. Low risk of ipsilateral stroke in patients with asymptomatic carotid stenosis on best medical treatment: a prospective, population-based study. Stroke J Cereb Circ. 2010 Jan;41(1):e11–17.

[21] Markus HS, Droste DW, Kaps M, Larrue V, Lees KR, Siebler M, et al. Dual antiplatelet therapy with clopidogrel and aspirin in symptomatic carotid stenosis evaluated using doppler embolic signal detection: the Clopidogrel and Aspirin for Reduction of

http://dx.doi.org/10.5772/57156

Emboli in Symptomatic Carotid Stenosis (CARESS) trial. Circulation. 2005 May 3;111(17):2233–40.

[22] Hobson RW 2nd, Weiss DG, Fields WS, Goldstone J, Moore WS, Towne JB, et al. Efficacy of carotid endarterectomy for asymptomatic carotid stenosis. The Veterans Affairs Cooperative Study Group. N Engl J Med. 1993 Jan 28;328(4):221–7.

[23] Halliday AW, Thomas D, Mansfield A. The Asymptomatic Carotid Surgery Trial (ACST). Rationale and design. Steering Committee. Eur J Vasc Surg. 1994 Nov;8(6): 703–10.

[24] Endarterectomy for asymptomatic carotid artery stenosis. Executive Committee for the Asymptomatic Carotid Atherosclerosis Study. Jama J Am Med Assoc. 1995 May 10;273(18):1421–8.

[25] Rothwell PM. Carotid endarterectomy for recently symptomatic carotid stenosis: consistent results from two large randomized controlled trials. Eur Heart J. 1999 Aug;20(15):1055–7.

[26] Barnett HJ, Taylor DW, Eliasziw M, Fox AJ, Ferguson GG, Haynes RB, et al. Benefit of carotid endarterectomy in patients with symptomatic moderate or severe stenosis. North American Symptomatic Carotid Endarterectomy Trial Collaborators. N Engl J Med. 1998 Nov 12;339(20):1415–25.

[27] Mattos MA, Sumner DS, Bohannon WT, Parra J, McLafferty RB, Karch LA, et al. Carotid endarterectomy in women: challenging the results from ACAS and NASCET. Ann Surg. 2001 Oct;234(4):438–445; discussion 445–446.

[28] Matsumura JS, Gray W, Chaturvedi S, Yamanouchi D, Peng L, Verta P. Results of carotid artery stenting with distal embolic protection with improved systems: Protected Carotid Artery Stenting in Patients at High Risk for Carotid Endarterectomy (PROTECT) trial. J Vasc Surg. 2012 Apr;55(4):968–976.e5.

[29] Cloft HJ. Distal protection: maybe less than you think. Ajnr Am J Neuroradiol. 2008 Mar;29(3):407–8.

[30] Oteros R, Jimenez-Gomez E, Bravo-Rodriguez F, Ochoa JJ, Guerrero R, Delgado F. Unprotected carotid artery stenting in symptomatic patients with high-grade stenosis: results and long-term follow-up in a single-center experience. Ajnr Am J Neuroradiol. 2012 Aug;33(7):1285–91.

[31] Tallarita T, Rabinstein AA, Cloft H, Kallmes D, Oderich GS, Brown RD, et al. Are distal protection devices "protective" during carotid angioplasty and stenting? Stroke J Cereb Circ. 2011 Jul;42(7):1962–6.

[32] Baldi S, Zander T, Rabellino M, González G, Maynar M. Carotid artery stenting without angioplasty and cerebral protection: a single-center experience with up to 7 years' follow-up. Ajnr Am J Neuroradiol. 2011 Apr;32(4):759–63.

[33] Bonati LH, Ederle J, McCabe DJH, Dobson J, Featherstone RL, Gaines PA, et al. Long-term risk of carotid restenosis in patients randomly assigned to endovascular treatment or endarterectomy in the Carotid and Vertebral Artery Transluminal Angioplasty Study (CAVATAS): long-term follow-up of a randomised trial. Lancet Neurol. 2009 Oct;8(10):908–17.

[34] Levy EI, Hanel RA, Lau T, Koebbe CJ, Levy N, Padalino DJ, et al. Frequency and management of recurrent stenosis after carotid artery stent implantation. J Neurosurg. 2005 Jan;102(1):29–37.

[35] Skelly CL, Gallagher K, Fairman RM, Carpenter JP, Velazquez OC, Parmer SS, et al. Risk factors for restenosis after carotid artery angioplasty and stenting. J Vasc Surg. 2006 Nov;44(5):1010–5.

[36] Mayberg MR, Wilson SE, Yatsu F, Weiss DG, Messina L, Hershey LA, et al. Carotid endarterectomy and prevention of cerebral ischemia in symptomatic carotid stenosis. Veterans Affairs Cooperative Studies Program 309 Trialist Group. Jama J Am Med Assoc. 1991 Dec 18;266(23):3289–94.

[37] Randomised trial of endarterectomy for recently symptomatic carotid stenosis: final results of the MRC European Carotid Surgery Trial (ECST). Lancet. 1998 May 9;351(9113):1379–87.

[38] Brott TG, Hobson RW 2nd, Howard G, Roubin GS, Clark WM, Brooks W, et al. Stenting versus endarterectomy for treatment of carotid-artery stenosis. N Engl J Med. 2010 Jul 1;363(1):11–23.

[39] Simons JP, Goodney PP, Baril DT, Nolan BW, Hevelone ND, Cronenwett JL, et al. The effect of postoperative stroke and myocardial infarction on long-term survival after carotid revascularization. J Vasc Surg. 2013 Feb 8;

[40] Aburahma AF, Mousa AY, Stone PA. Shunting during carotid endarterectomy. J Vasc Surg. 2011 Nov;54(5):1502–10.

[41] Cho J, Lee KK, Yun W-S, Kim H-K, Hwang Y-H, Huh S. Selective shunt during carotid endarterectomy using routine awake test with respect to a lower shunt rate. J Korean Surg Soc. 2013 Apr;84(4):238–44.

[42] Müller-Schunk S, Linn J, Peters N, Spannagl M, Deisenberg M, Brückmann H, et al. Monitoring of clopidogrel-related platelet inhibition: correlation of nonresponse with clinical outcome in supra-aortic stenting. Ajnr Am J Neuroradiol. 2008 Apr;29(4):786–91.

[43] Minarik M, Kopeckova M, Gassman M, Osmancik P, Benesova L. Rapid testing of clopidogrel resistance by genotyping of CYP2C19 and CYP2C9 polymorphisms using denaturing on-chip capillary electrophoresis. Electrophoresis. 2012 Apr;33(8): 1306–10.

[44] Deshaies EM, Eddleman CS, Boulos AS. Handbook of Neuroendovascular Surgery. Handb Neuroendovascular Surg. New York, New York: Thieme Medical Publishers, Inc.; 2012. p. 181–3.